Critical Th

TACTICS
for Nurses

ACHIEVING THE IOM COMPETENCIES

THIRD EDITION

M. Gaie Rubenfeld, RN, MS
Professor Emerita
School of Nursing
Eastern Michigan University
Ypsilanti, Michigan

Barbara K. Scheffer, RN, EdD
Professor Emerita
School of Nursing
Eastern Michigan University
Ypsilanti, Michigan

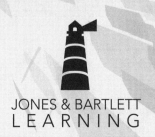

JONES & BARTLETT
LEARNING

World Headquarters
Jones & Bartlett Learning
5 Wall Street
Burlington, MA 01803
978-443-5000
info@jblearning.com
www.jblearning.com

Jones & Bartlett Learning books and products are available through most bookstores and online booksellers. To contact Jones & Bartlett Learning directly, call 800-832-0034, fax 978-443-8000, or visit our website, www.jblearning.com.

Substantial discounts on bulk quantities of Jones & Bartlett Learning publications are available to corporations, professional associations, and other qualified organizations. For details and specific discount information, contact the special sales department at Jones & Bartlett Learning via the above contact information or send an email to specialsales@jblearning.com.

Production Credits

Executive Publisher: William Brottmiller
Senior Editor: Amanda Martin
Associate Managing Editor: Sara Bempkins
Production Editor: Amanda Clerkin
Marketing Communications Manager: Katie Hennessy
VP, Manufacturing and Inventory Control:
   Therese Connell
Composition: Cenveo Publisher Services
Cover Design: Kristin E. Parker
Cover Image: © VikaSuh/ShutterStock, Inc.
Printing and Binding: Edwards Brothers Malloy
Cover Printing: Edwards Brothers Malloy

Library of Congress Cataloging-in-Publication Data
Rubenfeld, M. Gaie, author.
  Critical thinking tactics for nurses : achieving the IOM competencies /
M. Gaie Rubenfeld and Barbara K. Scheffer. — Third edition.
    p. ; cm.
  Includes bibliographical references and index.
  ISBN 978-1-284-04138-5
  I. Scheffer, Barbara K. author. II. Title.
  [DNLM: 1. Nursing Process. 2. Clinical Competence. 3. Thinking. WY 100.1]
  RT42
  610.73—dc23
                            2013047424

6048

Printed in the United States of America
18 17 16 15 14   10 9 8 7 6 5 4 3 2

Contents

Preface

This text is written for clinicians in various areas of practice, nursing students, and educators in clinical and academic settings who want to hone their critical thinking abilities and help others do the same. Although we come from a nursing perspective, our ideas are applicable in any healthcare discipline. Healthcare delivery is in dire need of critical thinkers, and all too often, books and articles note the need but provide few concrete suggestions for how to improve thinking. Most critical thinking resources are aimed at academic audiences and settings. Our aim is to bring *critical thinking* (called *CT* throughout this text) into the real world of healthcare delivery and education by offering practical suggestions for CT-promoting activities.

Because CT is a tool that must be implemented within a context of problems or issues, this text addresses the CT needed to achieve five healthcare competencies outlined by the Institute of Medicine (IOM) in their *Quality Chasm* series. Those competencies—*quality improvement, patient-centered care, work in interdisciplinary teams, evidence-based practice*, and *using informatics*—will, in the IOM's vision, improve healthcare delivery in the United States. These and very similar competencies have been foci of healthcare improvement plans in many other countries as well. The international literature supporting moves in these directions is growing daily. Informatics has made our world accessible as it never has been before. Not only do we need to work in interdisciplinary teams in our own institutions, but teamwork now crosses borders as all nations strive to improve health for their citizens.

The conceptualization of CT throughout this text comes from our years of research in this area, most notably our Delphi study to find a consensus description for CT in nursing. Through that research, an expert panel of 55 nurses from 9 countries and 23 U.S. states described 17 dimensions of CT in nursing—10 habits of the mind (affective dimensions) and 7 cognitive skills. The habits of the mind are *confidence, contextual perspective, creativity, flexibility, inquisitiveness, intellectual integrity, intuition, open-mindedness, perseverance*, and *reflection*. The skills are *analyzing, applying standards, discriminating, information seeking, logical reasoning, predicting*, and *transforming knowledge*. With those 17 dimensions, CT may be broken into manageable units as we describe thinking within the competency contexts.

Throughout this text, we often use the terms *critical thinking* (CT) and *thinking* interchangeably. We acknowledge that these terms are not synonymous in other contexts; however, within health care, we believe that all thinking is critical. Our readers may have seen comments in the literature implying that CT in nursing should be called something else, but no matter what it is called, thinking is a critical part of nursing that must be studied. Critical thinking by any other name is still critical thinking!

Keeping a focus on concrete, active learning strategies to promote CT, we have several strategies (called *TACTICS* to mirror our title) or practice activities throughout all chapters, except the last chapter. These activities will help readers reflect on their personal and professional thinking styles while practicing CT-enhancing strategies. Some TACTICS are for educators to use in academic or practice settings; others are directed toward clinicians.

We believe you may now be able to see where the book's title comes from. Obviously, the idea of *tactics* comes from our desire to provide practical strategies. As an acronym, it stands for several activities important to promoting CT: **T**racking, **A**ssessing, and **C**ultivating **T**hinking to **I**mprove **C**ompetency-based **S**trategies (TAC-TICS). *Tracking* alludes to following thinking paths, making them visible and therefore open for study and enhancement. *Assessing* denotes discerning the quality of thinking. *Cultivating* implies a growth-enhancing process; CT is not a concrete end point, but a process that may be enhanced. *Thinking*, as we described earlier, is defined as critical thinking with 17 dimensions. *Improve* is just what it says; we want to promote better CT. *Competency-based* strategies comes from the IOM competencies that serve as the context for our CT discussions. Competency-based implies performance of CT in the real world, as opposed to an academic checklist. *Strategies* are those means by which CT is practiced and enhanced so that healthcare quality may be enhanced.

Adding to what we hope are practical qualities of this text for busy clinicians, students, and educators, we have written in user-friendly language with short segments and set off specific ideas in easily visible boxes, tables, and figures. Although our focus has been on thinking, we have needed to provide information on the contextual issues. Out of necessity, our descriptions of subjects such as informatics, evidence-based practice, and quality improvement are only one chapter long and not meant to be primary references on those subjects. We hope we have provided enough context for our readers to focus on the CT parts.

We appreciate the value of humor and visual variety to thinking and have therefore enlisted the aid of two superb artists, Mark Steele and Jesse Rubenfeld, to render cartoons here and there to make some of our ideas come alive. Our intention is to keep you visually stimulated so your thinking stays at its peak and piqued.

We start this text with a chapter titled "*Why* Critical Thinking?" in keeping with our belief that most CT journeys start best with questions. We also want you to appreciate, right from the start, why CT is so important. Unfortunately, the label *critical thinking* has become a bit hackneyed over the past few years. Because many groups have stated the need to address CT, it seems that everyone talks about it. We have found, however, that there are lots of things labeled *critical thinking* that really do not address thinking per se.

Chapters 2, 3, and 4 set the stage for understanding CT in a *what, who, why, how, where*, and *when* format. Chapter 2, "*What* Is Critical Thinking?," provides the framework of the 17 dimensions, how they were developed, and their special place as one of the few conceptualizations of CT that was based on evidence from nurses and linked to health care. Chapter 3, "*Who* Are the Critical Thinkers?," shows the importance of individual, cultural, and environmental factors that define us as thinkers. We specifically address our intended audience of clinicians and educators as we provide various strategies for CT self-reflection. Chapter 4 combines the *how, when*, and *where* of CT because those factors are too intertwined to be addressed separately. This chapter introduces the five IOM competencies as the context for CT and becomes one of two bookends for the following chapters, each of which focuses on one competency. This chapter suggests specific strategies for educators to promote CT in their teaching and strategies for clinicians to practice CT reflection in action.

Chapters 5–9 focus on the five IOM competencies. Chapter 5, "Critical Thinking, Quality Improvement, and Safety," describes the risk-laden state of affairs in health care, traces the history of quality improvement schemes, and justifies the need for reform. That reform is framed as a move toward enhanced CT. Chapter 6, "Critical Thinking and Patient-Centered Care," describes the shift from the old style of provider-centered care and explores patients' and significant others' CT as they interface with providers' CT. Chapter 7, "Critical Thinking and Interdisciplinary Teams," differentiates individual and team CT and shows how both are vital to quality health care. Chapter 8, "Critical Thinking and Evidence-Based Practice," demonstrates how important CT is to the various phases and tasks in this shift from basing practice on traditions and authority to practice based on the best evidence. Chapter 9, "Critical Thinking and Informatics," explores this burgeoning field and how various dimensions of CT are used to deal with information technology. We acknowledge the special challenges that the rapidly changing field of informatics holds for nurses like us who are "old"—primarily in their 40s, 50s, and 60s.

Chapter 10 explores a popular but frustrating topic in nursing—that is, "Assessing Critical Thinking." Clinicians and health educators are being asked to show how their CT, and that of students, is improving. Because that assessment need has been so strong, especially in academic settings, most evaluation plans and instruments have been taken from other disciplines and have questionable validity in healthcare arenas. Or they have been created without a clear description of CT or how it works. We offer suggestions for assessment methods, including one based on our research, Assessing Critical Thinking (ACT). Having established validity with our research-based 17 CT dimensions, we have shown respectable interrater reliability in limited testing of a method that is efficient, without compromising assessment of all the complexities of CT. We also discuss the CT Inventory in Appendix A as a means to assess CT.

Chapter 11 is the other bookend for the previous chapters, which placed CT in the context of competencies and assessment. Originally, we envisioned this chapter as a look at the day-to-day realities, but as we finished with the previous chapters, we realized how strong the theme of complex change was throughout the book, so we titled the chapter "Thinking Realities of Yesterday, Today, and Tomorrow." We described the dynamic nature of CT and how it fits perfectly with complex adaptive systems and their constant state of flux. Chapter 11 concludes with some of our latest brainstorms. The first is a preliminary report on our current research into synthesis, which is our attempt to elucidate the CT dimension of *transforming knowledge*. The second brainstorm is a brief summary of our discussions with expert nurse educators who teach CT at undergraduate and graduate levels.

This edition includes two appendices. Appendix A is the CT Inventory that we developed. We have found that prompts, such as those in the inventory, help people think about their thinking, an essential prerequisite for improving CT. In this edition, we have added a research report from a colleague, who has studied RN students' reflections after using the CT Inventory. Appendix B provides resources for our ACT method of assessing CT.

We hope you will find this text practical and CT stimulating. The complex healthcare system has no choice but to change to meet the needs of society today. Clinicians must use their CT to contribute their part to that change, and educators must change their teaching to prepare better critical thinkers. Those changes, as outlined by many, including the IOM, must occur so clinicians come to practice with visions of a future with higher-quality care.

Because we are primarily educators these days, we solicited stories from our nurse colleagues in practice settings to make sure we have well represented the clinician side of this text. We hope that stories from the "swampy lowlands" (to borrow a phrase from Schon) have counterbalanced our ivory tower views. We hope our clinician readers agree. Enjoy your thinking journey as you read and reflect. We look to you to continue making CT a natural process within health care, today and tomorrow.

Acknowledgments

As with the first and second editions, this third edition would not have come to life without the assistance of many people. We would like to thank our nursing colleagues who gave us positive feedback on our previous writing projects, as well as the honor of the *AJN Book of the Year* award for the first edition. Thanks to Dr. George Allen, whose writing expertise we continue to envy; you taught us much about research on critical thinking assessment methods. To Drs. Margaret Lunney, Joanne Profetto-McGrath, and Marsha Fonteyn, who have for years advocated for the importance of critical thinking in nursing and supported our work, you remain an inspiration to us.

We extend our sincere gratitude to our contributors whose critical thinking insights have brought life to our words:

To our clinician contributors:

Sherry Bumpus, who shared her story of evidence-based practice

David Caraballo, who allowed us to use one of his student reflection assignments

Jane Duerr, who shared her approaches to reflection in action and her description of interdisciplinary practice

Kate Kimmet, who shared her story about informatics

Kari Szczechowski, from the Michigan Oakwood Healthcare System, who shared her story of patient-centered care

Jose Valderrama, who shared insight on his Hispanic cultural perspective

To our nurse educator contributors:

Elizabeth Bucciarelli, Eastern Michigan University's health sciences librarian, who shared her experiences of working with students to promote their use of informatics

Sandra Hines, who shared her research with the CT Inventory in Appendix A.

The Brainstorm Session on Teaching CT group, who shared their teaching strategies:
- Laurie Blondy
- Sherry Bumpus
- Marguerite DeBello
- Sandra Hines
- Martha Tanicala

To our coresearchers on the synthesis project:

Ann Blakeslee

Laurie Blondy

Brenda Cronin

Rose Luster-Turner

We would also like to thank our nursing students at Eastern Michigan University, who are good natured about our frequent critical thinking discussions and our creative attempts to teach thinking in innovative ways. To Mark Steele and Jesse Rubenfeld, our cartoonists, who constantly amaze us with their creative ability to capture our ideas in humorous sketches, we say thanks for sharing your talents.

Last, but not least, we'd like to thank our families, who again tolerated endless hours of viewing only the backs of our heads against the computer screen, who understood our absence from significant events, and who survived our mood swings. We love you and are so grateful that you do the household chores, feed us, run errands, and provide emotional support continually. Tyler, thanks for your support and words of wisdom. Jesse and Amber, thanks for the ongoing "Go Mom!" Rich, as always, thanks for your editorial wisdom, cheering, and household maintenance during these writing marathon times. Dan and Anna, Amanda and Ryan, thanks for always asking how things are going with "the book." Thank you Drew Allie, Penelope, and Cassandra, for just being you; your presence continues to put smiles on our faces. Kenn, thanks for ongoing support and praise for doing this again!

Contributors

Mark Steele, artist, contributor of cartoon art
(www.MarkSteeleArt.com)
Jesse Rubenfeld, illustrator, contributor of cartoon art
(www.jesserubenfeld.net)

CHAPTER 1

Why Critical Thinking?

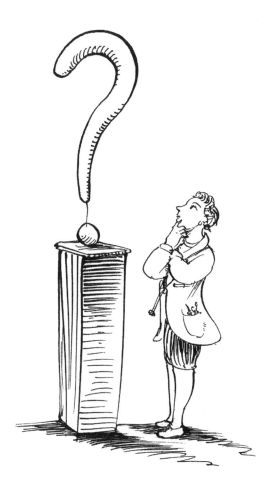

© Mark Steele. Reprinted by permission.

Healthcare delivery, and nursing in particular, is in dire need of critical thinkers. If you don't believe us, look at **Box 1-1** for the words of other authors. The ever-changing healthcare system is becoming increasingly complex and fraught with decision points where mistakes can occur. Clinicians make a jillion decisions every day. Most of those decisions are made in microseconds but can have very serious consequences. Some decisions allow for more thinking time, consultation with others, and a search of other resources

1

Box 1-1 *Why* Critical Thinking Is Essential in Nursing

"To provide quality care in this environment, nurses need to develop critical thinking (CT) skills that will provide them with expertise in flexible, individualized, situation-specific problem-solving" (Brunt, 2005, p. 60).

"Other reasons why nurses must be competent critical thinkers include the dramatic changes happening in health care related to information technology, fiscal cutbacks, human resource limitations, and the acuity of many patient care situations" (Carter & Rukholm, 2008, p. 134).

"Critical thinking is an integral part of clinical decision making and therefore a routine part of nurses' work" (Daly, 2001, p. 121).

"To deal effectively with rapid change nurses need to become skilled in higher-level thinking and reasoning . . . There is not always theoretical evidence to support practice, therefore, nursing needs to incorporate into its practice critical thinking processes to provide new answers to practical questions . . . Every day nurses sift through an abundance of data and information to assimilate and adapt knowledge for problem clarification in an attempt to find solutions" (Edwards, 2007, p. 303).

"As health care systems become more complex . . . it is important for nurses to develop critical-thinking, problem-solving, and reflective practice techniques" (Rogal & Young, 2008, p. 28).

"Increasingly complex needs and expanding roles in the delivery of health care require professional nurses to be capable critical thinkers and self-directed learners" (Worrell & Profetto-McGrath, 2007, p. 420).

"Given the undoubted global health issues, the need for critical thought and action is paramount" (Morrall & Goodman, 2012, conclusion).

"As the discipline evolves alongside societal needs, the complexity of health care, increased use of technology, and increased patient acuity requires nurses with well-developed critical thinking" (Raymond-Seniuk & Profetto-McGrath, 2011, p. 49).

---

before a conclusion is reached. But all decisions must be accurate and made in a timely manner.

There are many resources—books, articles, speeches—out there telling us what needs to be done to improve the quality of health care. Many of them allude to the need for critical thinking (CT), but few provide concrete suggestions for how to improve thinking. That's because it's not simple to improve thinking; it's not even simple to study it. Even a definition of nursing CT is hard to find. As complex as the healthcare system is, so too is CT.

The place of nurses in the healthcare system is also complex and getting increasingly so. Nurses are expanding their roles, taking on more responsibility, and learning to adapt to constant change. The kind of thinking that nurses do is convoluted and usually occurs in what Schon (1983) called the "swampy lowlands" (p. 43). The thinking of nurses is much more complex than most people realize.

It is within this complex context that we explore CT in nursing. We want to impress upon our readers why CT is so vital. We start this text with why, even before we tell you what CT is, because we want you to let your curiosity and questioning attitude lead the way into this exciting adventure.

Why Questions and Thinking

Why questions imply a search for reason, purpose, meaning, and value. The word *why* is frequently used to initiate inquiry, provide logic, justify conclusions, and find causes. *Why* demonstrates one of the first forms of thinking and exploration we used as children (Why is the sky blue?). Those of you with young children who constantly ask why might want the word banned from the dictionary on some of your tired days. But *why*, and the thinking connected with *why*, has triggered many important discoveries over the years. The discovery of penicillin, Einstein's theory of relativity, the exploration of space, and even the discovery of Viagra all followed *why*. (In fact, according to a personal communication with a pharmaceutical industry research scientist, it was a nurse who asked the question that led to the discovery of Viagra as a treatment for erectile dysfunction. During clinical trials of a pharmacological treatment of cardiovascular problems, she noticed that the volunteers were reluctant to return unused trial medications. She asked *why*, and the rest is history!)

For many, the natural tendency to ask *why* has diminished after years of traditional schooling. That is sad and also a bit frightening because *why* questions are powerful instigators of thinking. Even Einstein emphasized the value of *why* questions when he said, "The important thing is to never stop questioning. Curiosity has its own reason for existing" (Brainy Quote, 2013).

Why is also the favorite word of many educators who encourage students to provide rationales for their nursing interventions. *Why* is used by clinicians when they work as preceptors and mentors for new staff or when they question their own practice. Questioning why something is happening with a patient can be a life-saving inquiry. Clinicians and educators alike believe that *why* questions encourage CT (Scheffer, 2001). We will tease your brain to consider why in this first stop at action learning, **TACTICS 1-1**. As discussed in the preface, TACTICS for clinicians and educators will be used throughout this text to engage you in activities that will stimulate your CT and move thinking from abstract concepts to practical contexts.

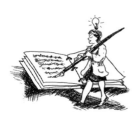

© Jesse Rubenfeld

TACTICS 1-1: Exploring Your Use of *Why*

Clinicians and Educators

With a colleague or on your own, think about the last time you asked *why*. How many times a day do you ask it? Enough times to learn what you want to know? Too many times? And what does it lead to? Are you simply asking out of habit, or do you then pursue the answers that prompt you to ask more questions and delve even deeper? How do colleagues react to your *why* questions? What motivates you to ask *why*?

Discussion

The answers to these questions should stimulate reflection. Are you satisfied with your answers? *Why* questions that stimulate reflection can prompt searches for purpose, meaning, and value. The great philosophers asked all these classic questions: *Why* are we here? *Why* do we exist? *Why* do we care? On a less esoteric level, reflecting on *why* helps us understand and appreciate the value of thinking. So *why* does CT benefit health care? To answer, we will look at *why* there has been so much interest in thinking in recent years. We will also respond to *why* thinking is so important.

Asking *why* questions will inevitably lead one to ask more questions, such as *who*, *what*, *when*, and *where*. It is this questioning stance that is essential to studying CT. We'd like our readers to begin their CT journey with questions for two reasons. First, we know this approach works because that's how we began our travels through the CT maze. Many years ago we knew why CT was important in nursing, and we asked how we could help nursing students become better thinkers; our exciting exploration of reading, researching, talking, and writing about CT took off. We want to share our discoveries so you can build on what we have learned. Second, we'd like you to think about your questions, and the questions that they lead to, because they are the essence of great thinking.

The great educational philosopher Paulo Freire (1998) wrote:

> To stimulate questions and critical reflection about the questions, asking what is meant by this or that question, is fundamental to curiosity. Otherwise, all we have is the passivity of students in the face of the discursive explanations of the teacher and answers to questions that have not been asked. (p. 80)

Although we cannot hear your questions, we'd like you to imagine a dialogue with us. Think about your questions and jot down your reflections on them in the margins as you read along. Even though we have been immersed in the teaching of CT in nursing for 2 decades, we are frequently faced with new questions. What is your most burning question about CT in nursing? Write it here, and after you complete your study, look back and see if that question was answered. My burning question is:

Why the Interest in CT in Health Care and Healthcare Education over the Past Two Decades?

Thinking has been a topic of discussion for philosophers for centuries, but other disciplines have also been concerned about thinking. Schon (1983) explored thinking in medicine, engineering, law, business, and education. Dreyfus and Dreyfus (1986) described the importance of thinking in the aviation industry.

Hundreds of thousands of articles and thousands of books have been written about CT in all disciplines. There are courses, whole curricula, and even institutes designed to improve thinking. We taught a required undergraduate nursing course called Critical Thinking in Nursing for several years. The National League for Nursing (NLN) highlighted the importance of promoting thinking in nursing curricula (NLN, 2006). An Australian website provides up-to-date information on colleges, universities, forums, and ongoing research on CT (Austhink, 2013). In health care, accrediting bodies, policy makers, and others promote CT. The Institute of Medicine (IOM, 2004) addressed CT across disciplines for improving national health care. Obviously, many people and organizations think CT is very important; some of their statements about the benefits of thinking are shown in **Box 1-2**.

Box 1-2 The Benefits of CT

"Professional knowledge is mismatched to the changing characteristics of the situation of practice—the complexity, uncertainty, instability, uniqueness, and value conflicts, which are increasingly perceived as central to the world of professional practice" (Schon, 1983, p. 14).

Problems encountered in practice "are not in the book" (Schon, 1983, p. 16).

"Knowledge is discovered by thinking, analyzed by thinking, organized by thinking, transformed by thinking, assessed by thinking, and most importantly acquired by thinking" (Paul, 1992, p. xi).

Thinking helps us recognize beliefs and assumptions that our minds consider to be facts (Brookfield, 1995).

Knowledge, facts, and information are frequently equated with intelligence. But the ability to use knowledge in logical, ethical, and moral ways is not always equal to the quality of the knowledge, facts, and information. Thinking provides the screening mechanism for converting knowledge, facts, and information into practical application in the real world (Schon, 1983).

There is "no way to create a neat and tidy step-by-step path to knowledge that all minds can mindlessly follow" (Paul, 1992, p. xi).

Pure logic and analytical reasoning is inadequate for expert decision making. Expert decision making is a blend of careful analysis, intuition, and the wisdom

(continues)

Box 1-2   The Benefits of CT (continued)

---

and judgment gleaned from experience. Human thinking and decision making continues to exceed that of machines (artificial intelligence) because of three key factors: awareness of the environment, the ability to discriminate, and tolerance for ambiguity (Dreyfus & Dreyfus, 1986).

"Only by changing how we think can we change deeply embedded policies and practices" (Senge, 1990, p. xiv).

"The deepest insight usually comes when they [people] realize that their problems, and their hopes for improvement, are inextricably tied to how they think" (Senge, 1990, p. 53).

Self-regulation, critical thinking, and creative thinking are probably the most important dimensions influencing learning (Marzano & Pickering, 1997),

True understanding comes from the ability to think and act flexibly, distinguish nuance, appreciate context, and use reflection (Wiggins & McTighe, 2001).

Our conceptualization of CT comes from years of practice and research in this area—most notably our Delphi study, which sought to find a consensus description for CT in nursing. Through that research, an expert panel of 55 nurses from 9 countries and 23 U.S. states described 17 dimensions of CT in nursing: 10 habits of the mind (affective dimensions) and 7 cognitive skills (Scheffer & Rubenfeld, 2000). The habits of the mind are *confidence, contextual perspective, creativity, flexibility, inquisitiveness, intellectual integrity, intuition, open-mindedness, perseverance,* and *reflection.* The cognitive skills are *analyzing, applying standards, discriminating, information seeking, logical reasoning, predicting,* and *transforming knowledge.* These 17 dimensions show CT broken down into manageable units. Because CT is complex, studying its pieces makes it more understandable, allowing you to see the thinking within various contexts. (Throughout the remainder of this text, every time we use one of the 17 dimensions, you will see them in italics to reinforce the language of thinking that you can begin to incorporate into your practice. **Box 1-3** gives you a quick list of these 17 dimensions.)

So why has there been so much emphasis on CT in health care over the past few decades? One has to only pick up a newspaper or magazine or listen to the news to learn the answer. Some of the key matters that require more or better thinking are the information and technology explosions; dwindling resources; cost containment; third-party payer gatekeeping; demographics; morbidity and mortality data; global economics and potential epidemics, patient safety, and failure to rescue; and emergent ethical dilemmas such as the right to life, prolongation of life without quality, and stem cell research.

Box 1-3   Quick List of the 17 Dimensions of Critical Thinking in Nursing

CT Habits of the Mind	*CT Skills*
Confidence	Analyzing
Contextual perspective	Applying standards
Creativity	Discriminating
Flexibility	Information seeking
Inquisitiveness	Logical reasoning
Intellectual integrity	Predicting
Intuition	Transforming knowledge
Open-mindedness	
Perseverance	
Reflection	

All healthcare disciplines are recognizing the need to pool their thinking to come up with better ways to deal with such complex issues. A notable example of such pooled thinking is the IOM project (2003). The project's charge was to tap into the thinking energy of an interdisciplinary group—nurses, physicians, pharmacists, physical therapists, social workers, and others—to identify new directions for health care. Past solutions clearly do not address the growing complexity of our current problems. If it's not working today, it surely will fail tomorrow. To quote from Einstein again, "We cannot solve our problems with the same thinking we used when we created them" (Brainy Quote, 2013).

One outcome of the IOM (2003) work was the development of five competencies—patient-centered care, interdisciplinary teams (IDTs), evidence-based practice, informatics, and quality improvement. These competencies were developed to help guide the thinking of all healthcare disciplines toward a unified plan of practice, education, and research to promote safe, effective, and efficient patient care. Let's look at some of the basic benefits of thinking in health care and who benefits from it. In **TACTICS 1-2** we'll start with a simple nursing situation and help Joyce, a novice clinician, who had trouble with a colostomy dressing.

TACTICS 1-2: Exploring Joyce's Thinking

Now wait a minute! I've done colostomy dressing changes a dozen times; I followed all the steps of the protocol exactly as I always do. Afterward I even checked out the textbook

the nursing student left on the unit, and it says to do exactly what I did. So I'm asking myself, why didn't it work?

Now refer to Box 1-1 and Box 1-2 and see if you can find any thinking clues that would help Joyce with her dilemma.

Discussion

The second statement in Box 1-2, "Problems encountered in practice are not in the book" (Schon, 1983), is a good match for what happened to Joyce. Do other statements also fit? "Not in the book" is the key here. One problem with a practice discipline such as nursing is that the real world seldom, if ever, looks like the book world. The book learning gets you started, but only started; it's never the whole solution. Nurses must rely on something else to deal with the many problems encountered in practice. Everything about nursing is contextual. Thinking is the only constant that will go from context to context.

The Context of Thinking

Studying CT by itself, outside context, is like studying how to take care of a colostomy without ever seeing a patient with a colostomy. There's only the abstraction of the idea, not the actual day-to-day reality of the concept. We can tell you why CT is important, but you won't fully appreciate that importance until you see CT in action. Studying CT by itself is a wonderful philosophical activity, but as nurses we must look at CT in action. CT is a tool to be used in the muddy world of health care.

Other authors have identified how important it is to address context. For example, Tesoro (2012) presented a Developing Nurses' Thinking (DNT) model showing CT within a context of nursing and nursing education. Four constructs were combined: "(a) patient safety, (b) domain knowledge, (c) critical thinking processes, and (d) repeated practice" (p. 436). Lunney's work (2008, 2010) put CT into the context of diagnostic accuracy. Without the necessary CT, diagnoses may be inaccurate and therefore affect the quality of health care as the nurse heads down the wrong path in patient care.

Because CT must be implemented within the context of specific problems or issues, this text addresses the CT needed to achieve five healthcare competencies outlined by the IOM in its Quality Chasm series. These competencies—patient-centered care, work in IDTs, evidence-based practice, using informatics, and quality improvement—will, in the IOM's vision, improve healthcare delivery in the United States (IOM, 2003). These and very similar competencies have been the foci of healthcare improvement plans in many other countries as well, and the international literature supporting movement in this direction is growing daily. Indeed, we have much to learn from clinicians, researchers, and educators in countries such as Canada, the United Kingdom, Australia, and the Netherlands, especially in the area of evidence-based practice. Informatics has made the world accessible as it never has been before. Not only do we need to work in IDTs in our own institutions, but teamwork now crosses borders as all nations strive to improve the health of their citizens.

The Big Picture of *Why* Thinking Is Important

We've learned that the purpose of asking *why* is to find meaning and value or benefit. To focus on benefits, we need to explore who benefits and what is the benefit—*why* is thinking important to them? We will use the term *stakeholders* to describe the individuals and groups who have a stake (something to gain or lose) in some endeavor. Stakeholders may gain or lose power, control, money, and—yes—health. They are also thinkers who gain or lose from thinking or not thinking. And their thinking has an effect on the whole as well. Do you see how complex this is?

To use a two-dimensional analogy, consider all the stakeholders in health care as being in a sequence of concentric circles. The innermost circle in the healthcare system contains the primary stakeholders. We classify them as primary because they benefit directly from the thinking of healthcare providers and, it is hoped, they contribute their thinking as well. This primary group includes patients and their significant others.

The concentric circle of thinkers closest to the primary stakeholders includes clinicians, educators, and other providers in the IDT. The thinking of these people directly affects patient outcomes. If done properly, the thinking of the individuals in this circle merges smoothly with the thinking of the primary stakeholders of the innermost circle. The results of that merged thinking are quality patient outcomes.

Moving outward, the next circle in this image would include unit managers, administrators, third-party payers, healthcare organizations, government groups, and healthcare professions. These stakeholders experience less direct effects of thinking in the swampy lowlands of care, but they are still essential stakeholders because their thinking has both positive and negative outcomes as well. Their impact has broader, long-lasting, and longer-term consequences as a result of legislation, policies and procedures, and guidelines.

Now let's take this two-dimensional image of concentric circles and make it three-dimensional. Visualize the primary stakeholders (patients and significant others), along with clinicians, educators, and the IDT, as the very center or nucleus. Take all those concentric circles full of other stakeholders' thinking and spin them around so they are on different planes. Picture the images from grade school of the rings of electrons rotating around the spinning nucleus of an atom. Are you getting the idea of the complexity and dynamic nature of thinking among the stakeholders?

Don't get overwhelmed by this complexity. We are going to help you dissect, or unpack, things to get a better look at the thinking involved. Or, if you want us to sound more professional, we are going to do some *analyzing* to better understand the pieces of thinking and the impact they have on stakeholders, and then we will move to synthesis to find new meaning.

Major Stakeholders and Critical Thinking

This next section focuses on CT with the major stakeholders. The major stakeholders in health care include two basic groups. Patients and significant others are the primary stakeholders group because they experience the direct consequences of thinking or nonthinking care. Clinicians, educators, and IDTs make up the second major group. This group is closest to the recipients of care and see and feel the up-close and personal results of thinking or nonthinking. These two groups and their thinking have the most impact on patient outcomes.

Quality patient outcomes require multiple levels of thinking from all stakeholders, even beyond the major ones. Patients and significant others are thinkers themselves and often struggle to coordinate their thinking with that of the healthcare team.

Why *Is CT Important to Patients and Significant Others, the Primary Stakeholders?*

Explaining why CT is important to patients and significant others is a bit of a no-brainer. Patients and significant others are at the center of the healthcare system. They are the primary stakeholders in quality care. They are dependent on the thinking and actions of those who work in health care to receive quality care. For now, we will simply say that the delivery of safe, effective, and efficient care has always been the underlying goal of good nursing care. CT is essential to achieving these goals.

The exercise in **TACTICS 1-3** highlights how nursing staff using (or not using) CT affects the primary stakeholder, the patient. This exercise could be used by clinicians or educators to emphasize why thinking is important to safe, effective, and efficient patient care.

TACTICS 1-3: Exploring Safe, Effective, and Efficient Care for Mr. Stone

1. Read the scenario about Mr. Stone.
2. As you read, consider whether better thinking could have prevented the extended hospital stay.

Scenario 1-1: Mr. Stone

Mr. Stone is a 60-year-old male. He was admitted to the hospital 3 days before the Christmas holiday for emergency surgery after his left arm was severed midway between his wrist and elbow in an industrial accident. He was in good health prior to the accident but had smoked one to two packs of cigarettes per day for 40 years. The surgery to remove the severed portion of his arm and prepare for a prosthesis was successful. Nursing care included administration of pain medications, monitoring for infection at the wound site, and assistance with activities of daily living. Mr. Stone was expected to be discharged in 2 to 3 days. On the second day after surgery, he developed pneumonia, and his hospital stay was extended 6 more days.

Discussion

Your answers about better thinking may be more general, but we'll start using the language of the dimensions of CT that we described earlier in this chapter (in Box 1-3). Consider thinking dimensions that possibly were not used. If the nurses were *applying standards*, they would have designed care to include coughing, incentive spirometry, and precise assessment of respiratory status when developing their postoperative care plan, not just medications and wound care. If the nurses were using *contextual perspective*, they would have more carefully assessed Mr. Stone's smoking habits and any history of respiratory problems. If the nurses were *discriminating*, they would have identified Mr. Stone as a very high-risk patient for postoperative pulmonary complications because of his smoking. If the nurses were *predicting*, they would have recognized the serious consequences of not developing a rigorous plan for postoperative coughing and deep breathing. They might even have made a referral to respiratory therapy to institute such a prevention plan.

Of course, Mr. Stone might have developed pneumonia in spite of all those nursing interventions; however, with better CT, the chances of this outcome would have been greatly reduced. Not only did Mr. Stone suffer the physical and emotional pain of the loss of an arm and early retirement, but because of his potentially preventable pneumonia, he also was hospitalized over the Christmas and New Year's Day holidays, a time of year that he would have enjoyed with family and friends at home.

In addition to safe care, CT is important for effective and efficient care. Effective care is individualized and accurate. It employs the correct interventions for the health situation at hand. Efficient care requires timely thinking so that resources are used appropriately. If Mr. Stone's nurses had been more effective in their thinking, they would have individualized their assessment, accurately diagnosed his risk for pneumonia right from the start, and implemented proper interventions. In addition, if Mr. Stone's nurses had used more CT, his hospital stay would have been shorter, thus saving time, money, and energy. In short, his care would have been more efficient. This scenario demonstrates the impact that thinking has on patients and their significant others. CT makes a huge difference in patient care outcomes!

The group of stakeholders in the next circle includes the clinicians, the educators, and the IDT. The stakeholders in this circle have the most direct impact on outcomes for patients.

Why Is CT Important to Clinicians?

Clinicians who think critically have more *confidence* in their reasoning. *Confidence* in reasoning allows nurses to speak their minds, to openly identify potential errors and near misses, to contribute to team meetings, and to provide solid rationales for their decisions. *Confidence* empowers them to make valid contributions and decisions related to patient care and unit concerns.

CT is important to job satisfaction because it helps the clinician attain and maintain a professional nursing self-image. Even when parts of the nursing role are uncomfortable, good clinicians rely on professional ethics and *intellectual integrity* to reinforce their thinking. They derive job satisfaction from knowing that their thinking was actively engaged and the job was done to the best of their ability. One strategy to achieve such satisfaction is through *reflection* (Gustaffsson & Fagerberg, 2004). The scenario in **TACTICS 1-4** illustrates how CT empowers decision making and enhances job satisfaction.

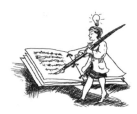

TACTICS 1-4: Enhancing Decision-Making Skills and Job Satisfaction through Professional Integrity

1. Read Scenario 1-2.
2. Where did Juan use his best thinking?
3. How do you think Juan felt about the situation?
4. How did Juan's CT affect both decision making and job satisfaction?

Scenario 1-2: *Juan's Home Visit*

Juan is a community health nurse. His home-care patient load today included 17-year-old Jenny and her 3-week-old newborn, Billy. This was Juan's first home visit with Jenny, following up on a referral from the pediatrician's office because Billy had not gained weight since birth. Jenny was an unwed mother living with her parents in a spacious, professionally decorated home in an upper-middle-class neighborhood. Jenny looked tired and interacted only minimally with Juan, and she rarely looked at the baby, who was restless and fussy in his bassinet. Jenny's mother was home, and she did most of the talking, explaining how she expected Jenny to take full responsibility for Billy's care. In fact, Jenny's parents both worked and were frequently out of town on business, but because of Juan's visit, Jenny's mother stayed home to assure the nurse that though the visit was well intentioned, it was certainly not necessary.

Juan examined Billy and found some disturbing data. Billy had lost another 3 ounces, and there were several dark areas on his back and legs. These markings had not been noted on the referral information.

Juan asked more questions. Jenny's mother assured him that Jenny was doing a fine job; they would be sure Billy got an extra feeding to gain his weight back; and all her children bruised easily, so Billy probably inherited that trait.

Juan, however, had to make a tough decision. He didn't want to believe the baby was being abused; this was a normal-looking family in a decent neighborhood. But he couldn't ignore the data: indications of ineffective maternal bonding, failure to thrive, and the apparent recent bruising all pointed to possible abuse. He also knew he was legally obligated to report suspected abuse. He was not comfortable with his decision to file a formal report, but he was confident it was the correct decision and that he could justify his reasoning. Juan found out later that the nurse at the pediatrician's office had similar concerns, but she only had the original weight loss data to go on. She told Juan that she didn't want to bias his thinking, so she didn't share her suspicions with him until after his visit.

Discussion

The key thinking areas that Juan used in this situation were *intellectual integrity* (although he did not want to believe that the infant was being abused, he had to consider the evidence), *applying standards* (he was legally required to report suspected abuse), *confidence* (he trusted his reasoning ability), and *logical reasoning* (he believed he had adequate evidence to support his suspicions).

Juan very likely also felt shocked, uncomfortable, and annoyed: shocked and uncomfortable that an upper-middle-class family might be abusing a child, and annoyed that the nurse in the pediatrician's office had not been open about her suspicions before the visit. He believed that he would have been *open-minded* enough to collect accurate information even if he had known of the nurse's hunch.

When Juan reflected on the situation, he could justify and support his decisions. He knew his judgment was sound. As an individual and a professional, he derived satisfaction from knowing that he may have saved a life and provided an opportunity for a family to become more functional. He became a nurse because he wanted to help people, and that goal was accomplished. By doing his job with compassion and *intellectual integrity*, his behavior matched his role expectations, leading to job satisfaction.

Another way that CT benefits clinicians is by helping them move from novice to advanced beginner to competent to proficient and, ultimately, to expert (Benner, 1984). Throughout this process, the clinician moves away from the context-free rules of novice decision making to more sophisticated levels of thinking. Thinking is essential to expert nurses, who can imagine the whole of a situation from a few details. They use *reflection* in action; they have learned to trust their *intuition*. And they do all of this consistently. Expert nurses engage all CT dimensions so naturally and with such ease that their decisions look effortless. The hard work of the thinking behind their actions is rarely apparent unless they have recognized how important it is to think out loud. Many experts don't recognize how fine-tuned thinking is, but they couldn't be experts without it. This level of thinking benefits patients as well as nurses.

Why *Is CT Important to Educators?*

Nurse educators derive all the benefits that clinicians do from CT, and more. CT helps novice (and experienced) educators accept the reality that they do not need to know everything. This acceptance usually comes harder to the novice educator. Most experienced educators come to realize that their brains do not have enough random-access memory (RAM) to store all needed information and that the information they need to store keeps changing. With good CT habits of mind and skills, educators can be comfortable saying, "Let's go look that up," or "That's a good question, but I'll have to get back to you with an answer," or "Gee, I don't know, but let's see if we

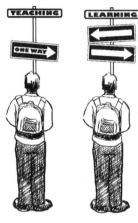

© Jesse Rubenfeld

can figure it out." Thinking helps educators accept that they don't know it all, but because of their CT, they have effective strategies to search for the best information.

CT helps both service-based and academic-based educators promote learning processes. Notice that we said learning, not teaching (see **Box 1-4**). Teaching can be simply imparting information to a passive recipient. Learning requires active engagement among the learner, the content, and the educator. CT helps the educator design such interactive learning processes, illuminating the connection between pieces of information and allowing learners to discover answers through their own use of CT. For example, instead of simply sharing the latest evidence-based guidelines on the use of a

---

Box 1-4 Comparing Learning and Teaching to Promote Critical Thinking in Nursing

Focus on Learning		*Focus on Teaching*	
The Teacher	Strong knowledge of content and the information needed for CT	**The Teacher**	Strong knowledge of content and information needed for CT
	Shares expertise with real-world examples		Shares expertise with real-world examples
	Designs active learning opportunities to engage learner and teacher in multiple levels of higher-order thinking skills		
	Strong emphasis on processes of learning, thinking, communication necessary to apply CT		Strong emphasis on content knowledge; for example, lab values, disease entities, etc.
	Integrates essential content knowledge with essential processes; for example, communication, CT, the nursing process		

Box 1-4 Comparing Learning and Teaching to Promote Critical
Thinking in Nursing (continued)

Focus on Learning		*Focus on Teaching*	
Assessment/ Evaluation	Designs multiple mini formative evaluation points to check for understanding throughout the course of study to assess thinking and learning	**Assessment/ Evaluation**	Uses either instructor-developed or standardized assessment options (quizzes, examinations, papers, projects) given to students throughout and at end of course
	Engages writing consultants, librarians, and peers in designing both formative and summative evaluation activities; for example, writing assignments, projects, vignettes to assess for CT, etc.		
	Reflects on outcomes of assessment tools and explores options for improvement		Reflects on outcomes of assessment results
The Learner	Actively engages in thinking and problem solving with content knowledge	**The Learner**	Passive recipient of information
	Moves from memorization to integration of knowledge and application of higher-order thinking		Highly skilled in memorization
Student Learning Outcomes	Learner is able to repeat back information during assessment	**Student Learning Outcomes**	Learner is able to repeat back information during assessment
	Learner is consistently able to appropriately apply classroom and laboratory knowledge into practice arena		Learner is usually able to apply classroom and laboratory knowledge in practice arena
	Learner is successfully able to integrate both content knowledge and process knowledge in a variety of practice settings		

new heparin-lock device with her staff, the staff development specialist provides time and a place for focused dialogue, exploring the advantages and disadvantages of this new device. What are the challenges of using it? How is it best used in patient care? Does it meet guidelines? CT is important to create learning processes that maximize real behavior change and transform information into useable knowledge.

CT also helps educators assess learning outcomes. For example, rather than selecting prepackaged assessment tools or educator-created competency checklists for evaluation of learning, the critically thinking educator will examine existing tools to see how well they match what needs to be learned. CT is needed to make those comparisons. For example, a nursing practice laboratory coordinator will anticipate how students should demonstrate competency in intramuscular injections. She will think about the answers to the following questions before she facilitates learning:

- What principles must the student articulate?
- What level of psychomotor skill must the student achieve?
- How can learning be designed to achieve the desired outcomes?
- What is the best way to assess that learning?

These questions must be answered before the actual laboratory learning (and thinking) occurs with the students. This preteaching CT helps the coordinator design assessment tools that do the job they are intended to do. Without thinking about the assessment, as well as the learning, educators do only half of their thinking jobs. Thinking is the common denominator for service-based and academic-based educators if they want to promote learning that results in behavior change.

Why Is CT Important to Interdisciplinary Teams?

Effective IDTs (1) are made up of members from more than one discipline or professional group, (2) are expected to pool their CT skills and habits of the mind to expand on ideas, and (3) consider all members as equal partners in thinking, including patients and significant others. Current evidence indicates that functional IDTs are the ideal for achieving desired health outcomes (IOM, 2003, 2011), and experts have noted the need to improve team thinking and actions (Halpern, 1998; Sanderson, 2003).

Other teams—multidisciplinary teams, for example—also benefit from CT, of course. But because CT is so important to IDTs, let us distinguish them from other healthcare teams. Multidisciplinary teams typically provide their discipline's perspective on patient situations but do not necessarily engage in collective problem identification and decision making. IDTs do all of this, and more.

So what is different about CT in IDTs, and why is this thinking so important? To pique your interest, we have selected just three reasons why CT is so important to IDT.

First, the thinking of the individual team members provides a wide range of raw material on which team thinking can be built. Their CT, combined with their individual knowledge base and paradigms for problem identification and decision making, is an essential contribution to the team's overall functioning.

Second, the team can examine, discuss, and select options from a larger pool of information and mix and match options before making decisions. It is this pooling of ideas that leads to the synergistic thinking so valued in health care.

Third, team thinking is also important to group cohesion. Starting in the 1960s, the literature on group work and teamwork consistently identified group cohesion as essential to effective outcomes (Massello, 1998). Team thinking provides opportunities for developing trust and respect, both of which contribute to this group cohesion and, thus, to more effective outcomes—the goal of IDT work.

Why *Is CT Important to the Other Stakeholders?*

The thinking of stakeholders who are less directly involved in care also can have a profound effect on the care of patients. Their CT is also important to the stakeholders themselves because CT affects their more immediate goals, such as unit functioning, survival of the organization, social policy, and professional responsibilities. We have selected unit managers; healthcare administrators and third-party payers; and a collective of healthcare organizations, governments, and professions as examples of these indirect stakeholders. As you read, see if you can think of additional reasons why CT might be important to them, and consider other such stakeholders who might be involved.

Why Is CT Important to Unit Managers?

Unit managers benefit from their own CT and the CT of others in many ways, including better use of resources, achieving unit goals, and demonstrating quality of care on the unit. The thinking unit manager (and thinking staff) might use *creativity* to rethink how clean linen is delivered to the unit to save money, or *flexibility* to schedule IDT meetings at convenient times to develop goals and strategies. He or she might model *inquisitiveness* by working with staff to identify new safety policies and procedures to improve quality on the unit. He or she might use *reflection* to mentor peers and improve consistency in management approaches (Hyrkas, Koivula, Lehti, & Paunonen-Ilmonen, 2003). Managers' CT abilities have a huge impact on all other stakeholders.

Why Is CT Important to Healthcare Administrators?

Administrators in charge of organizations such as hospitals, long-term care facilities, home-care agencies, trauma centers, and outpatient clinics are primarily responsible for maintaining and developing their organizations and promoting quality service in a cost-effective way. CT is the only way to find solutions to what some view as polarized interests. For example, quality and cost-effectiveness are frequently viewed as opposites, yet CT can help reframe that perspective. Polarity management is one strategy for using CT to *analyze* commonalities and then find *creative* ways to deal with other issues (Yoder-Wise, 1995). *Transforming knowledge* is another CT essential for administrators whose organizations are moving toward more patient-centered care (Miller, Galloway, Coughlin, & Brennan, 2001). Hansten and Washburn (1999) noted that administrators must have "advanced abilities to think critically . . . to improve clinical systems, decrease errors and sentinel events, and engage staff involvement to refine patient care systems" (p. 39).

Administration in health care is not confined to the practice setting. Administrators in institutions of higher education who teach health providers also need and benefit from CT. The setting may be different, but the needs are the same; CT is important in finding the balance between quality education and its cost. We don't have to tell you that healthcare education—particularly in medicine, nursing, pharmacy, and dentistry—is expensive. Remember the bumper sticker that says, "If you think education is expensive, try ignorance!" Maybe we should make a bumper sticker that says, "If you think thinking time is expensive, try health care without it!"

Why Is CT Important to Third-Party Payers?

Speaking of cost, this is where thinking is important to third-party payers—insurance companies, Medicare, and Medicaid. Remember Mr. Stone, who developed pneumonia because of inadequate CT? Fortunately, his insurance covered the cost of his prolonged hospitalization, but that cost was unnecessary and a waste of resources.

Third-party payers must rely on CT to maintain their ability to pay for health care and keep their stockholders happy. They particularly depend on *analyzing* and *predicting* to do their jobs. They also recognize the importance of changing their thinking from a focus on short-term goals to what will occur over the long term. The Affordable Care Act in the United States is making all third-party payers devote attention to the costs of care and quality (Legislative Council, 2010).

Why Is CT Important to Healthcare Organizations, Governments, and the Healthcare Professions?

The outermost circle of stakeholders contains the most complex organizations. CT at this level is very challenging and equally essential. Although at first glance these stakeholders may seem to have little impact on the day-to-day activities of healthcare organizations, in reality, their CT is very important to clinicians and educators. The CT of healthcare organizations, governments, and the healthcare professions influences the policies, legislation, and standards that guide both practice and education. It has long-term effects on the day-to-day activities and thinking of all stakeholders. Because these stakeholders have such a broad span of influence, they can use CT to see the big picture and the details, allowing them to design and implement policies that affect many people. Does this sound like *contextual perspective* or what?

Healthcare organizations need to use CT consistently to function effectively and achieve their missions and goals while maximizing their resources. For example, *creativity* helps them find better ways to organize staffing patterns. *Analysis* and *logical reasoning* help them examine infection patterns or track the rising costs of supplies. *Flexibility* helps them redirect services to meet changing customer needs.

All government organizations—be they international, national, provincial, state, or local—that are mandated to protect the public welfare need at least *analysis, logical reasoning*, and *contextual perspective* to help accomplish their goals while balancing the demands of other activities that are all competing for the same tax dollars. For example, *analysis* and *logical reasoning* can be used to determine why a state's mental health system is ranked lowest in the nation. *Contextual perspective* helps government groups understand how weather conditions affect the air conditioning needs of the growing number of citizens with chronic obstructive pulmonary disease. As the world gets smaller, the context of healthcare thinking must be global.

Other healthcare professions also rely on all 17 CT dimensions to meet the criteria for their professional status. Those criteria vary, depending on the source you use, but the basics of any profession include a code of ethics, a body of knowledge, higher education, and self-regulation (Haynes, Boese, & Butcher, 2004). How could one achieve a code of ethics without *reflection* and *logical reasoning*? How could one develop a body of knowledge without *analysis* and *inquisitiveness*? How could a professional organization design guidelines for a university curriculum without *perseverance* and *information seeking*? How could one manage self-regulation and accreditation standards without *applying standards, discriminating*, and *intellectual integrity*? *Contextual perspective* is essential as healthcare professions move toward interdisciplinary teamwork, learning from one another while maintaining their autonomous bodies of knowledge. You can probably cite examples for all the remaining CT dimensions.

Summary of the Impact of Stakeholders' CT on Quality Patient Outcomes

That's a whole lot of folks who need to recognize the impact of their thinking (or nonthinking) and the aspects of their thinking dimensions. We have summarized why CT is important for these various stakeholder groups in **Box 1-5**. This is only a very brief overview that we hope you will be able to expand on as you continue your thinking journey.

Box 1-5   *Why* Is CT Important for Various Stakeholders?

Why is CT important to:

   1. Patients and significant others?
     Thinking promotes safe care.
     Thinking enhances effective care.
     Thinking increases efficient care.

(continues)

Box 1-5   Why Is CT Important for Various Stakeholders? (continued)

---

2. Clinicians?
   Thinking empowers decision-making skills.
   Thinking enhances job satisfaction through professional integrity.
   Thinking achieves expertise in practice.
3. Educators?
   Thinking makes it OK to not know it all.
   Thinking promotes learning processes.
   Thinking enhances assessment of learning.
4. IDT?
   Individual thinking provides the IDT with raw material for problem
      identification and problem solving
   Team thinking provides synergy to create ideas that individuals would
   not achieve independently.
   Team thinking enhances group cohesion.
5. Unit managers?
   Thinking allows better use of resources.
   Thinking promotes achieving unit goals.
   Thinking demonstrates the quality of care on the unit.
6. Healthcare administrators?
   Thinking promotes quality service in a cost-effective way.
   Thinking is the way to find solutions to what some view as polarized
      interests, such as quality and cost-effectiveness.
   Thinking promotes safe, quality, patient-centered care.
7. Third-party payers?
   Thinking maintains their ability to pay for health care.
   Thinking keeps their stockholders happy.
   Thinking keeps them in business.
8. Healthcare organizations, governments, and the healthcare professions?
   Thinking allows them to see the big picture and the details.
   Thinking allows them to design and implement policies that affect
      many people.
   Thinking helps maximize resources.
   Thinking forms professions' codes and bodies of knowledge.

What Else Is Needed to Emphasize *Why* CT Is Important?

Something is important only if we value it. Words on paper do not create value. As Fullan (1993) said, "You can't mandate what matters" (p. 21). CT can never be mandated; the only successful activity is using mandates "as catalysts to reexamining"

(p. 24) the current state of affairs, which can lead to value changes. This applies to the nursing and healthcare sectors very clearly. Clinicians who are expected to promote CT but don't value it may give lip service to its importance and will not (1) commit the energy necessary for CT or (2) experience the role satisfaction that CT produces. Educators who expect to teach nursing and CT but do not value thinking will experience the same dilemmas.

So how can we help people learn to value CT? We start with Fullan's (1993) catalysts—words in mission statements, accreditation standards, and textbooks—and then we have to bring the words to life. We do this by talking about CT every day to nurture and cultivate our own CT and the CT of others. Consider the following scenario, in which a graduate student is explaining to his instructor how he modeled CT for a nursing student he was preceptoring on an inpatient medical–surgical unit.

This scenario demonstrates why talking about your thinking makes it more real for your students (if you are an educator) or your staff (if you are a clinician). Because they cannot see your neurons firing, you have the responsibility to make CT overt. When CT becomes overt through specific language, its value can be recognized.

Scenario 1-3: Modeling CT

A patient was admitted to an inpatient medical–surgical unit for evaluation of cardiac arrhythmia. She also had a history of mental illness. Her recent symptoms included nausea, diarrhea, and a low-grade fever. This was the *reflection* the graduate student teaching assistant shared with his instructor detailing how he had modeled his CT for an undergraduate nursing student:

I wanted the student to see how I was thinking through this problem and that it was OK to not have all the answers. The patient had a long history of bipolar disorder and had been taking lithium for several years, successfully managing her disease. The staff told us she was also a bit of a hypochondriac and that this was the second time this month she was complaining of the flu. I told the student, "We have to be careful and not let our perceptions affect our data collection; we have to be open-minded from the beginning. Let's use some inquisitiveness *here and find out from the patient what is happening. We need a little more* contextual perspective, *so we need to get some historical information, a sense of what has been going on in her life recently, food allergies, and so on. I'm also wondering about the possibility of lithium toxicity. Go grab a drug book and let's check that out. What do you think? How do her lab values compare to the norms? Let's do some analysis here and look at all the pieces and then think about how they do or don't fit together. Think about it for a minute and tell me what dimensions of our thinking will be needed next." We discovered that the patient was, in fact, having a toxic reaction to lithium. Her blood levels were over 1.5 mEq/L. She wasn't just being a hypochondriac. I really tried to use my CT words so that the student could see inside my brain. I had to figure this out all on my own—I want my student to have a head start.*

The challenge is to really talk about thinking, not just talk about doing! It takes practice, *reflection*, and peer feedback to get things rolling. The TACTICS activity

activity in **TACTICS 1-5** was designed to help clinicians and educators stimulate, cultivate, and nurture their talking about thinking.

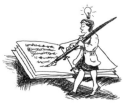

TACTICS 1-5: Verbalizing CT So Others Will See the Value

Clinicians and Educators

This activity requires three people, paper and pencil, and maybe some colored highlighters. One person assumes the role of the educator, one person assumes the role of the staff member or student, and one person assumes the role of the observer. Ideally this activity could be videotaped, but it works equally well without taping. The activity can be repeated by exchanging roles after the first time around.

Part I (5–10 minutes)

EDUCATOR: Your job is to select a teaching situation that will help your staff or students learn some aspect of nursing care but will also allow you to model your thinking as you are modeling your explanation of care.

　　STAFF/STUDENT: Your job is to listen for the educator's CT messages and jot them down as you are learning.

　　OBSERVER: Your job is to listen for both the educator's and the staff or student's thinking. Take notes that can be shared with the others later. Note: What words were used that reflect thinking? How many thinking words (*open-mindedness, confidence, analyzing, predicting,* and so on) were used in comparison with action words ("Next I need to flush the tubing")? Be as specific as possible as you take notes.

　　Begin the exercise. After 5–10 minutes, have each participant rate the educator, using the following scale of 1–10, with 10 being the total teaching activity.

　　What proportion of teaching focused on doing?　　　1 2 3 4 5 6 7 8 9 10
　　What proportion of teaching focused on thinking?　　1 2 3 4 5 6 7 8 9 10
　　Which specific CT descriptors were used? _____

　　What might the educator do differently next time to more explicitly model thinking with CT words? _____

　　If you have highlighters, use them to mark the actual CT descriptors.

Part II (10–15 minutes)

OBSERVER: Share your notes and your rankings with the others.
STAFF/STUDENT: Share your notes and your rankings with the others.
EDUCATOR: Share your notes and your rankings with the others.

Discussion

How did everyone do? What did you discover about how your modeling of thinking can be used the next time you teach CT?

Educators in any setting are expected to teach thinking. Teaching CT, however, requires one to accept that CT is a process, not simply more content. For example, when teaching the process of communication, we don't simply lecture on it; we model it, provide lots of opportunities to practice it, and have students overtly identify skills such as restatement, clarifying, and open-ended questions. We use process recordings to help students see those skill labels and patterns of use. Teaching CT must also be process oriented. *Reflection* journals serve this purpose and are valuable tools to make thinking more overt.

Talking about thinking, as in the previous TACTICS exercise, helps us and others visualize thinking. Talking about thinking helps us recognize why CT is important to us and to our students, patients, organizations, and professions. Talking about CT using CT terminology can help us accomplish what organizational and professional mandates can only serve as catalysts for—valuing thinking.

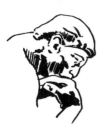

© Jesse Rubenfeld

PAUSE *and Ponder*

Why Do You Think CT Is Important?

By now we hope you appreciate why CT is so important to health-care stakeholders, particularly why thinking is so important to clinicians and educators. CT is that important bridge that transforms information to useful knowledge on which patients and all the stakeholders can act. Without CT, any attempts for safe, effective, efficient health care are meaningless.

REFLECTION CUES

- *Why* questions imply a search for reason, purpose, meaning, and value.
- *Why* and the thinking connected with *why* have triggered many important discoveries over the years.
- Many disciplines believe that CT is important: medicine, engineering, law, business, education, aviation, and health care.
- Current healthcare situations that require more or better CT include the information explosion; dwindling resources; cost containment; morbidity and mortality data; patient safety; and emergent ethical dilemmas, such as prolongation of life without quality and stem cell research.
- Many stakeholders experience the consequences of thinking and not thinking: patients and significant others, clinicians, educators and IDTs, unit managers, healthcare administrators, third-party payers, healthcare organizations, governments, and healthcare professions.
- CT leads to safe, effective, and efficient care for patients.
- CT leads to empowered decision making, job satisfaction, and expertise in practice for clinicians.
- CT leads to a focus on learning more than teaching.
- Clinicians and educators must begin to vocalize their CT to cultivate and nurture it in others.

References

Austhink. (2013). Tools for critical thinking, better writing, and decision making. Retrieved from http://austhink.com/

Benner, P. (1984). *From novice to expert: Power and excellence in nursing practice*. Menlo Park, CA: Addison-Wesley.

Brainy Quote. (2013). Curiosity quotes. Retrieved from http://www.brainyquote.com/quotes/keywords/curiosity.html

Brookfield, S. (1995). *Becoming a critically reflective teacher*. San Francisco, CA: Jossey-Bass.

Brunt, B. A. (2005). Critical thinking in nursing: An integrated review. *Journal of Continuing Education in Nursing, 36*, 60–67.

Carter, L. M., & Rukholm, E. (2008). A study of critical thinking, teacher-student interaction, and discipline-specific writing in an online educational setting for registered nurses. *Journal of Continuing Education in Nursing, 39*, 133–138.

Daly, W. M. (2001). The development of an alternative method in the assessment of critical thinking as an outcome of nursing education. *Journal of Advanced Nursing, 36*, 120–130.

Dreyfus, H. L., & Dreyfus, S. E. (1986). *Mind over machine: The power of human intuition and expertise in the era of the computer*. New York, NY: Free Press.

Edwards, S. L. (2007). Critical thinking: A two-phase framework. *Nurse Education in Practice, 7*, 303–314. doi: 10.1016/j.nepr/2006/09/004

Freire, P. (1998). *Pedagogy of freedom: Ethics, democracy, and civic courage* (P. Clarke, Trans.). Lanham, MD: Rowman & Littlefield.

Fullan, M. (1993). *Change forces: Probing the depths of educational reform*. Bristol, PA: Falmer Press.

Gustaffsson, C., & Fagerberg, I. (2004). Reflection, the way to professional development? *Journal of Clinical Nursing, 13*, 271–280.

Halpern, D. F. (1998). Teaching critical thinking for transfer across domains: Dispositions, skills, structure training, and metacognitive monitoring. *American Psychologist, 53*, 449–455.

Hansten, R. I., & Washburn, M. J. (1999). Individual and organizational accountability for developing critical thinking. *Journal of Nursing Administration, 29*(11), 39–45.

Haynes, L., Boese, T., & Butcher, H. (2004). *Nursing in contemporary society: Issues, trends, and transition to practice*. Upper Saddle River, NJ: Pearson Prentice Hall.

Hyrkas, K., Koivula, M., Lehti, K., & Paunonen-Ilmonen, M. (2003). Nurse managers' conceptions of quality management as promoted by peer supervision. *Journal of Nursing Management, 11*, 48–58.

Institute of Medicine. (2003). *Health professions education: A bridge to quality*. Washington, DC: National Academies Press.

Institute of Medicine. (2004). *Keeping patients safe: Transforming the work environment for nurses*. Washington, DC: National Academies Press.

Institute of Medicine. (2011). *The future of nursing: Leading change, advancing health*. Washington, DC: National Academies Press.

Legislative Counsel. (2010). Patient Protection and Affordable Care Act: Health-related portions of the Health Care and Education Reconciliation Act of 2010. Retrieved from http://housedocs.house.gov/energycommerce/ppacacon.pdf

Lunney, M. (2008). Critical need to address accuracy of nurses' diagnoses. *Online Journal of Issues in Nursing, 13*(1). doi: 10.3912/OJIN,Vol13No01PPT06

Lunney, M. (2010). Use of critical thinking in the diagnostic process. *International Journal of Nursing Terminologies and Classifications, 21*(2), 82–88. doi: 10.1111/j.1744–618X.2010.01150.x

Marzano, R., & Pickering, D. (1997). *Dimensions of learning teacher's manual* (2nd ed.). Alexandria, VA: Association for Supervision and Curriculum Development.

Massello, D. J. (1998). Operations management: Administering the program. In K. J. Kelly-Thomas (Ed.), *Clinical and nursing staff development: Current competent, future focus* (2nd ed., pp. 337–364). Philadelphia, PA: Lippincott.

Miller, J., Galloway, M., Coughlin, C., & Brennan, E. (2001). Care-centered organizations, Part I: Governance. *Journal of Nursing Administration, 31*(2), 67–73.

Morrall, P., & Goodman, B. (2012). Critical thinking, nurse education and universities: Some thoughts on current issues and implications for nursing practice. *Nurse Education Today.* Retrieved from http://dx .doi.org/10.1016/j.nedt.2012.11.011

National League for Nursing. (2006). *Excellence in nursing education model.* New York, NY: Author.

Paul, R. (1992). *Critical thinking: What every person needs to survive in a rapidly changing world.* Santa Rosa, CA: Foundation for Critical Thinking.

Raymond-Seniuk, C., & Profetto-McGrath, J. (2011). Can one learn to think critically?—a philosophical exploration. *Open Nursing Journal, 5,* 45–51.

Rogal, S. M., & Young, J. (2008). Exploring critical thinking in critical care nursing education: A pilot study. *Journal of Continuing Education in Nursing, 39,* 28–33.

Sanderson, H. (2003). Implementing person-centered planning by developing person-centered teams. *Journal of Integrated Care, 11*(3), 18–25.

Scheffer, B. K. (2001). Nurse educators' perspectives on their critical thinking: Snapshots from their personal and professional lives. *Dissertation Abstracts International: 62*(02B), 786.

Scheffer, B. K., & Rubenfeld, M. G. (2000). A consensus statement on critical thinking in nursing. *Journal of Nursing Education, 39,* 352–359.

Schon, D. A. (1983). *The reflective practitioner: How professionals think in action.* New York, NY: Basic Books.

Senge, P. M. (1990). *The fifth discipline: The art and practice of the learning organization.* New York, NY: Doubleday.

Tesoro, M. G. (2012). Effects of using the developing nurses' thinking model on nursing students' diagnostic accuracy. *Journal of Nursing Education, 51*(2), 436–443. doi:10.3928/01484834–20120615–01

Wiggins, G., & McTighe, J. (2001). *Understanding by design.* Upper Saddle River, NJ: Merrill Prentice Hall.

Worrell, J. A., & Profetto-McGrath, J. (2007). Critical thinking as an outcome of context-based learning among post RN students: A literature review. *Nurse Education Today, 27,* 420–426. doi: 10.1016 /jnedt.2006.07.004

Yoder-Wise, P. S. (1995). *Leading and managing in nursing.* St. Louis, MO: Mosby.

CHAPTER 2

What Is Critical Thinking?

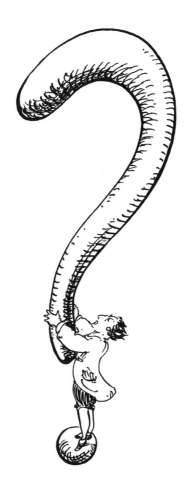

© Mark Steele. Reprinted by permission.

To emphasize the importance of this chapter's title question, we will pose some challenges for you. Consider how you would respond to these requests:

- Describe the thinking you use as a nurse.
- Improve your critical thinking.
- Tell us what critical thinking is.
- Explain how critical thinking is supposed to be practiced in nursing.

We would venture to guess that even though you consider yourself a good critical thinker, you'd be hard pressed to provide quick, simple responses. And, if you were then asked to describe how you became a nurse who thinks critically, it might be even more challenging. Don't be concerned: first, you're not alone; and second, that's what this text is designed to help you do—respond to requests such as those just mentioned.

Most people have difficulty describing their thinking processes, even expert clinicians and faculty who teach critical thinking (CT). That's not because they aren't good thinkers; it's just that, until recently, few people asked each other about their thinking, and we simply haven't developed a vocabulary to describe such heady things. When asked to describe their thinking, many people pause and say, "I just do!" When they are pressed to elaborate, you may get a variety of emotional responses. Many people will act frustrated because the request is unusual, they don't have ready answers, and they're too busy to think about it anyway.

If they're really frustrated, they might respond, "Why is it even important to try to describe thinking? Aren't actions more important in the big scheme of things?" The answer is yes, but actions are only as good as their appropriateness to the problem or condition that prompted the action. In today's healthcare arena, those conditions change constantly. What you did yesterday might not work tomorrow or even an hour from now. You must keep abreast of new information and changing patient data and consistently make those things work together. And new information is being discovered and refined daily, if not hourly.

So what is a nurse to do? There's all this existing information, there's a constant flow of new information, and then there's the need to turn it all into working knowledge so you can provide safe, effective, efficient nursing actions. You need to bridge the gap between the ever-growing information and the actions it requires. You need a series of steps or a process to convert information into knowledge. Finally, you must translate that knowledge, which is very abstract, into practice actions, which are very concrete. That transition works best if you can recognize those steps or processes; otherwise, you are less likely to arrive at predictable and consistently successful actions.

We can't all be like Indiana Jones in the movie *Indiana Jones and the Last Crusade* (Lucas et al., 1989). He stepped off into the chasm as a leap of faith. After he found himself on firm footing, he threw pebbles back to define the bridge that was camouflaged by its surroundings. Think of CT as that bridge. We will provide some pebbles ahead of time; once you see that CT bridge, your mind will more easily transform information into knowledge, and that knowledge, albeit abstract, will be the basis of the best workable course of action. We're hoping your curiosity is so stimulated that you are bursting to learn the details that we alluded to when we used the term *CT*.

The Critical Thinking "Bridge"

CT is the metaphorical bridge between information and action, but what are those pebbles for? They're going to do for you exactly what they did for Indiana Jones: they're going to turn something that is invisible from one perspective into something visible from a new perspective. But first it might be helpful to look at the three reasons why the bridge (CT) is invisible in the first place. Reason Number 1: CT is intangible; you can't study it under a microscope, hold it, smell it, or examine it for a pulse. Reason Number 2: CT is very individual—no two people think in the same way, nor do they broadcast their thoughts, so it's impossible to learn how to think critically by watching only actions. Reason Number 3: CT requires effort. Many of us assume CT will just happen over time as we gain knowledge and experience, so we just wait and don't worry about it. This may have worked in the past, but time is a luxury these days. We need to use CT today, not tomorrow.

So how can you start to see this previously invisible CT? Can you do it without pebbles? To some extent, yes, you probably can. For example, think about the opposite of CT. We'll bet you can easily identify people who don't use CT. What do they do? Now think of a nurse you consider to be a great thinker. She's the person you want to work with, especially if you're a novice. If something new comes up, she's the one who can figure out how to deal with it. She's creative, open-minded, logical. Now, with this positive image, the next question is, Can you learn to get to that expert level of thinking? How, and how quickly? Can you help other nurses get there too? The good news is yes, you can. However, this is where the pebbles come in. The pebbles are the three tools that will make the process of becoming a great CT nurse easier.

Pebbles on the Metaphorical Bridge

First, you need to be clear on just what CT in nursing is—for that, you need a definition. Second, you need to know how to describe what it looks like, using words to elaborate on the definition. Both of these tasks require a vocabulary. Once you can use specific words to describe your thinking processes, you can more easily discover what you're good at and where you need to improve. With a definition and words, you can also help others identify, describe, and improve their critical thinking. Third, you will need to visualize what CT words look like in action, particularly as CT is practiced in nursing. Addressing these three points—a definition, a vocabulary, and translating words to actions—will help us figure out the *what* of CT.

Pebble #1: Defining CT

Let's start by tackling the issue of defining and describing CT in nursing. We can't do justice to that task without some contextual and historical perspective. There are many descriptions of critical thinking in the literature; however, because many of those definitions are borrowed from other disciplines, they vary in terms of usefulness to

© Jesse Rubenfeld

nursing. Let's focus on the historical context of CT so you can appreciate how essential this concept is to us, our patients, our students, and our society.[1]

---

[1] With our apologies to the historians and philosophers in our audience who are already aware of this history, we will give only a quick overview of CT's philosophical roots. For those of you who yearn for more, check out some philosophy books or go to this website, which we used for much of the information in this section: http://www.philosophypages.com (Kemerling, 2001). Being Westerners, we will also apologize to other cultures, such as those from Asia, whose CT roots could be traced, for example, to the teachings of Lao Tzu and Confucius.

For those of you who find descriptions of history a bit boring, we've inserted a box of highlights in the historical evolution of CT (see **Box 2-1**).

Box 2-1   Tracking the Historical Evolution of CT

5th century BC	Pre-Socrates
Early 4th century BC	Socrates and the Socratic method of answering questions with questions
Mid-4th century BC	Plato and Aristotle
16th–17th century AD	Sir Francis Bacon and systematic study
Early 17th century AD	Descartes and systematic doubt
18th century	Immanuel Kant's *Critique of Pure Reason*
Early to mid-20th century	John Dewey: Thinking as part of human nature
Mid-20th century	Jean Piaget encouraged openness to multiple points of view
1986 and 1984	Dreyfus and Dreyfus *Mind over Machine* and Benner *From Novice to Expert*
1990s	Higher order thinking skills in the K–12 education system
1990	APA Delphi Study to define critical thinking
1990s	Postsecondary education and nursing, healthcare delivery
2000	Nursing Delphi Study (Scheffer & Rubenfeld)

In Western history, CT can be traced back to Socrates and his Socratic method, or answering questions with questions. Actually, Socrates emphasized deep questioning of ideas that were accepted as fact but that may simply have been beliefs. For example, everyone then believed that the earth was flat, but this did not make it a fact. Later, Plato and Aristotle expanded on Socrates's ideas to emphasize that things are not always what they seem and that sound reasoning takes into account objections to accepted ideas. During the Renaissance, Francis Bacon focused on empirical information gathering, establishing our modern research standards of systematic study. That empirical, or fact, base was important to overcome the natural biases that our minds use to understand our world and our place in it. René Descartes promoted systematic doubt: all thinking should be questioned and tested. (It may be comforting to those who spend lots of time thinking about thinking that Descartes acknowledged our existence as thinking beings to be the most factual thing to know. Even if we doubt that anything else exists, we must exist to do the doubting. Now, think about that!) In the 18th century, Immanuel Kant's *Critique of Pure Reason* examined the conundrum of using principles for thinking that cannot be empirically tested. Consider this statement: We are "burdened by questions ... prescribed by ... reason itself ... [which we] are not able to ignore, but which ... [we are] also not able to answer" (Kant, 1787/1965, p. 7).

John Dewey, the often-cited CT promoter in educational circles, took CT into the 20th century with his pragmatic view of thought as part of human behavior. And Jean Piaget, cautioning about the dangers of egocentric and sociocentric characteristics of human thought, emphasized the need to be open to multiple points of view. In the 1980s, the aviation industry began designing strategies to help pilots progress from novice to expert levels more quickly (Dreyfus & Dreyfus, 1986). That industry was very interested in the CT of human pilots because an aircraft's autopilot could not be programmed to react to all the dynamic events that occur when taking off, flying, and landing an airplane. As advanced as artificial intelligence is, it cannot yet replace the human thinking required in emergency situations. Patricia Benner (1984), a well-known nursing theorist, collaborated with Dreyfus and Dreyfus in the development of her Novice to Expert Model of nursing care. It is not surprising that the aviation industry and professional nursing are equally concerned about critical thinking—both deal with split-second decision making to keep people safe.

Thinking, how the brain works, and how learning takes place became dominant themes in education in Western society in the early 1980s (Hart, 1983). Initially, the focus was on teaching CT in kindergarten through grade 12, with books such as *Developing Minds: A Resource Book for Teaching Thinking* (Costa, 1985). In the early 1990s, the movement to improve thinking spread to postsecondary education. Assessment of all students' CT skills is now part of college and university accreditation standards in the United States. For example, criterion 4 of the Higher Learning Commission's Institutional Accreditation Guidelines (2010) cited the importance of "fostering and supporting inquiry, creativity, practice, and social responsibility" (p. 6).

Since the 1990s, critical thinking has become a focus in nursing and nursing education. The American Association of Colleges of Nursing's *Essentials of Baccalaureate Education for Professional Nursing Practice* (2008) lists the use of clinical/critical reasoning as one of its assumptions for a baccalaureate generalist graduate, and its accreditation arm—the Commission on Collegiate Nursing Education (CCNE)—required nursing programs to address all the components in the essentials document, including CT (Commission on Collegiate Nursing Education, 2013). The American Nurses Association also emphasized CT in its *Nursing: Scope and Standards of Practice* (2010). The language of CT is addressed in the association's scope statement and is incorporated throughout all the standards.

Outside of healthcare clinical settings, a seminal work by the American Philosophical Association (APA), under the direction of Facione (1990), defined CT using a Delphi method to survey academicians. Philosophers composed roughly half of his 46-member panel; others were from fields such as education, physics, computer science, and psychology. They arrived at this consensus statement: "We understand critical thinking to be purposeful, self-regulatory judgment which results in interpretation, analysis, evaluation, and inference as well as explanation of the evidential, conceptual, methodological, criteriological, or contextual considerations upon which judgment is based" (p. 2). This definition of CT has been used extensively in nursing but, because no nurses or healthcare providers participated in the APA study, there is some question as to whether its findings are the best fit for nursing.

Because of the growing need for CT in nursing, some practitioners found it necessary to develop nursing-specific conceptualizations of CT so we could teach it better (e.g., Rubenfeld & Scheffer, 1999). In recent years, nurses have used research to describe CT and its components so that we have stronger evidence of CT in our profession. Of note is Fonteyn's work to describe thinking strategies for nursing practice (1998). Using a "think aloud" method, Fonteyn and her team studied 14 expert registered nurses from a variety of specialty areas. Twelve predominant thinking strategies were identified (see **Box 2-2**).

Following a method similar to that used by Facione for the APA, we conducted a comprehensive study to find consensus on a description of critical thinking in nursing in the mid-1990s (Scheffer & Rubenfeld, 2000). In this three-year study, we also employed a Delphi method to gain consensus from a geographically dispersed group of expert nurses through successive rounds of questions, answers, data analysis, and voting (Goodman, 1987). Our panel of 55 expert nurses was culled from practice, education, and research settings and from nine countries and 23 U.S. states. During five rounds of questions and responses, we identified and defined 10 habits of the mind and 7 cognitive skills of critical thinking in nursing.

Box 2-2   **Thinking Strategies of Expert Registered Nurses**

- Recognizing a pattern
- Setting priorities
- Searching for information
- Generating hypotheses
- Making predictions
- Forming relationships
- Stating a proposition
- Asserting a practice rule
- Making choices
- Judging the value
- Drawing conclusions
- Providing explanations

Source: Fonteyn, 1998.

We started our consensus rounds with a broad question: What are the skills and habits of the mind of critical thinking in nursing? Our choice of words was deliberate; we wanted to get at not only the cognitive skills, but the affective component as well. Numerous authors (e.g., Tanner, 1997) have identified the importance of this affective component, which Facione (1990) named "dispositions." After a most helpful discussion with Dr. Pete Facione (a philosopher–scholar) and his wife, Dr. Noreen Facione (a nurse–scholar), we chose the label "habits of the mind" because we wanted to get away from some of the stereotypical views of traits or dispositions as being static. Because habits can be initiated and changed, this term seemed to be more dynamic.

For every round of our Delphi process, we analyzed data and returned reports to participants explaining what we had done with their information and asking a new set of questions based on the revised configuration of the data. By the end of five rounds, we were ready for voting on the final statement and definitions of the 10 habits of the mind and 7 skills. There was 88.2% consensus on the final statement and similar consensus on the definitions of the dimensions. (For the full report of the research method and consensus voting, see Scheffer & Rubenfeld, 2000.) The final consensus statement is as follows:

> Critical thinking in nursing is an essential component of professional accountability and quality nursing care. Critical thinkers in nursing exhibit these habits of the mind: confidence, contextual perspective, creativity, flexibility, inquisitiveness, intellectual integrity, intuition, open-mindedness, perseverance, and reflection. Critical thinkers in nursing practice the cognitive skills of analyzing, applying standards, discriminating, information-seeking, logical reasoning, predicting and transforming knowledge. (p. 357)

See **Box 2-3** for definitions of the 10 habits of the mind and 7 skills. These dimensions of CT in nursing will be used as a framework for discussing CT throughout this text, so you will want to refer to them frequently.

Box 2-3   Critical Thinking Skills and Habits of the Mind for Nursing

CRITICAL THINKING SKILLS

Analyzing: Separating or breaking a whole into parts to discover their nature, function, and relationships

Applying standards: Judging according to established personal, professional, or social rules or criteria

Discriminating: Recognizing differences and similarities among things or situations and distinguishing carefully as to category or rank

(continues)

Box 2-3 Critical Thinking Skills and Habits of the Mind for
Nursing (continued)

Information seeking: Searching for evidence, facts, or knowledge by identifying relevant sources and gathering objective, subjective, historical, and current
data from those sources
Logical reasoning: Drawing inferences or conclusions that are supported in or
justified by evidence
Predicting: Envisioning a plan and its consequences
Transforming knowledge: Changing or converting the condition, nature, form,
or function of concepts among contexts

CRITICAL THINKING HABITS OF THE MIND

Confidence: Assurance of one's reasoning abilities
Contextual perspective: Consideration of the whole situation, including relationships, background, and environment, relevant to some happening
Creativity: Intellectual inventiveness used to generate, discover, or restructure
ideas; imagining alternatives
Flexibility: Capacity to adapt, accommodate, modify, or change thoughts, ideas,
and behaviors
Inquisitiveness: An eagerness to know by seeking knowledge and understand-
ing through observation and thoughtful questioning in order to explore pos-
sibilities and alternatives
Intellectual integrity: Seeking the truth through sincere, honest processes, even
if the results are contrary to one's assumptions and beliefs
Intuition: Insightful sense of knowing without conscious use of reason
Open-mindedness: A viewpoint characterized by being receptive to divergent
views and sensitive to one's biases
Perseverance: Pursuit of a course with determination to overcome obstacles
Reflection: Contemplation upon a subject, especially one's assumptions and
thinking for the purposes of deeper understanding and self-evaluation

---

Republished with permission of Slack Incorporated, from Journal of Nursing Education, Gale Rubenfeld and Barbara Scheffer, 39, 2000, p. 358; permission conveyed through Copyright Clearance Center.

In the years since 2000, the consensus definition has provided a framework for
several studies related to CT in nursing and other disciplines. For example, Fogler
and LeBlanc (2014), teaching engineers, used several CT dimensions from our study
to illustrate thinking activities to determine why fish were dying in a river. In nursing,
for example, Lunney has used the CT dimensions to focus on thinking for diagnostic
reasoning (2001, 2008, 2010). A cogent exploration of CT within the philosophical

views taken in nursing was revealed by Raymond-Seniuk and Profetto-McGrath (2011). These authors reminded us of the need not to be complacent in our use of CT words without thinking of the complexities of CT through multiple lenses. We are happy to report that the dimensions of CT as defined by Scheffer and Rubenfeld's 2000 consensus statement were well represented in this thoughtful analysis.

Comparison of the Nursing Delphi Study to the Philosophical Delphi Study

Box 2-4 compares the results of our study with those of Facione and his group. The definitions of CT skills are from Facione's 1990 Delphi study. The dispositions descriptions are taken from Facione, Sanchez, Facione, and Gainen (1995). In Facione's original work, he found 19 dispositions that fit into two types—approaches to life and living in general, and approaches to specific issues, questions, or problems.

Box 2-4   Comparison of Nursing and APA Components of CT

Nursing Skills (Scheffer & Rubenfeld, 2000, p. 358)	*APA Skills* (Facione, 1990)
Analyzing: "separating or breaking a whole into parts to discover their nature, function and relationships"	**Analysis:** "to identify the intended and actual inferential relationships among statements, questions, concepts, descriptions or other forms of representation intended to express beliefs, judgments, experiences, reasons, information, or opinions" (p. 14) (Its subskills are identified as "examining ideas, identifying arguments and analyzing arguments" [p. 12].)
Applying Standards: "judging according to established personal, professional or social rules or criteria"	**Evaluation:** "to assess the credibility of statements or other representations which are accounts or descriptions of a person's perception, experience, situation, judgment, belief, or opinion; and to assess the logical strength of the actual or intended inferential relationships among statements, descriptions, questions or other form of representation" (p. 15)

(continues)

Box 2-4 Comparison of Nursing and APA Components of CT (continued)

Nursing Skills	*APA Skills*
(Scheffer & Rubenfeld, 2000, p. 358)	(Facione, 1990)
Discriminating:	**Interpretation:**
"recognizing differences and similarities among things or situations and distinguishing carefully as to category or rank"	"to comprehend and express the meaning or significance of a wide variety of experiences, situations, data, events, judgments, conventions, beliefs, rules, procedures or criteria" (p. 13) (Its subskills are categorization, decoding sentences, and clarifying meaning.)
Information Seeking:	**Inference subskill:**
"searching for evidence, facts or knowledge by identifying relevant sources and gathering objective, subjective, historical and current data from those sources"	querying evidence: "to identify and secure elements needed to draw reasonable conclusions" (p. 16)
Logical Reasoning:	**Explanation:**
"drawing inferences or conclusions that are supported in or justified by evidence"	"to state the results of one's reasoning; to justify that reasoning terms of the evidential, conceptual, methodological, criteriological and contextual considerations upon which one's results were based; and to present one's reasoning in the form of cogent arguments" (p. 18)
Predicting:	**Inference subskill:**
"envisioning a plan and its consequences"	conjecturing alternatives: "to formulate multiple alternatives for resolving a problem … to draw out presuppositions and project the range of possible consequences of decisions, positions, policies, theories, or beliefs" (p. 17)
Transforming Knowledge:	**No comparable skill**
"changing or converting the condition, nature, form or function of concepts among contexts"	
No comparable skill; **see Habit of the Mind, Reflection.**	**Self-regulation**

Box 2-4   Comparison of Nursing and APA Components of CT (continued)

Nursing Habits of the Mind (Scheffer & Rubenfeld, 2000, p. 358)	**APA Dispositions** (Facione, Sanchez, Facione, & Gainen, 1995)
Confidence: "assurance of one's reasoning abilities"	**CT Self-confidence:** "to trust the soundness of one's own reasoned judgments and to lead others in the rational resolution of problems" (p. 8)
Contextual Perspective: "consideration of the whole situation, including relationships, background and environment, relevant to some happening"	**Maturity:** "approach[ing] problems, inquiry, and decision making with a sense that some problems are necessarily ill-structured, some situations admit more than one plausible option, and many times judgments must be made based on standards, contexts, and evidence which preclude certainty" (p. 9)
Flexibility: "capacity to adapt, accommodate, modify or change thoughts, ideas and behaviors"	
Creativity: "intellectual inventiveness used to generate, discover, or restructure ideas; imagining alternatives"	**No comparable disposition**
Inquisitiveness: "an eagerness to know by seeking knowledge and understanding through observation and thoughtful questioning in order to explore possibilities and alternatives"	**Inquisitiveness:** "one's intellectual curiosity and one's desire for learning even when the application of the knowledge is not readily apparent" (p. 6)
Intellectual Integrity: "seeking the truth through sincere, honest processes, even if the results are contrary to one's assumptions and beliefs"	**Truthseeking:** "being eager to seek the best knowledge in a given context, courageous about asking questions, and honest and objective about pursuing inquiry even if the findings do not support one's self-interests or one's preconceived opinions" (p. 8)
Intuition: insightful sense of knowing without conscious use of reason	**No comparable disposition**

(continues)

Box 2-4 Comparison of Nursing and APA Components of CT (continued)

Nursing Habits of the Mind	APA Dispositions
(Scheffer & Rubenfeld, 2000, p. 358)	(Facione, Sanchez, Facione, & Gainen, 1995)
Open-mindedness:	**Open-mindedness:**
a viewpoint characterized by being receptive to divergent views and sensitive to one's biases	"being tolerant of divergent views and sensitive to the possibility of one's own bias" (p. 6)
Perseverance:	**Systematicity:**
pursuit of a course with determination to overcome obstacles	"being organized, orderly, focused and diligent in inquiry" (p. 7)
Reflection:	**No comparable disposition but comparable to APA skill: Self-Regulation:**
contemplation upon a subject, especially one's assumptions and thinking, for the purposes of deeper understanding and self-evaluation	"self-consciously to monitor one's cognitive activities, the elements used in those activities, and the results educed, particularly by applying skills in analysis and evaluation to one's own inferential judgments with a view toward questioning, confirming, validating, or correcting either one's reasoning or one's results" (Facione, 1990, p. 19)
No comparable habit of the mind.	**Analyticity:**
	"prizing the application of reasoning and the use of evidence to resolve problems, anticipating potential conceptual or practical difficulties, and consistently being alert to the need to intervene" (p. 7)

Those 19 dispositions were later consolidated to form seven dispositions in a factor analysis by Facione, Facione, and Sanchez (1994) as they began to develop a CT dispositions test.

Although the comparisons are not direct, there are striking similarities between the two study results. However, a significant difference is also apparent. Two habits of the mind and one skill were not identified by the APA group—*creativity, intuition,* and *transforming knowledge*. Are these dimensions unique to nursing? Or are they unique to applied sciences or to health professions? We believe our comparison shows that there are quite likely some discipline-specific dimensions of CT and some that are possibly universal.

Pebble #2: CT Language/Words

If these 17 dimensions represent CT in nursing, let's see how your thinking fits with them. Think about your thinking. Ask yourself, for example, how strong your CT *confidence* is or how you use *analyzing* in your clinical practice. (See **TACTICS 2-1**.)

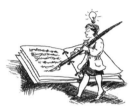

TACTICS 2-1: CT Self-Checklist

Look at **Box 2-5** and mark where you think you fall on each of the thinking continua.

This TACTIC can be used by both clinicians and educators.

Discussion

Are you beginning to see where your strengths and weaknesses lie? Let's take this further. At the beginning of this chapter, we asked how you would describe the thinking you use. Now how would you describe your thinking? Is it different now that you have the words to use? Is it easier to describe your thinking now that you know the words? Have you ever had to do this? In fact, most of us haven't been asked to describe our thinking—at least not until recently. These days, clinicians are being asked to show how they think because CT is recognized as being tied to quality of

---

Box 2-5 Critical Thinking Self-Checklist

1. How confident am I in my reasoning ability?
   Not very confident ←—————————————————→ Very confident

2. Do I tend to look at situations with their context in mind, or do I tend to see things as separate compartments?
   Compartmentalized thinking ←—————————→ Contextual thinking

3. How creative am I in my thinking?
   Not very creative ←—————————————————→ Very creative

4. How flexible is my thinking?
   Rigid ←—————————————————————————→ Very flexible

5. How inquisitive am I?
   Not naturally curious ←—————————————→ Innately inquisitive

6. How much *intellectual integrity* do I have?
   Go with my assumptions ←——————→ Seek the truth no matter what

(continues)

Box 2-5   Critical Thinking Self-Checklist (continued)

7. How intuitive am I?
   Not very intuitive   Always go with my gut

8. How open-minded am I?
   Quite biased   Open to all possibilities

9. How much *perseverance* do I have in my thinking?
   Once I have problems I'll stop   Keep at it no matter what
                                               gets in the way

10. How reflective am I? Do I think about my thinking?
    Not very reflective   Always striving for deeper
                                               understanding of self

11. How good am I at *analyzing* situations?
    I don't break things down much   I always pick things apart
                                               to understand them

12. How much do I pay attention to standards with my thinking?
    Not used much for judgments   Always use criteria for
                                               judgments

13. How finely do I discriminate among things?
    Don't recognize small   Always recognize small
    differences/similarities   things

14. How good am I at seeking out information?
    I think about what's right there   I dig for all possible evidence

15. How strong is my *logical reasoning*?
    I can't always justify my conclusions   I can always trace my
                                               conclusions to evidence

16. How good are my abilities to predict consequences in situations?
    Don't see much farther than my nose   I always think, What would
                                               happen if ... ?

17. How well do I transform knowledge from one situation to the next?
    Prefer textbook situations   Can adapt concepts to meet
                                               situation

care. We need a new language of thinking—and a mutual understanding of what the words in that language mean.

Do you remember the first time you used a computer, ran into problems, and asked for help? Depending on your age or how long ago that was, if your helper was like most computer-literates, he or she probably used words like *booting, Windows, drivers, defragging, cookies, encryption, beta testing,* and *right click.* Did you sit there with your mouth hanging open, feeling foolish? Were you at a loss for what to say because you didn't know the language? Eventually, you probably learned enough computer lingo to function in today's technological world. Well, learning how to describe CT is a similar process. Without the words, it's impossible to even ask useful questions.

When we first started to teach CT and asked students to describe how they were thinking, they would tell us what they were thinking about. After trying several tactics to get our point across, we finally realized that the communication problem was very basic. Very few of our students had a vocabulary to use; they were not accustomed to describing something so abstract. As we used words to describe CT in nursing more and more, eventually it became clear that a list of descriptors would help students describe their thinking. Look at **Box 2-6** and see how many of those words and phrases you use and when and where you've heard or seen others using them.

Box 2-6   Words to Describe Critical Thinking

DESCRIPTORS FOR CT HABITS OF THE MIND

Confidence

My thinking was on track, decisive; I reconsidered and still thought I made the best decision; I knew my conclusion was well founded; My thinking was clear, unambiguous, trustworthy; I was secure in my thinking

Contextual Perspective

I could see the whole picture; I considered [reflected on, reconsidered] other possibilities; I took other things [surrounding issues] under consideration; I redefined the situation in view of ... ; Considering the circumstances, I ... ; I broadened my view/perspective/mind

Creativity

I let my imagination go; I was inspired to think of ... ; I stretched my mind; I took my thinking outside the box; I envisioned/dreamed up/invented ... ; I tried to be visionary; My mind was fertile ground; I used the artistic side of my brain

Flexibility

I changed directions in my mind; I gave up on that idea and went on to ... ; I moved away from my traditional thinking; I redefined the situation and started again; I questioned what I was thinking and considered another path; I tried to be adaptable in my thinking; I let my thinking go with the flow

(continues)

Box 2-6   Words to Describe Critical Thinking (continued)

Inquisitiveness

I had a strong desire for more knowledge; I itched to know more about ... ; I was eager to know more; I took a lively interest in ... ; I pricked up my ears, stuck my nose in ... ; I burned with curiosity; I was really interested in ... ; My mind was buzzing with questions

Intellectual Integrity

I was not satisfied with my conclusion, so I ... ; Although it went against everything I believed ... ; I need to get at the truth; I tried to find the bottom line; I racked my brain; I questioned my biases; I asked myself difficult questions; I dug to the bottom; I reflected on my inferences; I examined why I thought that ...

Intuition

I felt it in my bones; I couldn't put my finger on why, but I thought ... ; Instinctively I knew ... ; My hunch was that ... ; I had a premonition/inspiration/ impression ... ; My natural tendency was to ... ; Subconsciously I knew that ... ; Without thought, I figured out ... ; Automatically I thought that ... ; While I couldn't say why, I thought immediately ... ; My sixth sense said that I should consider ...

Open-mindedness

I tried to be receptive to new ideas; I tried not to judge; I listened to reason; I looked at both sides of the issue; I tried to be objective and unprejudiced; I questioned why I thought that ... ; I weighed the pros and cons; I tried to be neutral

Perseverance

I was single-minded in my determination to ... ; I persistently kept at it; I plodded on through my thoughts; I was stubborn and tireless in my pursuit; I kept going, trying this and that; I would not accept that for an answer; I had to overcome so many obstacles

Reflection

I pondered my reactions; I mulled it over in my mind; I ruminated over what I had thought and done; I had to reexamine/rethink/reconsider/review things; I evaluated my thoughts; I wondered what I could have done differently; I concentrated on my thinking process; I talked to myself about ... ; I deliberately meditated on what I was thinking

Box 2-6 Words to Describe Critical Thinking (continued)

DESCRIPTORS FOR CT SKILLS

Analyzing

I dissected the situation; I broke things down so I could understand them better; I tried to reduce things into manageable units; I detailed a schematic of ... ; I sorted things out; I took the whole situation apart so I could see ... ; I looked for the parts; I made sure each component was addressed; I set it out, one, two, or three; I looked at each piece individually; I studied it bit by bit; I thought of it piecemeal instead of all together; I tried to see the trees instead of just the forest

Applying Standards

I knew I had to ... ; There are certain things you just have to account for; I thought of the bottom line that is always ... ; I know that some things are just right or wrong; As a professional, I knew I had to ... ; I knew it was unethical to ... ; I considered what my license allowed and expected me to do; I thought of/studied the policy for ... ; I compared this situation to what I knew to be the rule; I judged that according to ...

Discriminating

I grouped things together; I put things in categories; I tried to consider what the priority was; I rank ordered the various ... ; I stood back and tried to see how those things were related; I wondered if this was as important as ... ; I thought of the discrepancies in the story; I could distinguish the pieces; What I was hearing and what I was seeing was consistent [inconsistent]; I wondered what I should do first; When I focused on the finer details, I could see ... ; This was different from [the same as] that

Information Seeking

I made sure I had all the pieces of the picture; I knew I needed to look up/study ... ; I wondered how I could find out ... ; I went back to look more closely at ... ; I asked myself if I knew the whole story; I kept searching for more data; I wanted [needed] to have all the facts [knowledge]; I looked for evidence of ...

Logical Reasoning

I deduced from the information that ... ; I could trace my conclusion back to the data; My diagnosis was grounded in the evidence; I considered all the

(continues)

Box 2-6   Words to Describe Critical Thinking (continued)

information and then inferred ... ; I could justify my conclusion by ... ; I moved down a straight path from initial data to the final conclusion; I had a strong argument for ... ; I made a good case for ... ; There was sound evidence to support ... ; My rationale for the conclusion was ... ; Putting two and two together, I inferred ... ; I brought reason to bear in the situation by ...

Predicting

I could imagine that happening if I did ... ; I anticipated ... ; I was prepared for ... ; I tried to be farsighted in my view; I made provisions for ... ; I envisioned the outcome to be ... ; I had a feeling that would happen; I could foresee ... ; My prognosis was ... ; I figured the probability of   ; I could tell that down the line ... ; I tried to go beyond the here and now; The immediate plan was this, but the long term needed to be ...

Transforming Knowledge

I knew I'd have to individualize; Although this situation was somewhat different, I knew ... ; I wondered if that would fit in this situation; I thought this would be a textbook case, but it wasn't; I took what I knew and asked myself if it would work; I tried to translate that into this; I adapted my knowledge about ... ; I could accommodate ... ; I improved on the basics by adding ... ; I figured if this was true, then that would be too; At first I was puzzled, then I saw that there were similarities, too; It was easy to cross over ...

You need the vocabulary to describe your thinking. If you think you're ready, you can go to Appendix A and look at the CT Inventory. It's a more detailed version of the checklist in Box 2-5 and can be used in a variety of situations. (You may find the descriptors in Box 2-6 helpful when answering the questions it poses.) This inventory has been used to help nurses and nursing students describe their thinking and to evaluate growth in CT. Once you take the time to complete that inventory, we think you'll have a better sense of how you think, and you will really be able to answer someone who asks, "How would you describe your thinking as a nurse?"

If, at this point, you are really excited by CT, you can tease your brain by considering the CT ironies in **Box 2-7**. If you can spend enjoyable time pondering these more esoteric points, you have the makings of a philosopher!

 ### *Pebble #3: Visualizing CT in Action*

And now for CT in action: What does it look like? Can you see it? Some argue that we cannot see or measure CT because it is only manifested in actions. That is somewhat true, but there are problems with just

---

Box 2-7   CT Ironies to Ponder

- If I teach you what CT is, I'm actually discouraging you from using CT to figure it out for yourself.
- If I argue that CT is impossible or unnecessary, I'm actually being contradictory because posing such argumentation demonstrates CT.
- If CT truly requires a *contextual perspective*, then I must always adapt to the context to promote CT; does then CT itself change with the context?

---

looking at actions. Some "right" actions are pure luck; you can't count on them happening the next time. Some right actions are based on sloppy thinking. And some right actions are based on keen CT. Which kind of thinking do you want to count on? Sometimes it's easier to see the consequences of not thinking well than to see the results of carefully considered actions. Things go wrong when nurses don't use CT. To fully appreciate CT in action, one really needs to combine descriptions of thinking with the actions that thinking produces. **TACTICS 2-2** and **TACTICS 2-3** both illustrate that combined approach.

TACTICS 2-2: *What Do Great Thinkers Look Like?*

Clinicians

Think of the people you work with; rank them in terms of their thinking. One or two people probably stand out as great thinkers. What makes you put them in the great thinker category? It's probably their actions and their communication. Now, list those characteristics and see if you can picture great thinking in action.

Educators

Have your students or staff do the preceding exercise and write down their descriptions of a great thinker they know personally, either as a formal paper or as an informal list of characteristics. Then have them share their descriptions and look for commonalities.

Discussion

In our workshops, students who do this exercise report the characteristics of great thinkers as follows: this person "always explains what he's doing ... is always asking questions ... can always stand up for herself when she's questioned ... teaches every patient and family member he comes in contact with ... rarely takes things at face value ... rechecks everything ... is the one we all go to for help with medication calculations ... says what's on her mind ... is the one we like to work with."

TACTICS 2-3: Talking and Thinking: A Patient Scenario

Clinicians

Consider this scenario:

You are working on a medical unit. Mrs. Franks, 79 years old with a history of alcoholism, was admitted 2 days ago for heart failure. Two hours before your shift began, she was moved to your unit from the telemetry unit. According to your shift report, she has been alert and oriented, has some minor lower extremity edema, has gone from many to a few crackles in her lungs, had her Foley removed this morning, and has urinated once in the past 6 hours. Her weight has decreased 4 kg since admission. She is not on a fluid restriction and has been eating and drinking small amounts. She has used her prn oxygen rarely. You walk into the room to find a very agitated Mrs. Franks trying to get out of bed, saying, "I have to got to the store before it closes because I have company coming for dinner." Speaking in a calm voice, you ask her to tell you how she feels. Meanwhile, you check her pulse and find it at 92 but regular. You remember that she's on a beta-blocker.

Now, finish this scenario. What would you think? What would you do and why?

Educators

Use this same case or find one that works with your setting and that matches the level of knowledge of your students or staff. Service-based educators should select a unit-specific case. Set up some parameters for responding to this scene; for example, if you are trying to promote better assessment skills among one unit's staff, have the nurses list their answers and place them in a centrally located box for a drawing later. Give a prize for the best answer, or post all the answers anonymously and have the staff rate them.

Discussion

What would exemplify the best thinking in this situation with Mrs. Franks? We'll give you an idea of what an expert nurse would do. Obviously, novices would not necessarily come up with these responses.

We'd expect the nurse to assess respiratory rate, lung sounds, pulse oximetry, blood pressure, temperature, cognitive function, glucose (if there's any history of hypo- or hyperglycemia), hemoglobin level to consider if she's anemic, medications and side effects, and additional information about her alcoholism (e.g., how long since drinking last, amount consumed) and her past history of alcoholic behavior via her chart or family report, if possible. We'd also want the nurse to check patterns to see if her pulse of 92 is normal according to her baseline.

We'd expect each of those things to be assessed in just about that order. We'd expect the nurse to speak softly and confidently to the patient, ask her if she needs the bathroom or is in pain, orient her to her surroundings, help her stay in bed, and make sure she is safe before leaving her alone in the room.

That nurse should be entertaining reasonable hunches of what might be going on and ruling them in or out, such as decreased oxygen saturation, increased pulmonary congestion, cardiac event, infectious process (such as pneumonia or urinary tract infection), medication side effect, and anxiety over the new environment. We'd expect that nurse to be considering his or her knowledge of such things as normal aging, for example, and that responses are usually blunted in elders. Other knowledge would be in such areas as typical heart failure signs, symptoms, and complications. We'd expect that nurse to communicate with the healthcare team about this event. We'd expect a nurse who has worked in that environment for several months to have some intuitive response to this situation but not jump to premature conclusions. Finally, we'd expect any nurse to take the situation seriously.

Some variations on this exercise are to have staff or students discuss such scenarios in a group, write similar scenarios, and project what "wrong" things nurses might do in such situations.

The patient scenario in TACTICS 2-3 should remind you of the nursing process, and we would like to take a little detour to discuss CT as it relates to the nursing process.

Back to Pebble #3: *Visualizing CT in Action*

A disheartening part of our work with critical thinking over the years has been to read and hear that critical thinking is a buzzword that nurses don't understand or use—that it is too vague and undefined to have practical applications. To some extent we understand that, especially coming from folks who don't spend time studying the defined parts of critical thinking or look at it out of context. We even wrote an editorial, years ago, titled *Critical Thinking: A Tool in Search of a Job* (Scheffer & Rubenfeld, 2006).

One of the jobs is the everyday reality of CT within the context of the nursing process, that is, what nurses do every day in patient encounters. When we first started to teach and study CT many years ago, it was in the context of the thinking and doing of the nursing process. We described great nursing as the following formula:

Patient + You + Thinking Skills + Knowledge + Nursing Process = Great Nursing

These many years later, with research-based, honed descriptions of the thinking part, we still come back to this formula. Now, obviously, nothing in nursing is as linear as this formula, but the pieces are there in every messy nursing encounter.

Speaking of formulas, some folks have said that the nursing process—the now-familiar assessing, planning, implementing, and evaluating—is just that, a recipe or formula that can be followed blindly, without thought. If one goes back to the roots of nursing process, however, it becomes clear that thinking was always integral to the process. In the late 1960s, Helen Yura and Mary Walsh, at The Catholic University of America in Washington, DC, got a group of nurses together to define what nurses do. They wrote the first edition of their book, *The Nursing Process: Assessing, Planning, Implementing, Evaluating*, in 1967 and, because of its popularity, they went on to write four more editions (Yura & Walsh, 1988). This description of the nursing process has become so familiar that few people go back to the original work. Thinking was always a part of this process, and it was never envisioned as a linear recipe. The nursing process and the thinking required to achieve it was designed to be iterative and recurrent. Nurses jump into this process at various points. What nurse starts an intervention with a patient without doing some assessing at the same time? Sometimes, as the nurse is evaluating the effectiveness of actions, it becomes clear that the actions should have been planned more completely. And on it goes.

Let's delve into the thinking within the parts of the nursing process. Assessment, which on face value is just collecting information, is much more than that. The skilled nurse is a health detective with a keen level of *inquisitiveness* for seeking relevant data. Even during data collection, the nurse has first impressions. Think *intuition* for starters. The nurse's knowledge comes into play as those data are compared to norms. Think *applying standards*. Is a 20-pound weight loss normal over a 2-week period, even if the patient had the flu? Initial hunches about what is going on start popping into the nurse's head as the *analysis* part of assessment kicks in. Being *open-minded* and *contextual*, the nurse combines those initial hunches with further *information seeking* as the nurse clusters bits and pieces of information, looking for patterns and critical indicators. We call this search for relevant data *directed data collection* because there is a need to be *open-minded* and aware of biases while getting details that might support a hunch while avoiding premature conclusions.

The nurse, as the health detective in these situations, digs deeper and deeper to find out what's up. Clusters of relevant data are viewed with *discrimination* and further *inquisitiveness* before any conclusive assessment is reached.

At some point—in microseconds in some situations, and over a longer period of time in other situations—the nurse must come to a conclusion about what a patient's issues are. There are many possible conclusions; it may represent a patient's strength (e.g., supportive family, stable vital signs, intact skin, effective communication skills) or it may be a health concern. The health concern could be a problem for referral (e.g., a progressive hearing loss would call for a referral to an ears, nose, and throat physician), an inter-disciplinary problem (e.g., decreased strength and stamina would require work with physical therapy), or a nursing diagnosis of an actual problem or risk for a problem (e.g., chronic pain related to limited mobility; risk for injury related to poor balance and unstable transfers). See **Box 2-8** for conclusions of assessment.

Reaching a conclusion about a relevant nursing issue requires all 17 dimensions of CT. The complexities of that thinking are phenomenal at times. There are many diverse sources of data streamed into a nurse's consciousness; these data must be sorted, checked for validity, and clustered to make sense of the whole lot. It is so easy to forget about *intellectual integrity* and jump to a premature conclusion, shut off one's thinking and go with the obvious of what's in front of you. Look at the 6 strengths and 4 health concern conclusions of assessment and the supporting data clusters in **Box 2-9** and then consider how much thinking went into the nurse's 10 conclusions in this case of a patient in a nursing home environment. Also, con-sider that data gaps may be as relevant as data in the case of the problem for referral. Remember, a great health detective pays close attention to what is and isn't there. Arriving at any final conclusion is a process of ruling in and ruling out information

---

Box 2-8 Conclusions of Assessment

A. Strengths
    1. Physical
    2. Psychosocial
    3. Social
    4. Spiritual
    5. Environmental
    6. Cultural
B. Health concerns
    1. Nursing diagnoses
        a. Problem responses
           i. Actual
           ii. Risk for
        b. Wellness response
    2. Interdisciplinary problem
    3. Problem for referral

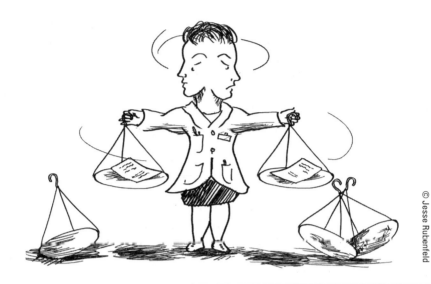

© Jesse Rubenfeld

Ruling in and ruling out.

Box 2-9 Conclusions of Assessment and Supporting Data Clusters

Strength Conclusions	*Supporting Data Clusters*
Vital signs stable	B/P 110/70, P 86, R 16, T 98.7
Adequate nutrition	Ht. 5'2," Wt. 105 lbs, follows 1800 cal diet, hair shiny
Adequate bowel elimination	BM every other day, soft, brown, drinks prune juice
Adequate sleep pattern	Sleeps through the night, feels rested in morning
Adequate health insurance	Has Medicare and supplemental insurance
Well groomed	Hair shiny, clean clothing, wears lipstick daily

HEALTH CONCERN CONCLUSIONS

    A. Nursing diagnoses
        1. Nursing diagnosis: Impaired skin integrity related to mobility deficits, urinary incontinence, fragile skin, and compromised circulation

Diagnostic Label

Impaired skin integrity   Coccyx and elbow reddened, ecchymosed left shin, skin tear left hand, complaints of discomfort and irritation of buttocks

Box 2-9   Conclusions of Assessment and Supporting Data
Clusters (continued)

Related Factors

Mobility deficits   Wheelchair bound, stiff joints,
                                      trouble getting out of bed, limited
                                      ROM right hip, hitting wheelchair
                                      during transfers, osteoarthritis,
                                      right hip ORIF 4 months ago

Urinary incontinence   Dribbles urine, wears diaper always

Fragile skin   Skin dry, thin, translucent

Compromised circulation   Sitting in wheelchair all day, Type
                                      2 diabetes, ankle edema

2. Nursing diagnosis: Social isolation related to sensory deficits

Diagnostic Label

Social isolation   Spends a lot of time alone in her
                                      room listening to the radio, cro-
                                      cheting (noninteractive activities),
                                      says she feels alone and different
                                      from others because she is almost
                                      blind, has made no friends, sees
                                      family once a year

Related Factor

Sensory deficits   Almost blind, hearing slightly
                                      diminished

B. Interdisciplinary problem: Physical therapy and nursing

Impaired physical mobility   Wheelchair bound, stiff joints, trou-
                                      ble getting out of bed, limited ROM
                                      right hip, hitting wheelchair during
                                      transfers, osteoarthritis, right hip
                                      ORIF 4 months ago

C. Problem for referral:

Vision deficits   Medical Dx: Type 2 DM, legally
                                      blind, neurological changes have
                                      already affected hearing; data gaps:
                                      actual visual acuity, use of glasses,
                                      last vision exam, patient's description
                                      of actual vision limits

and preliminary conclusions along the way. Our colleagues in medicine refer to this as the process of making differential diagnoses.

Assessment, and the thinking that goes along with it, is not ever finished; at some point the nurse and the patient need to agree on what the issues are and move on to what should be done about those issues. Of course, sometimes the patient is unable to participate in the determination of health issues and the nurse must do the thinking for both of them. Most times, however, the patient's thinking is as important as the nurse's. In deciding what the relevant issues are, the nurse and patient put their heads together. Those heads also need to be working together to decide on the priorities for planning and selecting actions for implementing care. This togetherness is called patient-centered care.

CT is as important to the planning phase of the nursing process as it is in the assessing phase. Once the nurse and patient have determined conclusions of assessment, they need to set priorities and realistic goals. Thinking dimensions of *contextual perspective*, *flexibility*, and *open-mindedness* are very important when planning care with patients. Consider the thinking that goes into setting priorities. Setting priorities, at first glance, seems to be simple. It is far from that. For example, a nurse working with Ms. Romero, who recently had an amputation, could identify the following conclusions of assessment:

- Nursing diagnosis: Body image disturbance related to feelings about recent below-the-knee amputation
- Interdisciplinary problem: Imbalanced nutrition—less than body requirements related to complexity of dietary needs and homelessness
- Problem for referral: Patient is homeless after mudslides and floods destroyed her home; she will be discharged tomorrow

At first glance, the problem for referral seems to be the highest priority, but the nurse would never know that if the patient's thinking and input weren't considered. Ms. Romero could have a large network of friends and extended family willing to have her live with them. In that case, something less obvious could become the priority.

The general guidelines for setting priorities are as follows:

1. Immediate life-threatening issues
2. Safety issues
3. Patient-identified priorities
4. Nurse-identified priorities (based on the overall picture of each health concern in relation to other concerns, the patient as a whole person, and availability of time and resources)

Guidelines 1 and 2 are often obvious, but 3 and 4 require CT by both the nurse and the patient.

Setting realistic goals or expected outcome indicators may highlight CT dimensions of *creativity*, *discriminating*, and *predicting*. A reasonable outcome for one patient will not be reasonable for another. A patient who had a stroke, for example, could not be expected to self-transfer within 1 week if that patient had severe mobility problems prior to the stroke, whereas another patient, who had been fully mobile pre-stroke, might be able to improve mobility quickly.

Planning interventions to meet expected outcomes is equally dependent on good thinking by both the nurse and the patient. If an expected outcome is self-administration of insulin, the interventions necessary to reach that outcome with a patient who cannot read, for example, will be very different than interventions needed with a patient who is a retired physician. Planning and implementing interventions call for the nurse to use CT dimensions of *transforming knowledge* to meet the *contextual perspective*; sometimes a large dose of *perseverance* and *creativity* are needed to move from textbook care plans to customized patient care.

The evaluation phase of the nursing process circles back to thinking and actions that are similar to assessing, except now *applying standards* becomes more obvious. First, the standard set in the planning of expected outcomes must be addressed. Was that outcome met? If not, why? Have the standards of quality and safety been met? The nurse looks at the evidence and uses *logical reasoning* to draw conclusions about the patient's progress toward achieving the expected outcomes.

This brief overview of the dimensions of thinking at play in the nursing process shows how complex the thinking during the simple-looking phases of assessing, planning, implementing, and evaluating really is. As we go back to our assertion that CT is a tool in search of a job, remember, there are many jobs that are part of nursing. The message is this: great nursing requires thinking and doing. One without the other either does not work or can be very dangerous.

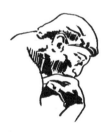

© Jesse Rubenfeld

PAUSE and Ponder

Conclusions About What CT Is

This chapter was necessary to set the stage. Now, when someone asks you about CT, we hope you will have something more to say than, that's a good question! Understanding the concept of CT is essential to nursing practice, but the ideas and words that describe the concept are only building blocks. Now we need to use those building blocks to nurture and expand CT in nursing.

REFLECTION CUES

- CT bridges the gap between knowledge and actions.
- The Western history of CT can be traced as far back as Socrates and up to recent nursing research.
- CT in nursing is exemplified by 10 habits of the mind (*confidence, contextual perspective, creativity, flexibility, inquisitiveness, intellectual integrity, intuition, open-mindedness, perseverance, reflection*) and 7 cognitive skills (*analyzing,*

applying standards, discriminating, information seeking, logical reasoning, predicting, transforming knowledge).

■ Dimensions of nursing CT that are not found in nonnursing descriptions are *creativity, intuition,* and *transforming knowledge.*

■ Verbalizing one's CT requires descriptive language not commonly used in the action-oriented discipline of nursing.

■ It is difficult to see the CT behind the actions. Actions must be combined with descriptions of thinking.

■ Although most of us can identify colleagues who are good thinkers, it is very difficult to tease out the thinking behind their actions.

■ Incorporating the language of thinking into our vocabulary increases our awareness of our own thinking, our awareness of the thinking of others, and our ability to describe our thinking to colleagues.

■ Critical thinking is a tool in search of a job.

■ The nursing process is a daily job of nurses that requires both thinking and doing.

■ Nurses, as health detectives, need to be aware of the multiple conclusions of assessment and how those conclusions are supported with the underlying thinking.

■ Conclusions of assessment are prioritized with conjoint thinking by the nurse and patient.

■ Planning, implementing, and evaluating care works best when nurses and patients think together.

REFERENCES

American Association of Colleges of Nursing. (2008). *The essentials of baccalaureate education for professional nursing practice.* Washington, DC: Author.

American Nurses Association. (2010). *Nursing: Scope and standards of practice* (2nd ed.). Washington, DC: Author.

Benner, P. (1984). *From novice to expert: Power and excellence in nursing practice.* Menlo Park, CA: Addison-Wesley.

Commission on Collegiate Nursing Education. (2013). *Standards for accreditation of baccalaureate and graduate nursing programs.* Retrieved from http://www.aacn.nche.edu/ccne-accreditation/standards-procedures-resources/baccalaureate-graduate/standards

Costa, A. L. (Ed.). (1985). *Developing minds: A resource book for teaching thinking.* Alexandria, VA: Association for Supervision and Curriculum Development.

Dreyfus, H. L., & Dreyfus, S. E. (1986). *Mind over machine: The power of human intuition and expertise in the era of the computer.* New York, NY: Free Press.

Facione, N. C., Facione, P. A., & Sanchez, C. A. (1994). Critical thinking disposition as a measure of competent clinical judgment: The development of the California Critical Thinking Disposition Inventory. *Journal of Nursing Education, 33,* 345–350.

Facione, P. A. (1990). *Critical thinking: A statement of expert consensus for purposes of educational assessment and instruction.* Millbrae, CA: California Academic Press. (ERIC Document Reproduction Service No. ED315423)

Facione, P. A., Sanchez, C. A., Facione, N. C., & Gainen, J. (1995). The disposition toward critical thinking. *Journal of Nursing Education, 44,* 1–25.

Fogler, H. S., & LeBlanc, S. E. (2014). *Strategies for creative problem solving* (3rd ed.). Upper Saddle River, NJ: Pearson Education.

Fonteyn, M. E. (1998). *Thinking strategies for nursing practice*. Philadelphia, PA: Lippincott.

Goodman, C. N. (1987). The Delphi technique: A critique. *Journal of Advanced Nursing, 12*, 729–734.

Hart, L. A. (1983). *Human brain and human learning*. New York, NY: Longman.

Higher Learning Commission. (2010). *Institutional accreditation: An overview*. Retrieved from http://www.ncahlc.org

Kant, I. (1965). *Critique of pure reason* (N. K. Smith, Trans.). New York, NY: St. Martin's Press. (Original work published 1787)

Kemerling, G. (2001). *History of western philosophy*. Retrieved from http://www.philosophypages.com/hy/index.htm

Lucas, G., Marshall, F., Repola, A. F., & Watts, R. (Producers), & Spielberg, S. (Director). (1989). *Indiana Jones and the last crusade* [Motion picture]. U.S.: LucasFilm.

Lunney, M. (2001). *Critical thinking & nursing diagnosis: Case studies & analyses*. Philadelphia, PA: North American Nursing Diagnosis Association.

Lunney, M. (2008). Critical need to address accuracy of nurses' diagnoses. *Online Journal of Issues in Nursing, 13*(1). doi: 10.3912/OJIN,Vol13No01PPT06

Lunney, M. (2010). Use of critical thinking in the diagnostic process. *International Journal of Nursing Terminologies and Classifications, 21*(2), 82–88. doi: 10.1111/j.1744-618X.2010.01150.x

Raymond-Seniuk, C., & Profetto-McGrath, J. (2011). Can one learn to think critically?—a philosophical exploration. *Open Nursing Journal, 5*, 45–51.

Rubenfeld, M. G., & Scheffer, B. K. (1999). *Critical thinking in nursing: An interactive approach* (2nd ed.). Philadelphia, PA: Lippincott.

Scheffer, B. K., & Rubenfeld, M. G. (2000). A consensus statement on critical thinking in nursing. *Journal of Nursing Education, 39*, 352–359.

Scheffer, B. K., & Rubenfeld, M. G. (2006). Critical thinking: A tool in search of a job. *Journal of Nursing Education, 45*, 195–196.

Tanner, C. (1997). Spock would have been a terrible nurse (and other issues related to critical thinking in nursing). *Journal of Nursing Education, 36*, 3–4.

Yura, H., & Walsh, M. B. (1988). *The nursing process: Assessing, planning, implementing, evaluating* (5th ed.). Norwalk, CT: Appleton & Lange.

Who Are the Critical Thinkers?

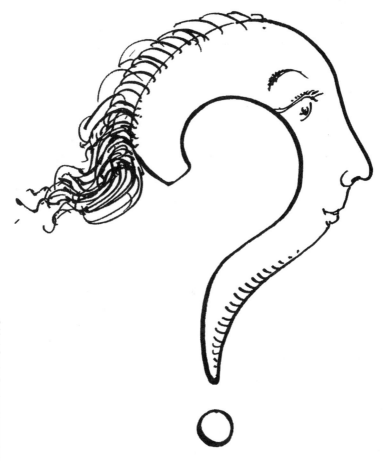

When characterizing people who work in health care, we usually focus on what they do, not how they think. However, people in the health professions, especially nurses, are some of the best critical thinkers in the world. Nurses have a wide breadth and deep depth of knowledge; they must apply that knowledge in a huge variety of contexts; and they must recognize and evaluate variations from the norm in every patient. As health care becomes increasingly complex, the thinking needed becomes even more sophisticated. Those who do the thinking must become even more cognizant of the thinking they employ to do the work of health care.

Who are you? Most of you are probably nurses or nursing students, but because these ideas are relevant to all healthcare providers, some of you may be from other disciplines. We hope so, because, as we will discuss later, we are big believers in the necessity of interdisciplinary practice. Are you a clinician or an educator, or does your position combine both roles? Perhaps you are a researcher, a manager, or an administrator in a practice setting. Nurses' roles and positions are often complex because they embrace multiple thinking tasks throughout the day.

We needed to develop an organized way to address you that also fits with our critical thinking–enhancing TACTICS. As we see it, you want to improve your critical thinking (CT) or help others improve theirs; therefore, we classified you as being in one of two categories: clinicians or educators. For clinicians, much of what we say focuses on how you can improve your CT; for educators, the focus is on strategies to promote CT in others. We're aware that in the real world, these two roles are not mutually exclusive. Clinicians often try to help others improve CT, and educators often work to improve their personal CT. Still, for ease of communication, we have divided you, our readers, into two groups: clinicians and educators.

A major reason we've chosen to write to this audience is that we want to promote a unified view of CT as a vital but complex clinical and educational issue. We are quite aware that the literature on CT in nursing is primarily oriented toward those in academic settings: students and teachers. Indeed, most things we've written are academically slanted. However, the bottom line is that we all want to improve CT in clinical practice. If we don't start viewing this from both perspectives simultaneously, we'll be building an ivory tower version and a digging-out-a-trench version. Neither will be adequate to meet the thinking demands of health care today or tomorrow.

Clinicians

We envision clinicians at multiple points in their professional practice careers and in a variety of healthcare settings. Those multiple career points span from that of a novice who is learning in the clinical setting (i.e., nursing students or orientees) to that of a nurse who is considered an expert in practice. Many challenges tax your thinking skills in the practice arena, not least of which is the seemingly constant change in the demands and responsibilities of your positions. Complex changes are occurring in all healthcare delivery systems (Erickson, Ditomassi, & Jones, 2008; Falise, 2007; Institute of Medicine, 2011; Redman, 2006; Rossen, Bartlett, & Herrick, 2008). Kelly-Thomas (1998) referred to the "re-do" words typically heard in healthcare environments these days—reengineering, restructuring, retooling, revisioning. These re-do issues require, above all else, nurses to be *confident, contextual, creative, open-minded*, and *flexible* in their thinking strategies. We will return often to the subject of complex change.

Educators

We envision educators in various settings as well, primarily as service based (staff development specialists, preceptors, continuing education directors, and so on) or academic based (nursing school faculty). We expect that some of our clinicians and educators are graduate students pursuing one or both roles. Whichever kind of educator you are, you deal with many complex problems that affect how you see yourself as a thinker and how you'll be able to promote CT in your students and staff. Academic-based educators may be more familiar with CT language because much of what has been written about CT has been for traditional educational settings. We hope you will find this text to be helpful because it presents a practical view of CT, not just an academic view.

Other Thinkers Who Interact with Clinicians and Educators

Although for this discussion we've delineated two *who* groups and acknowledged that all people are thinkers, here is an important point: no one of us thinks in isolation. To view CT as an individual process will take us down a disastrous path where we waste time and money and possibly do harm. Other thinkers must also be considered, including patients, patients' significant others, and additional members of the healthcare team. Remember that everything we say about CT applies to all the thinkers around you—other nurses, students, healthcare providers, patients and their significant others, administrators, politicians, and many others. The thinking of stakeholders also has an impact.

Selected Factors That Affect Critical Thinkers

Many factors influence us as thinkers. For example, clinicians may be viewed as facing enormous challenges because their work is traditionally action oriented, taking place in settings that rarely sanction thinking time. Educators, on the other hand, are usually viewed as actively working when they sit with furrowed brows. In addition to these environmental factors, many other things influence one's thinking—genetics; self-concept; feelings, especially anxiety; generation or age; knowledge; and personal and organizational culture. See **Box 3-1** for a synopsis of these factors.

Genetics as an Influence on CT

Let's look at genetics, or basic wiring, first. No two people think in the same way. (That's great, isn't it?) Whether those differences stem from genetics or one's upbringing is frequently debated. In reality, it's both, but we do know that some differences are

Box 3-1 Selected Factors Influencing Critical Thinkers

Factor	Key Issue
Genetics	Your brain's hard wiring. Some adjustments over time, but if you are a right-brain thinker it is very challenging to think like a left-brain thinker.
Self-concept	Appears to be a direct relationship between self-concept and critical thinking. The CT habit of the mind *confidence* comes into play here.
Feelings (especially anxiety)	Very strong inverse relationship between anxiety and critical thinking. The higher the anxiety, the lower the critical thinking.
Generation or age	Values, work ethic, and communication style vary by generation.
Knowledge	You need knowledge to apply critical thinking habits and skills. You can't think in a vacuum! Knowledge is complex, contextual, and constructed, and it may help or hinder CT.
Culture (personal)	
▪ Communication style	▪ Verbal, nonverbal, and written styles impact thinking and vice versa
▪ Time orientation	▪ Past, present, future, mixed viewpoints may guide thinking
Culture (organizational)	This is the context in which thinking occurs. It can be supportive or toxic to critical thinking.

inborn. Some people have the ability to remember numerous esoteric facts but can't figure out how to solve simple everyday problems such as how to boil water! Others never seem flustered when things go wrong but can't remember when they last went to the bathroom. Acknowledging differences in thinking without judging that one way is better than another is a challenge, but a necessary one, especially for educators who are trying to individualize teaching strategies to nurture thinking.

If you haven't thought about your natural, inborn thinking abilities, do that now. If you can articulate your personal hard wiring, it will make you a better learner. Are you a visual thinker? (You need to see it to understand it.) Are you an auditory thinker? (Once you hear it, you remember it.) Do you have to do something with information—perform an action—before it stays in your brain? If you can describe to a teacher what works best for you, you will be a better learner. You will also be more sensitive to the learning and thinking styles of others and therefore be a better educator. Keep in mind that it is rare to have only one of these learning styles; most of us have combinations but find one that is our preferred style.

Consider this example from an author–educator:

My son has attention deficit disorder, and although his intelligence test results showed him to be above average, he could not learn how to add columns of numbers. When given a fourth-grade assignment to copy a list of numbers and add them, he would write the numbers in what seemed to be a random pattern so the tens or hundreds were never above and below each other. I kept saying to him, "Line them up!" and he would repeatedly do this random thing. Finally, in total frustration, I drew lines on the sheet of paper. Then he had no trouble at all. It made me realize that he has no patterning ability in his mind remotely close to what I have in mine. Once we moved to graph paper with big squares, he was fine with addition of long sets of numbers. (By the way, this boy moved to the advanced math classes in high school.)

This boy's situation, in addition to illustrating how vastly different thinking styles can be, shows us that intelligence is not a simple construct. Howard Gardner deftly illustrated thinking complexity in his description of multiple intelligences (1983, 1993, 1999, 2006). Refer to Gardner's list in **Box 3-2**. Can you relate to some of

---

Box 3-2 Gardner's Multiple Intelligences

- **Spatial:** the mind's eye: preference for use of images, pictures, graphical representations
- **Logical-Mathematical:** use of an entire range of reasoning skills, preference for factual data, and both inductive and deductive reasoning
- **Linguistic:** embracing speaking and listening, reading, writing, and other forms of communication
- **Musical:** patterned rhythms of the mind, learning and knowing by sharing, expressing, perceiving, and creating pitch and patterns
- **Bodily-Kinesthetic:** using the body as a conduit for the mind, using action and motion
- **Interpersonal:** using the give and take of communication with intonation and punctuation with a goal of understanding, empathy, and learning from one another
- **Intrapersonal:** focusing on knowing self with a goal of internalizing learning through thoughtful connections and transformation of knowledge into meaning
- **Naturalist:** the ability to recognize and differentiate characteristics and phenomena of the plant and animal world as well as inorganic material immersion in a work of art

---

Source: Frames of Mind: The Theory of Multiple Intelligences by Howard Gardner, Copyright (c) 1983 by Howard Gardner. Reprinted by permission of Basic Books, a member of The Perseus Books Group.

those intelligences more than others? We'd guess yes. Gardner believed that we have varying proportions of each of these intelligences but that some of them come more naturally to us than others. That may be due to genetics or because some groups and cultures value some traits over others. Our self-concept of our thinking style is largely based on our dominant intelligences.

Self-Concept as an Influence on CT

Think about this statement: I am a great thinker. Do you believe it? If yes, why? If no, why? You can probably imagine a philosophy professor saying this. That's because we traditionally associate great thinking with fields such as philosophy. Nursing is traditionally associated with doing and actions. Both of these traditional associations are too limited, especially the nursing one. Expert nursing care requires expert levels of thinking for actions to be safe.

Obviously, culture influences self-concept, but there's more to it than that, such as life circumstances and how much positive (or negative) feedback you get for your thinking ability. If your 10th-grade math teacher told you that girls are never any good at math (and yes, teachers still say such things), the girls in that class would need some other equally dramatic evaluation of their math skills to counter that attitude and develop a positive concept of themselves as mathematical thinkers. If you were always praised for your problem-solving abilities, you'd be proud of your analytical skills, thereby promoting a positive self-concept in that CT dimension.

The math example speaks to a very important point about the differences in how women and men think. Women and men are socialized differently, especially in relation to self-concept and thinking ability. This is not an all-or-nothing interpretation, however. Excellent research has been done on female thinking (Belenky, Clinchy, Goldberger, & Tarule, 1986; Gilligan, 1982), and there are many helpful suggestions for addressing gender differences in classrooms (Brookfield & Preskill, 1999). Though gender has a significant influence on self-concept and is definitely a force to be reckoned with in nursing, with its lopsided ratio of women to men, even the experts caution us not to assume that gender is the only factor that affects how we think.

Unfortunately, women are still trying to escape the negative connotations of descriptions like "she's really smart," which cause most of us to flash back to high school where that meant "she's not pretty." The implication was that looks were more important than brains. Think of how women are described in the media even today, and then consider how men are described; inevitably, women are described in terms of appearance, and men are described in terms of intelligence and accomplishments.

Although women have quite a few stereotypes working against them, men in nursing don't fare much better in how society views their thinking abilities. Because these men are nurses and not, for example, engineers, their thinking is considered less sophisticated. Unfortunately, people often judge a nontraditional career decision negatively, especially with respect to thinking ability. Why would a man be a nurse (when he could have been an engineer or a doctor)?

Sometimes the world doesn't view nurses as great thinkers and sees nurses through gender-biased eyes. Let's stop buying into those notions and work on what we do have control over—our self-concept as great thinkers. Simply reflecting on your thinking can help you improve your self-concept. After completing such *reflection* assignments, our students have said, "We never thought about our thinking before. We really do think a lot, don't we?" If we accept the stereotypical beliefs that we're not great thinkers, is it any wonder that we have self-concept problems about our thinking?

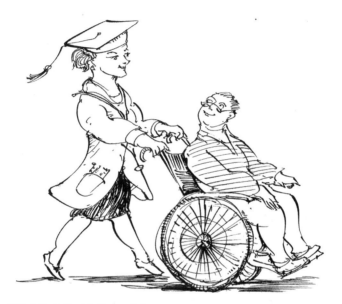

© Mark Steele. Reprinted by permission.

Suzanne Gordon (2005, 2010), a reporter who has studied nursing extensively, made some interesting comments about our image. Her contention is that the usual descriptions of nursing as a calling and as a caring profession do us more harm than good. Such descriptions emphasize virtue and devalue our skill, knowledge, and thinking ability. "Updating the image of nursing will involve applying some critical thinking to the sentimentalized virtue script that nurses so often rely on today" (2005, p. 440).

We need to value our brains and define ourselves as knowledge workers, not production workers. Kaeding and Rambur (2004) described knowledge work as

> based on assessment, judgment, problem-solving, and the generation of ideas. It is nonrepetitive, nonroutine, and dependent on cognitive activity. Manual work is integral but not dominant. Gender is valued equally. Professional knowledge is not hierarchical, and evidence of learning is important to safe and effective job performance. (p. 137)

Seago (2008) described how healthcare organizations are beginning to use the term *knowledge worker* as a new descriptor for healthcare providers to conceptualize the culture change needed for the 21st century. Maybe we should go back to wearing nursing caps, but this time we should make them in the shape of mortarboards representing the knowledge gleaned through education and experience.

Feelings, Especially Anxiety, as Influences on CT

Another major factor that influences thinking involves emotions. Intense feelings— love, hate, depression, elation—will always be factors shaping our cognitive skills. When we did our Delphi study to find consensus on CT, we specifically asked about habits of the mind in addition to cognitive skills. Most people, at least in nursing, acknowledge that CT has both affective (habits of the mind) and cognitive (skills) components. Those two components exist in tandem all the time. But when we add an extreme emotional response to a situation, affective components of CT exert a stronger influence.

Many mood states affect thinking, but anxiety is particularly important in the healthcare sector, which has more than its share of anxiety-producing situations. Most older nurses (age 50 and older) can tell horror stories about how they were so terrified by nursing school teachers that they couldn't think at all. Hart (1983) called that "reptilian" brain functioning, meaning that the higher-order thinking skills of mammals shuts down, and only basic survival thinking takes over. Teaching through terror, we hope, has gone the way of our nursing caps. Nevertheless, doing a nursing task for the first time, even with a nurturing teacher to help, still makes our hearts race and our palms dampen. And some nursing tasks continue to make us anxious even after we've done them many times.

There are many self-help books on how to deal with anxiety, so we're not going to give a short course here. However, we do encourage you to consider what happens to your thinking when you're anxious and what circumstances, in particular, make you anxious. Also, consider what Margaret Carson (2003) called the "emotional burden" of nursing. Carson studied nurses who had been in combat situations, but she also cautioned nurses to consider the psychological toll of other high-stress nursing situations. In our experience, nurses do not do a good job of taking care of themselves; we need to think about our emotional responses more, value things like lunch and bathroom breaks, and consider the importance of decreasing anxiety to sharpen our thinking skills.

If you teach others, orient new staff, or function as a preceptor, we have a special message for you: if you expect your students and staff to be good thinkers, you must guide them gently, acknowledge their anxiety, and employ teaching and mentoring strategies, such as humor, that reduce anxiety. It is both humbling and helpful to remember your first lecture or your first attempt to catheterize an uncooperative patient. Telling students about your fears or relating to new staff how you botched simple jobs in your first weeks on the unit can do wonders to help them relax and reassure them that they also will gain mastery. Most of all, we must approach teaching as a collaborative effort, not a game of one-upmanship in which you are the all-knowing expert and your students have blank slates for brains. Anxiety is a day-to-day reality of nursing. We need to acknowledge it, remember its influence on thinking, and constantly work to lessen it to help ourselves and others.

Generational and Age Influences on CT

The nursing profession contains five generations of workers; those age-related differences affect many important attributes—attitudes, beliefs, communication, work style, and, of course, thinking. There are several classifications of generations. Oblinger and Oblinger (2005) described them this way: "Matures," born between 1900 and 1945; "Baby Boomers," born between 1946 and 1964; "Generation X," born between 1965 and 1981; and the "Net Generation," born between 1982 and 1991. The newest generation, born in the 1990s, have been called the "Digital Natives" (Prensky, 2001) or "Shallows" (Carr, 2011); technology use has become natural for them. It seems their brains are physically changing, perhaps because of the constant use of modern information processing technology. Having five generations working together is a new phenomenon because nurses now remain in the workplace longer than they once did (Sherman, 2006). It behooves clinicians and educators to reflect on the significance of generational differences to avoid conflict and misunderstanding.

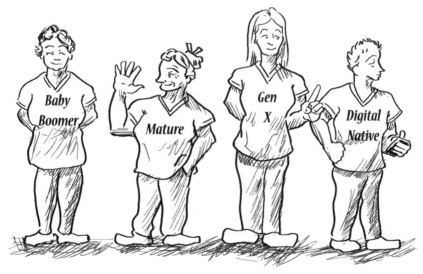

© Jesse Rubenfeld

Some believe that generational differences are more related to technology exposure than to age itself, so when reflecting on implications of those differences, an open mind is crucial. Although any generalizations will inevitably be incorrect in specific instances, it is helpful to consider how these generalizations could affect thinking. (See **Box 3-3**.) Continuing with Oblinger and Oblinger's (2005) descriptions, Matures were described as self-sacrificing, respectful of authority, and intolerant of waste and technology. Putting that in a thinking frame of reference, we might expect our older nurses' *information-seeking* and *applying-standards* CT skills to be manifested as seeking answers from authorities whom they respect. They may have less *flexibility* in their thinking, but they will have *perseverance*. They will not be *confident* when dealing with technology, but from their years of experience, they may have a larger *contextual perspective* and will likely be strong on *intuition* and *confident* in their *logical reasoning* in a wide range of situations.

Box 3-3 Generational Influences

Born Between	Label	Characteristics	Likely Key CT Habits of the Mind and Skills
1900 and 1945	Matures	Self-sacrificing, respectful of authority, intolerant of waste and technology	*Information seeking* *Applying standards* *Perseverance* *Contextual perspective* *Intuition* *Confidence*
1946 and 1964	Baby Boomers	Optimistic workaholics, strong work ethic and sense of responsibility, intolerant of laziness	*Confidence* *Predicting* *Discriminating* *Transforming knowledge*
1965 and 1981	Generation X	Independent, free, skeptical, multitaskers who value a balanced lifestyle; intolerant of red tape	*Flexibility* *Open-mindedness* *Information seeking* *Inquisitiveness* *Applying standards*
1982 and 1991	Net Generation/ Millennials	Hopeful, determined, use latest technology, intolerant of slowness	*Information seeking* *Creativity* *Contextual perspective*
1992 and the present	Digital Natives/ Shallows	Fast, parallel information processors, multitaskers, prefer graphics over text, thrive on instant gratification and frequent rewards	*Contextual perspective* *Creativity* *Intuition* *Transforming knowledge*

Baby Boomers were seen as optimistic workaholics with a strong work ethic and sense of responsibility; they are intolerant of laziness and believe they can do most things well (Oblinger & Oblinger, 2005). We might expect them to be *confident* in their thinking and have strong *predicting* and *discriminating* abilities. Like the Matures, they have years of experience to draw on as they think through situations and may do well with *transforming knowledge*. They may be less *open-minded* in their thinking, especially when they deal with Generation Xers, who are not workaholics.

Generation X was characterized as independent, free, skeptical, and comfortable with multitasking and as valuing a balance of life and work. They are intolerant of red tape and hype (Oblinger & Oblinger, 2005). They may be more *flexible* in their thinking and *open-minded* to divergent views as long as those views aren't seen as restrictive. They will likely *seek information* from a variety of sources, not necessarily from authorities. Because they are skeptical, they may be more independently *inquisitive*. When *applying standards*, they may use more personal standards than work-related standards.

The Net Generation, also called Millennials, are hopeful, determined, into the latest technology, and intolerant of anything slow (Oblinger & Oblinger, 2005). They don't know a world without the Internet, so their *information-seeking* skills are first and foremost oriented there. They may be impatient with older workers who are less adept at surfing, but they may work and think well in teams because they are used to networking. They are likely *creative* in their thinking, seeking their own approaches to knowledge rather than doing what they're told. They may have a wider *contextual perspective* because they are used to visual communication and experiential learning, but they may miss things that are not of interest to them.

The new generation, who have not known a world without the Internet, iPhones, instant messaging, and texting, have been called the Shallows by Carr (2011) and Digital Natives by Prensky (2001, 2012). These folks are so used to instant information that they can't imagine a world without it. It seems their brains, through neuroplasticity, are changing due to persistent digital input (Carr, 2011; Prensky, 2001, 2012). Their evolving brains process information in small chunks very quickly; they are used to reading snippets of information and do not like long passages of text. They are used to visual images in their digital world. Their brains have become trained to process information in parallel streams as opposed to a sequential flow. Carr's description captures these changes:

> With writing on the screen, we're still able to decode text quickly—we read, if anything faster than ever—but we're no longer guided toward a deep, personally constructed understanding of the text's connotations. Instead, we're hurried off toward another bit of related information, and then another, and another. The strip-mining of 'relevant content' replaces the slow excavation of meaning. (p. 166)

Although these labels seem negative at first glance, what we oldsters have to remember is that this new generation has assets to offer that we have yet to appreciate.

Obviously these generalizations are simplistic, but what is important to consider is that we cannot expect a young, recently graduated nurse to think in the same way that the older nurse would. Weston (2006) called this the generational "mental model." "Based upon world events that framed their youth and initial work experiences, members of each generation have develop [sic] somewhat unique mental models . . . logical and consistent with their lived experience" ("Sources of Multi-generational Misunderstandings," para. 1). We must promote tolerance of the differences among us and tailor teamwork and teaching and learning to the thinking style of each person. In the practice arena, we must acknowledge the strengths and contributions of each generation and link people together based on how they can help one another (Sherman, 2006).

Teaching and learning issues are especially challenging; because teachers, both in academia and in clinical settings, are primarily Baby Boomers, the teaching approaches that fit with their characteristics are a misfit for the learning needs of Generation X, the Net Generation, and the Digital Natives. Faculty who are used to sequential knowledge building, recall of information, and repetition must learn to appreciate the new generation of learners who are used to digital, interactive, and fast-paced learning (Skiba & Barton, 2006).

Knowledge Influences on CT

Just how important is a nurse's knowledge to CT? Well for starters, people in general and nurses specifically do not think in a vacuum. We need something to think about. So is it simply a matter of absorbing enough information and nursing content knowledge, and then nurses can be good critical thinkers? This idea is way oversimplified. Thus, the issue of knowledge bears exploration. Just how does knowledge influence CT? And how do we conceptualize that knowledge and its influence?

Lechasseur, Lazure, and Guilbert (2011), using a grounded theory approach, studied knowledge as used by students of nursing in Canada. As a rationalization for their study, the authors stated that "the various types of knowledge involved must be better defined, as should the factors influencing their selection and mobilization" (p. 1931). Whereas eight types of knowledge (intrapersonal, interpersonal, perceptual, moral–ethical, scientific, practical, experiential, and contextual) identified in prior literature, starting with Carper's ways of knowing (1978), were identified, another type emerged. That was a contextualized type of knowledge. They coined a term for this new type as "combinational constructive knowledge" (p. 1930). It was difficult for students to verbalize the complexity of this knowledge that called for a higher level of critical thinking, including *creativity*, and a focus on the uniqueness of the patient situation.

This combinational constructive knowledge is quite intriguing. It resonates with the complex type of knowledge that we have gained in our many nursing years. Consider how complex our nursing knowledge base is the longer we practice. Bits and pieces of information are put together into lumps, patterns, schemes, and blobs in our minds. What do we do with that mixture of knowledge? Well, consider something as banal as constipation, a health issue nurses own for their patients' comfort. Think of the knowledge that constitutes constipation: Well, there's basic anatomy and physiology of the gut. Ah, but we know that varies by individuals, diet, time of the month, age, fluid intake, mobility, ethnicity, medications . . . shall we keep going? You get the idea, right? Even something as simple as taking care of constipation is based on combinational constructive knowledge if your aim is a patient's comfortable bowel elimination.

Although consideration of combinational constructive knowledge seems to help with our understanding of the influence of knowledge on CT, another study posed the question of whether knowledge could interfere with CT. The relationship between CT and knowledge emerged as a theme in the qualitative study of Chinese students by Chan (2012). That relationship was polarized as being a partnership or rivalry. "Some participants found knowledge a prerequisite for making a sound judgement [sic], while others argued that believing in established knowledge could prevent one from questioning the validity of arguments" (p. 563).

Aha, so is knowledge a good or bad influence on CT? Hmmm. We will let you ponder that some more. Consider your knowledge base. Is it fluid enough to be combined and reconstructed, or is it so standardized that it might interfere with your thinking? You might want to stop and reflect on your *intellectual integrity*. Can you reflect on your existing knowledge and reconstruct it if another piece of the knowledge picture seems contrary to your previous assumptions or beliefs?

Cultural Influences on CT

Unquestionably, we are influenced by our native culture and by the culture in which we live and work. Depending on your level of ethnocentrism or your exposure to different cultures, you may not realize how deeply societal and cultural norms affect your thinking and that of people around you.

Culture, as defined by Rose (2013), is "an integrated pattern of learned beliefs and behaviors that can be shared among groups, including thoughts, styles of communicating, ways of interacting, views on roles and relationships, values, practices, and customs" (p. 203). Culture is not static; it changes with time as cultural groups change the definitions of their parameters. Although we can trace almost everything we think and do back to some cultural influence, there are some aspects of culture that are especially relevant when it comes to CT, particularly communication and time orientation. We will also discuss the organizational culture of the healthcare work environment and how it affects CT.

Communication, Culture, and CT

Communication is the most obvious area where culture could affect CT. The term *communication* covers a broad range of topics about which numerous books are written. In this section, we focus on two: language and translation of meaning across cultures, and one's style for communicating thinking.

First, consider what language a person speaks. Is it the language of the majority? If not, consider what implications translation can have on the various components of CT. Words to describe thinking are complex and abstract and often have no direct translation in other languages. On a trip to Japan to present a paper on CT, we found that the phrase *habits of the mind* caused the most complex translation problem. There was no direct translation, so we tried to think of a synonym. In our research, we chose that phrase—*habits of the mind*—deliberately because we wanted to get across these finer points: The word *traits* often connotes static qualities, and we wanted to stay away from that. *Characteristics* was too broad, and *dispositions* was closely aligned with *traits*. As the translator tried these and other words, she became very frustrated. *Tendencies toward* seemed to work, as did *affinity for*, but ultimately, the complete meaning of *habits of the mind* was probably never effectively translated.

What did this do to our discussion about CT? In this case, the idea that habits of the mind can be enhanced and our suggestions on how to do that may literally have gotten lost in translation. Because language is the basis of understanding, the very words used to describe CT and its dimensions need to be clarified at the outset of any discussion. If we aren't using the same descriptors, we may not be talking about the same thing.

Second, consider the different styles of communication that exist among cultural groups. To study CT requires questioning, but how is questioning viewed in other cultures? Is it considered an impolite or a desirable activity? Group activities to enhance CT usually involve sharing thoughts about thinking style; such sharing can be seen as a very intimate process. Do some cultures have rules that prohibit such personal exchanges?

I (Gaie) will switch to singular first-person writing here for a moment because this observation is personal. I can think of two extremes to illustrate the differences in communication style among cultures. One occurred in my native Newfoundland, a small maritime province in Canada. The other occurred in Japan, where I recently did the presentation on CT to which I referred earlier. I have not lived in Newfoundland for many years, but I visit frequently. It seems that there is open debate on everything in my home province. I have never seen a place with so many radio talk shows! Everyone has an opinion on everything, and people freely express their opinions through whatever medium is available. Several people talking at once, using emphatic gestures, is more the norm than the exception. While doing a presentation on CT to nurses there several years ago, I had to stop frequently for discussion and questions from the audience. To someone unfamiliar with the culture, the questions might have seemed confrontational. I felt right at home!

In Japan, on the other hand, the large audience of nurses was extremely quiet. I was a bit intimidated when I walked into the auditorium to find 3000 nurses who were so silent. It reminded me of how the room sounded the day before while I rehearsed—but then it was completely empty. I'm used to the din that American and Canadian audiences make as they wait for programs to begin. In Japan, when I asked for questions, there were few. Those who spoke did not use hand gestures and began each interaction with a deferential comment, such as "excuse me." Japanese nursing faculty, who are very interested in promoting CT, told me they have to repeatedly encourage students to discuss issues and ask questions; students there are much more comfortable with lectures.

Extremes such as these, and all kinds of examples in between, occur in nursing practice and schools throughout North America as well. What do such differences mean to the educator or clinician? Because questioning is considered a desirable part of CT, the tendency is to believe that the assertive communicator is a better critical thinker. However, we must consider just what it is that we most value. Is it the communication of questions or the questioning itself that is important? Perhaps we need to think of ways beyond verbal means to encourage questioning. Perhaps quiet people are more comfortable sharing their questions in writing. Smaller group discussions that are not teacher led or Web caucuses might be more appropriate for those from cultures in which open questioning is seen as impolite.

Even words within the same language can assume different meanings and connotations (the underlying meanings). For example, some geographic regions have different meanings for the same word. In some parts of the United States, the word *dinner* means the noon meal, while in other parts of the United States it means the third meal of the day. Think about the teaching implications for patients learning about diabetic eating patterns. You have to consider where you are when you interpret words. Then, to make matters even more challenging, consider how some words have acquired stronger values than other words. Think about how those values have an impact on how all the healthcare stakeholders think and interact with each other. Have some fun with **TACTICS 3-1** to see how the value meaning attached to words cannot only vary but also impact your thinking and the thinking of other stakeholders.

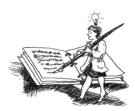

TACTICS 3-1: What's the Value Meaning Attached to These Words?

1. Read the following list of words one by one.
2. On a scale of 1–10, with 1 being the most negative value and 10 being the most positive value, rank each of these 10 words.

Critical thinking	Bias
Judgment	Nonjudgmental
Frequent flyer	Medicine
Children	Nursing
Noncompliant	Elderly

3. Compare your value ranking with a peer.
4. Discuss similarities and differences *and* propose how your values might impact both your thinking and your care.

Discussion

Which words had the highest values? Why do you think they did? Which words had the lowest values? How do you see your value (liking or disliking) of the word having an impact on how you think and how you practice nursing? Did you tend to give *judgment* and *bias* and *noncompliant* lower values? If so, why? Are there situations in which judgment and bias might be highly valued? And is *noncompliant* a useful label? Does it help in thinking and planning care or simply blame the patient? Share with your peer what you can do to look more deeply into the value behind words and become aware of how that value may impact both your thinking and your care.

Time Orientation, Culture, and CT

If communication styles seem culturally bound, what about other things, such as the cultural influence on time orientation? There is a certain expectation of a futuristic view in nursing descriptions of CT. Speaking generally, certain groups have one of three dominant time perspectives: past, present, or future. Of course, there are many exceptions to these broad generalizations, but we usually view Eastern cultures as more focused on the past, Hispanic and Native American or Aboriginal cultures as more focused on the present, and European American cultures as more focused on the future.

A Hispanic nurse once told us that he asks Hispanic patients if they'd like him to record appointment times on their cards half an hour earlier so they'd be on time for their appointments. He initiates that question with a comment about his own tendency for tardiness because he's not very future oriented.

Another example from Gaie: A friend and I stopped to visit a basket maker on a Mi'kmaq reservation in Cape Breton, Nova Scotia, a couple years ago. We were so fascinated with her exquisite weaving of a quill basket that we stayed longer than planned. Upon realizing the time, we jumped up, saying, "We'll be late getting to our friend's house. We need to get going." The basket maker looked at us, smiled, and said, "Just tell them you were on the res' and you're on Indian time." Clearly, her present-oriented perspective was so much a part of her culture that she was very comfortable making humorous references to it. Later I thought about what it would be like if she were a student in my CT class. What would she think when I stressed the importance of *predicting* (one of the CT skills we identified in our study) as part of CT? Would she adopt a futuristic thinking mode because it was expected? How would that affect other parts of her thinking, honed by years of her own culture's influence?

Another issue relative to time is the predominant U.S. value that time is money and its companion, time equals action. For vivid examples of this in health care, we only have to look at managed care approaches in which nurse practitioners and physicians are required to see large numbers of patients each hour to meet income quotas. Home healthcare nurses are given similar quota directives—ones that make quality care difficult. What happens to CT in a culture that clearly values the tangible results of work but not the process of improving quality through thinking? It takes time to think; some things take longer to think about than others, and some people think faster or slower than others. (See **TACTICS 3-2**.)

TACTICS 3-2: Cultural Influences on Thinkers

Clinicians

Using the checklist in **Box 3-4**, reflect on your culture and how it might affect your CT habits of the mind. Then think of someone you work with who comes from a culture different than yours. Think of a patient from a different culture. How do you think those persons would answer the questions?

Educators

Use the checklist in Box 3-4 as the basis for a group discussion. Consider whether your students and staff gain an awareness of other cultures.

Box 3-4   Cultural Influences on Thinking Habits of the Mind

Directions: Place an X on the line to indicate your self-rating.

My culture:
- values
  limited questioning of authority   open debate
  ←————————————————————————————→
- is primarily focused on the
  ❏ past   ❏ present   ❏ future
- values
  contemplation   actions
  ←————————————————————————————→

In my culture I am encouraged to:
- be confident of my reasoning ability
  never   always
  ←————————————————————————————→
- consider where someone is coming from when I interact
  never   always
  ←————————————————————————————→
- be as creative as possible
  never   always
  ←————————————————————————————→
- be flexible, even if it means changing my expectations
  never   always
  ←————————————————————————————→
- be openly inquisitive
  never   always
  ←————————————————————————————→
- seek the truth, even if it differs from my beliefs
  never   always
  ←————————————————————————————→

(continues)

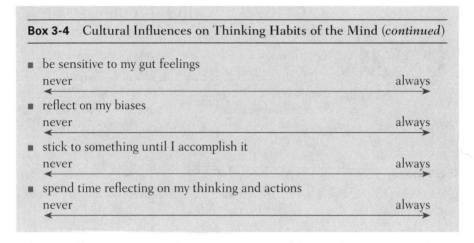

Box 3-4 Cultural Influences on Thinking Habits of the Mind (*continued*)

■ be sensitive to my gut feelings
   never   always

■ reflect on my biases
   never   always

■ stick to something until I accomplish it
   never   always

■ spend time reflecting on my thinking and actions
   never   always

Discussion

Did you learn anything about your culture? Other people's cultures? You've probably considered such things before, but have you put them into a CT frame of reference? We tend to think of cultural norms in terms of such things as eating, holidays, and dress, but we don't often associate them with our thinking.

Organizational Culture and CT

This brings us to a significant cultural influence on you as a thinker—the organizational culture of your work environment. Here we consider how much your employment environment defines you as a thinker. Much has been written about the influence of work environment on thinking (e.g., Chan, 2001; Senge, 1990; Senge, Smith, Kruschwitz, Laur, & Schley, 2010). In her study of nursing preceptorship, Myrick (2002) identified the work climate or environment as a key variable enabling CT.

Organizational cultures can be very powerful. There is a strong tendency to assume that behaving in accordance with one's organizational culture is the correct way to do things and avoid role conflicts. Such assumptions generally lead to a status quo environment that precludes thinking. After all, it's easy. Status quo thinking, however, is not healthy and eventually leads to the decline, entropy, and ultimate demise of the organization (Higgins, 1995).

Organizational cultures that promote a status quo existence are potentially dangerous to critical thinkers. Brookfield (1993) recognized this situation and warned critically thinking nurses about "cultural suicide" (being ostracized by coworkers as a result of challenging the status quo). Many critically thinking nurses are thought of as being on the fringes of mainstream thinking because they question, challenge, and annoy those who prefer to keep things the same.

Although few would admit to this, today's complex systems of healthcare practice and education often blatantly discourage CT. Mohr, Deatrick, Richmond, and Mahon (2001) addressed organizational values conflicts, painting a picture of troubled organizations. Some unhealthy traits they mentioned were excessive control, distraction with minutiae, repression, intolerance for new members and diversity, territorial behaviors, depression, submissiveness, and horizontal violence (passive–aggressive behavior). This is a culture that will certainly not contribute to the growth of its members' CT.

Organizational cultures that encourage CT and acknowledge the inevitability of change are called *learning organizations*, and they use *systems thinking* (Chan, 2001; Senge, 1990). Or, as Senge et al. (2010) said in their later writing, "learning journeys" are necessary for organizational growth. Members of these cultures that encourage CT exhibit traits of trustworthiness, autonomy, responsibility, and *reflection* (Mohr et al., 2001). They rely on resources such as books, computers, links to libraries, and librarians. They provide think time and emphasize language and description and share thinking. They give verbal credit and reward the thinking process, not just the end product. They welcome debate. If you are fortunate enough to work in that kind of environment, it is bound to positively influence you as a thinker. People like us, who spend a lot of time thinking about thinking, define such places as heaven, nirvana; we dream about such organizational cultures and hope to see them as the norm in nursing. (See **TACTICS 3-3**.)

TACTICS 3-3: Environmental Factors Influencing Thinkers

Clinicians

Think about your environment. Generally speaking:
1. Where does it fall on the continuum from status quo thinking to our description of thinking heaven?
2. What is your position in that environment?
3. Can you influence the working culture?
4. How could you influence it?
5. Make a list of things you can influence in your environment that would make it more thinking-friendly.

Educators

Think about your teaching style.
1. Complete the checklist in **Box 3-5**.
2. How would you rate yourself as a positive influence on the thinking of your learners?
3. Review one of your teaching plans; do you see evidence of strategies that promote thinking?
4. Can you or should you change anything in your plan?

Discussion

How does your environmental culture stack up? Are you doing a good job of promoting CT in your organization? Cultures that promote CT have members who think individually and collectively. Such organizations are not neat; indeed, they appear rather chaotic. They are in a constant state of change. Think about what kind of

---

Box 3-5 Thought-Promoting Teaching Style Checklist

In my teaching I:
- Evaluate and give credit for thinking processes (e.g., "good thinking!")
- Use multisensory techniques
- Encourage lots of questions
- Do not get defensive when questioned or challenged
- Help students find information resources
- Describe to students how I think
- Model my thinking
- Use deliberate methods to decrease anxiety
- Develop teaching objectives or expected competencies that go beyond recall of information and require transforming information into usable knowledge
- Use humor
- Create a thinking-friendly environmental culture that accepts mistakes as opportunities to grow
- Vary teaching methods and strategies throughout each session
- Engage students in peer review activities
- Provide written *reflection* time in class
- Ask students to expand on their answers (e.g., "tell me more")
- Promote students' positive self-concepts
- Emphasize collaborative learning between teacher and student (as opposed to authoritarian style)
- Allow or encourage the student to be the teacher

---

thinker you are and how much that part of you is defined by your work culture. What can you do to make your environment more conducive to CT?

This *reflection* process helps to identify who in your organization are potential CT mentors. Not all members of an organization strive to be great thinkers. The larger the numbers of critical thinkers in an organization, the better the quality of health care.

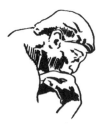

PAUSE and Ponder

Defining Ourselves as Critical Thinkers

In this chapter, we have focused on clinicians and educators who are the keys to promoting CT in nursing. Once again, let us caution you: CT is not just an individual phenomenon. Our CT is influenced by all the thinkers around us, and we influence their thinking, too. Repeatedly throughout this text, we assert the importance of this point. Today's healthcare delivery and educational systems are enormously complex. If clinicians and educators don't define themselves as critical thinkers, we will have unsolvable problems.

REFLECTION CUES

- This chapter specifically speaks to clinicians and educators about their identities as thinkers.
- Clinicians include everyone from beginning nursing students to expert nurses in the practice arena.
- Educators include everyone in all areas of teaching, from staff development to continuing education to the academic settings.
- Many factors influence one's development as a critical thinker.
- Genetics, or your natural thinking processes, influences *who* you are as a thinker.
- Gardner's multiple intelligences increase our awareness of different styles of thinking and processing information.
- Self-concept as an influence on CT is shaped by many factors, such as gender and social mores.
- Nurses are great thinkers, even though the world doesn't always see them as such or acknowledge their thinking as essential to their actions.
- Nurses are knowledge workers, not production workers.
- All emotions, especially anxiety, exert a huge influence on one's CT.
- The values, attitudes, and beliefs of different generations impact the teaching, learning, and thinking of healthcare providers.
- Knowledge influences CT in complex ways that could be both positive and negative.
- Both our native cultures and the cultures in which we live and work influence us as thinkers.
- Cultural differences in communication and time orientation affect *who* we become as thinkers.
- Cultures that discourage CT have traits such as intolerance, territorial behaviors, and repression.
- Organizational cultures that promote CT are called learning environments and use more systems thinking.
- We need to reflect on *who* we are as thinkers and how we promote a culture of thinking.

REFERENCES

Belenky, M. F., Clinchy, B. M., Goldberger, N. R., & Tarule, J. M. (1986). *Women's ways of knowing: The development of self, voice, and mind.* New York, NY: Basic Books.

Brookfield, S. (1993). On impostorship, cultural suicide, and other dangers: How nurses learn critical thinking. *Journal of Continuing Education in Nursing, 24,* 197–205.

Brookfield, S. D., & Preskill, S. (1999). *Discussion as a way of teaching: Tools and techniques for democratic classrooms.* San Francisco, CA: Jossey-Bass.

Carper, B. A. (1978). Fundamental patterns of knowing in nursing. *Advances in Nursing Science, 1,* 13–23.

Carr, N. (2011). *What the Internet is doing to our brains: The shallows.* New York, NY: W. W. Norton.

Carson, M. (2003, November). *There to care: A lesson from nursing history.* Paper presented at the 37th biennial convention of Sigma Theta Tau International, Toronto, Ontario, Canada.

Chan, C-P. C. A. (2001). Implications of organizational learning for nursing managers from the cultural, interpersonal and systems thinking perspectives. *Nursing Inquiry, 8,* 196–199.

Chan, Z. C. Y. (2012). Critical thinking and creativity in nursing: Learners' perspectives. *Nurse Education Today, 33*(5), 558–563. doi: 10.1016/j.nedt.2012.09.007. Epub 2012 Oct 9.

Erickson, J. I., Ditomassi, M. O., & Jones, D. A. (2008). Interdisciplinary institute for patient care: Advancing clinical excellence. *Journal of Nursing Administration, 38,* 308–314.

Falise, J. P. (2007). True collaboration: Interdisciplinary rounds in nonteaching hospitals—it can be done! *AACN Advanced Critical Care, 18,* 346–351.

Gardner, H. (1983). *Frames of mind: The theory of multiple intelligences* (10th anniversary ed.). New York, NY: Basic Books.

Gardner, H, (1993). *Multiple intelligences: The theory in practice.* New York, NY: Basic Books.

Gardner, H. (1999). *Intelligence reframed: Multiple intelligences for the 21st century* New York, NY: Basic Books.

Gardner, H. (2006). *Multiple intelligences: New horizons.* New York, NY: Basic Books.

Gilligan, C. (1982). *In a different voice: Psychological theory and women's development.* Cambridge, MA: Harvard University Press.

Gordon, S. (2005). *Nursing against the odds: How health care cost cutting, media stereotypes, and medical hubris undermine nurses and patient care.* Ithaca, NY: Cornell University Press.

Gordon, S. (Ed.). (2010). *When chicken soup isn't enough: Stories of nurses standing up for themselves, their patients, and their profession.* Ithaca, NY: Cornell University Press.

Hart, L. A. (1983). *Human brain and human learning.* New York, NY: Longman.

Higgins, J. M. (1995). Innovate or evaporate: Seven secrets of innovative corporations. *The Futurist, 29*(5), 42–48.

Institute of Medicine. (2011). *The future of nursing: Leading change, advancing health.* Washington, DC: National Academies Press.

Kaeding, T. H., & Rambur, B. (2004). Recruiting knowledge, not just nurses. *Journal of Professional Nursing, 20,* 137–138.

Kelly-Thomas, K. J. (1998). *Clinical and nursing staff development: Current competence, future focus* (2nd ed.). Philadelphia, PA: Lippincott.

Lechasseur, K., Lazure, G., & Guilbert, L. (2011). Knowledge mobilized by a critical thinking process deployed by nursing students in practical care situations: A qualitative study. *Journal of Advanced Nursing, 67*(9), 1930–1940. doi: 10.1111/j.1365-2648.2011.05637.x

Mohr, W. K., Deatrick, J., Richmond, T., & Mahon, M. M. (2001). A reflection on values in turbulent times. *Nursing Outlook, 49,* 30–36.

Myrick, F. (2002). Preceptorship and critical thinking in nursing education. *Journal of Nursing Education, 41,* 154–164.

Oblinger, D. G., & Oblinger, J. L. (2005). Is it age or IT: First steps toward understanding the Net Generation. In D. G. Oblinger & J. L. Oblinger (Eds.), *Educating the Net Generation* (chapter 2). Retrieved from www.educause.edu/educatingthenetgen/

Prensky, M. (2001). Digital natives, digital immigrants. *On the Horizon, 9*(5). Retrieved from http://www.marcprensky.com/writing/Prensky%20-%20Digital%20Natives,%20Digital%20Immigrants%20-%20Part1.pdf

Prensky, M. (2012). *From digital natives to digital wisdom: Hopeful essays for 21st century learning.* Thousand Oaks, CA: Corwin.

Redman, R. W. (2006). The challenge of interdisciplinary teams. *Research and Theory for Nursing Practice, 20,* 105–107.

Rose, P. R. (2013). *Cultural competency for the health professional.* Burlington, MA: Jones & Bartlett Learning.

Rossen, E. K., Bartlett, R. B., & Herrick, C. A. (2008). Interdisciplinary collaboration: The need to revisit. *Issues in Mental Health Nursing, 29,* 387–396.

Seago, J. A. (2008). Professional communication. In R. G. Hughes (Ed.), *Patient safety and quality: An evidence-based handbook for nurses* (pp. 2-247–2-269). Rockville, MD: Agency for Healthcare Research and Quality. (AHRQ Publication No. 08-0043)

Senge, P., Smith, B., Kruschwitz, N., Laur, J., & Schley, S. (2010). *The necessary revolution: Working together to create a sustainable world.* New York, NY: Broadway Books.

Senge, P. M. (1990). *The fifth discipline: The art & practice of the learning organization.* New York, NY: Doubleday.

Sherman, R. O. (2006). Leading a multigenerational nursing workforce: Issues, challenges and strategies. *Online Journal of Issues in Nursing, 11*(2). Retrieved from http://www.nursingworld.org/MainMenuCategories/ANAMarketplace/ANAPeriodicals/OJIN/TableofContents/Volume112006/No2May06/tpc30_216074.aspx

Skiba, D. J., & Barton, A. J. (2006). Adapting your teaching to accommodate the net generation of learners. *Online Journal of Issues in Nursing, 11*(2). Retrieved from http://www.nursingworld.org/MainMenuCategories/ANAMarketplace/ANAPeriodicals/OJIN/TableofContents/Volume112006/No2May06.aspx

Weston, M. J. (2006). Integrating generational perspectives in nursing. *Online Journal of Issues in Nursing,11*(2). Retrieved from http://www.nursingworld.org/MainMenuCategories/ANAMarketplace/ANAPeriodicals/OJIN/TableofContents/Volume112006/No2May06.aspx

Institute of Medicine Competencies as a Context for Thinking: The *How, When,* and *Where* of Critical Thinking

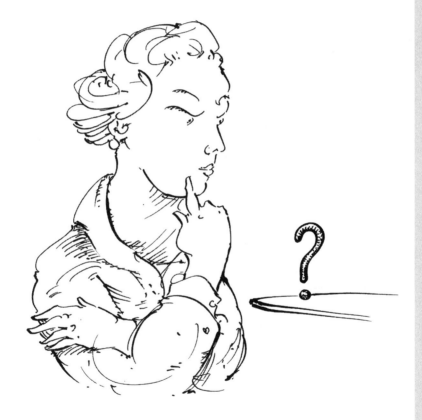

You can probably tell that our scheme of the *why, what, who,* and so on looks good to start with but gets very muddy as we move along. We gave up trying to keep them separated and have combined the last three of the six—*how, when,* and *where*—together. It was difficult to keep *who* separated from *what* and *why,* but it is virtually impossible to discuss these last three out of the context of the others. If nothing else, critical thinking (CT) is contextual in nature. No matter what crosses our minds, it does so because something (*what*), somewhere (*where*), at some time (*when*), triggered that thought. *How* one thinks about anything, therefore, is influenced by the context (*when* and *where*) of that thought. That thinking, in turn, affects *what* happens relative to that issue or problem. The process is dynamic and convoluted. CT must have a context; otherwise it's just an academic abstraction. CT is a "tool in search of a job" (Scheffer & Rubenfeld, 2006, p. 195).

Current Challenges and Solutions for Healthcare Delivery

Nowhere is the *how* of CT more needed than in the healthcare arena, and the *when* is definitely now. Health care is faced with many challenges these days. People are living longer and therefore acquire more chronic conditions. Increasing numbers of specialists have made great strides in helping people deal with these many conditions, but at the same time, care has become fragmented. The healthcare system is fraught with politics. In the United States, there are many citizens with no health care because they have no insurance, but the Affordable Care Act is a start in fixing that problem (Legislative Counsel, 2010). A nursing shortage of heretofore unseen proportions looms with no coordinated plan to correct it. We could go on and on; most of you could add issues that would make the list continue for pages.

The Institute of Medicine Quality Chasm Series

The challenges facing the U.S. healthcare system have been made very public by the Institute of Medicine (IOM), which, in 2000, produced the first of several reports: *To Err is Human: Building a Safer Health System*. The report's startling statement that perhaps as many as 98,000 Americans die yearly from medical errors drove home a picture of the healthcare system's dire situation. The IOM advocated an acceptance that error is inevitable and that blaming individuals is not the way to deal with those errors, and it recommended that errors be analyzed to determine ways to prevent them in the future.

In its 2001 report, *Crossing the Quality Chasm: A New Health System for the 21st Century*, the IOM called healthcare professionals to action to improve patient care quality and safety. Six aims were described: health care should be safe, effective, patient centered, timely, efficient, and equitable. One recommendation was to convene an interdisciplinary summit to recommend approaches to accomplish these aims. The culminated ideas from that summit, which met in 2002, were reported in *Health Professions Education: A Bridge to Quality* (IOM, 2003). The summit found that one major way we can affect practice is to change how we prepare healthcare practitioners. We need to lay better groundwork.

"All health professionals should be educated to deliver patient-centered care as members of an interdisciplinary team, emphasizing evidence-based practice, quality improvement approaches and informatics" (IOM, 2003, p. 3). The relationship among those five areas is shown in **Figure 4-1**.

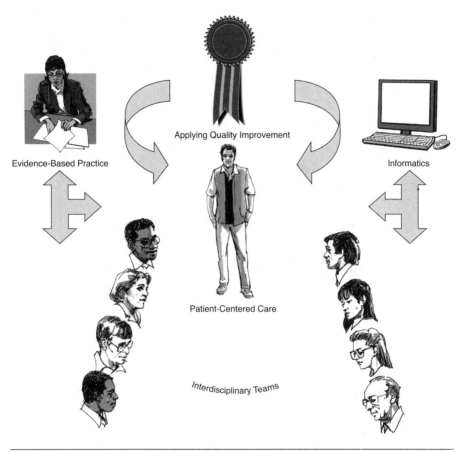

Applying Quality Improvement

Evidence-Based Practice

Informatics

Patient-Centered Care

Interdisciplinary Teams

Figure 4-1 Working in interdisciplinary teams and using evidence-based practice and informatics for patient-centered care and quality improvement.

It is important to note that the IOM has continued to produce reports that describe potential solutions to the dilemmas in health care. In 2004, *Patient Safety: Achieving a New Standard for Care* expanded on earlier ideas for studying and preventing errors (IOM, 2004b). The critical role of nurses in patient safety was the focus of another 2004 report, *Keeping Patients Safe: Transforming the Work Environment of Nurses* (IOM, 2004a). Sources of threats to safety in which "bundles of change" were needed were identified in "each of the four fundamental components of all organizations: (1) management and leadership, (2) workforce deployment, (3) work processes, and (4) organizational culture" (IOM, 2004a, p. 48). In a description of what nurses do, an important distinction was made between visible and invisible activities. Those "invisible" activities were thinking activities.

The invisible or cognitive work incorporates knowledge learned from formal education and subsequently acquired expertise. It includes such processes as assessing a patient's health condition, monitoring and detecting when a change in therapy is needed, and integrating an individual patient's health care needs with the interventions of a variety of different health care providers to formulate a plan of care tailored to the particular patient. While certain assessment, monitoring, and care planning actions may be visible (e.g., a nurse watching a cardiac monitor or listening to a patient's chest), these cognitive processes are not. Often when a nurse appears to be carrying out a visible activity . . . he or she is actually performing numerous invisible tasks… (IOM, 2004a, p. 89)

The IOM, in a joint effort with the Robert Wood Johnson Foundation, continued its focus on nursing with its 2011 report *The Future of Nursing: Leading Change, Advancing Health*. More than ever nurses are being called upon to take up their role as effectors of change in health care. "Nurses' regular, close proximity to patients and scientific understanding of care processes across the continuum of care give them a unique ability to act as partners with other health professionals and to lead in the improvement and redesign of the health care system and its many practice environments" (p. 3).

Four "key messages" for nursing were outlined:

Nurses "should practice to the full extent of their education and training . . . should achieve higher levels of education and training through an improved education system . . . should be full partners, with physicians and other health professionals, in redesigning health care in the United States . . . [and] effective workforce planning and policy making require better data collection and an improved information infrastructure." (IOM, 2011, p. 4)

We strongly recommend that our readers visit the IOM website (http://www.iom.edu) periodically to view the important work that is being done to promote a safer, higher-quality American healthcare system.

Nursing has risen to the challenges posed by the IOM. More and more publications are making reference to the IOM ideas in proposals for change in nursing. For example, the Agency for Healthcare Research and Quality (AHRQ) and the Robert Wood Johnson Foundation developed a handbook for nurses on patient safety and quality (Hughes, 2008). That three-volume set is a wealth of information for nurses, and indeed all health providers, providing background research and tools for improving the quality of care.

In 2008, the American Association of Colleges of Nursing (AACN) revised its *Essentials of Baccalaureate Education for Professional Nursing Practice*; early in the discussion of background influences on this document was reference to the IOM reports and the necessity of building a safer healthcare system (AACN, 2008). Many of the IOM recommended revisions to health education can be seen in the nine essentials.

The latest IOM report (2011) has instigated responses from many, both inside and outside the nursing profession. For example, Ellerbe and Regen (2012) responded with a view from their New Jersey healthcare system showing what they were doing to promote the key messages of the IOM report. Interestingly, from a CT perspective, they hire only baccalaureate-prepared nurses, reasoning that "the complexity of acute care patients . . . requires a baccalaureate-prepared nurse to ensure appropriate critical thinking and positive patient outcomes" (p. 214).

The Affordable Care Act (Legislative Counsel, 2010) also spurred nurses to consider new and expanded roles in health care that echo many of the messages of the IOM. Hassmiller (2010) outlined nine roles for nurses in healthcare reform: "use nurse-led innovations . . . generate evidence and engage in research . . . redesign nursing education . . . expand the scope of practice . . . diversify our workforce . . . embrace technology . . . foster interprofessional collaboration . . . develop leadership at every level . . . [and] be at the table" (pp. 68–69).

Core Competencies to Improve Healthcare

To live up to the vision of necessary changes in health professions education, the IOM advocated a set of five core competencies for all health professions. *Competency* was defined as "the habitual and judicious use of communication, knowledge, technical skills, clinical reasoning, emotions, values and reflection in daily practice" (Hundert, as cited in IOM, 2003, pp. 3–4). **Box 4-1** includes the definitions of the five competencies. As you can see, specific actions outlined in each definition fall into the communication, technical skills, clinical reasoning, emotions, values, and *reflection* categories of competence.

What Are Competencies?

We want to make sure that everyone understands what constitutes competencies or competency-based performance, because there are many misconceptions about these terms. By using the word *competencies*, the IOM was focusing on summative behaviors that they want, even expect, to see in practice. Competencies are very specific end points that can be assessed; they are more than just a general list of areas for improvement. The use of competency language in the IOM's recommendations makes a stronger statement than a mere focus shift in healthcare delivery and education. They expect providers to be consistently competent in their performance in these five areas. Note the phrase *habitual and judicious use* in the preceding quote.

Bargagliotti, Luttrell, and Lenburg, citing Lenburg's earlier work, provided this definition: "Competency-based performance evaluation is defined as a criterion-referenced, summative evaluation process that assesses a participant's actual ability to meet a predetermined set of performance standards under controlled conditions and

Box 4-1 Core Competencies for a New Vision for Health Professions Education

1. *Provide patient-centered care*—identify, respect, and care about patients' differences, values, preferences, and expressed needs; relieve pain and suffering; coordinate continuous care; listen to, clearly inform, communicate with, and educate patients; share decision making and management; and continuously advocate disease prevention, wellness, and promotion of healthy lifestyles, including a focus on population health.
2. *Work in interdisciplinary teams*—cooperate, collaborate, communicate, and integrate care in teams to ensure that care is continuous and reliable.
3. *Employ evidence-based practice*—integrate best research with clinical expertise and patient values for optimum care, and participate in learning and research activities to the extent feasible.
4. *Apply quality improvement*—identify errors and hazards in care; understand and implement basic safety design principles, such as standardization and simplification; continually understand and measure quality of care in terms of structure, process, and outcomes in relation to patient and community needs; and design and test interventions to change processes and systems of care, with the objective of improving quality.
5. *Utilize informatics*—communicate, manage knowledge, mitigate error, and support decision making using information technology.

Source: Reproduced with permission from *Health Professions Education: A Bridge to Quality*, 2003 by the National Academy of Sciences, Courtesy of the National Academies Press, Washington, D.C.

protocols" (1999, para. 4). They noted the difference between this type of evaluation and traditional check-off methods in which a set of steps is demonstrated. Competency-based evaluations focus on evidence of effective implementation of specified skills; critical elements are demonstrated, but not necessarily in a step-by-step format. It's a bottom-line, real-world view, not a set of textbook steps. In short, it's all about performance.

Critical Thinking and Competencies

Although the term *critical thinking* is never used in the IOM competencies, words that are close cousins certainly appear in these performance ideals. The definition of *competency*, cited previously, speaks directly to clinical reasoning, knowledge, values, and *reflection*. Looking at all competencies, we see phrases such as *sharing decision making for patient-centered care; integrating best research when employing evidence-based practice; understanding quality and designing interventions in applying quality improvement; managing knowledge and supporting decision making with informatics* (IOM, 2003). In short, CT seems to be a necessary prerequisite to meeting the core competencies and is threaded throughout each of the five competencies. Let's consider some underlying approaches that will need to change for the IOM competencies to become a reality.

A Picture of Changes in Healthcare Delivery and Education

Clearly evident in the IOM's vision is a move away from status quo behavior in healthcare education and practice and toward a focus on context-bound thinking (the *how*, *when*, and *where*). The quality of clinical practice will improve, and there will be more collaboration among providers and with patients. Decisions will be based on evidence found through current informatics rather than on tradition. In the IOM's view, these practice changes will occur through changes in health professions' education practices. We will begin our discussion of the *how* and *where*; then we'll discuss changes in education, but we'd like you to take a broad view of education. The education of health professionals doesn't just occur in educational institutions; it occurs in the practice setting as well. Because nursing and other health professions deal with a rapidly changing body of knowledge, all professionals must be lifelong learners.

There are many driving forces for change in practice arenas, such as cost containment, consumer demands, and new information. However, without a concomitant change in health professions education, that change will take longer (an important *when* consideration) and be less embedded in the values of clinicians. In addition, because of the immediate demands of the practice arena, service-based educators will very likely feel the pressures to change more quickly than academic-based educators.

Changes in Teaching and Learning within a Thinking Framework

Let's consider how teaching and learning are approached in service settings as compared with academic settings because, although teaching and learning principles and approaches are used in both, the nature of the settings (*where*) sometimes makes a difference to the related issues. **Box 4-2** compares some of those key differences.

Service-based educators often have to fit their teaching of required updated information into short, variable time slots to accommodate various shifts of nurses. Academic-based educators generally have structured class or clinical time that lasts anywhere from 1 to 8 hours. Time and schedules certainly make a difference in the techniques used to teach clinicians as compared with nursing students.

Service-based educators often deal with very heterogeneous groups—experienced nurses, novice nurses, and unlicensed assistive personnel. This creates additional challenges, because the language used in teaching and the expectations of the group must be modified, and leveling information must play a part. In spite of these differences, both practice- and academic-based educators use some similar teaching

Box 4-2 Differences between Academic-Based and Service-Based Education

Factor	Academic-Based	Service-Based
Time blocks for teaching	Structured	Variable
Amount of time in blocks	Hours	Minutes
Mix of novice to expert	More homogeneous	More heterogeneous
Mix of students	Nursing students	Nursing and unlicensed personnel
Focus on knowledge	Knowledge more than practice	Practice more than knowledge
Context	More noncontextual	More contextual
Teaching environment	Mostly classrooms	Variable spaces

and learning approaches; thus, change in educational offerings, and delivery, will occur in both settings. Service-based educators, with their less-structured teaching situations, may find these changes easier to deal with. Educators in academic settings may experience more challenges because of traditions.

How these changes in education occur is where CT comes in; we must change our thinking. To meet the five core competencies, education cannot be carried out in the tradition of educators handing down information to learners. Instead, academic faculty and service-based educators will need to help students become active knowledge seekers rather than passive information receivers. This type of teaching and learning is a collaborative effort, not the one-up, one-down configuration of the traditional authoritarian teaching. Giddens and Brady (2007) advocated a change from our traditional content-saturated nursing education to a concept-based approach. In the latter, students are active learners instead of passive recipients of content.

The National League for Nursing (NLN) has called for a paradigm shift in nursing education, away from teacher-centered, content-delivery approaches to one that "encourages student-centered learning and the development of critical thinking skills" (Stanley & Dougherty, 2010, p. 378). "Content in schools of nursing must reflect the dynamic changes of today's health care system. It must be current, relevant, and based on evidence, and it must be examined critically, with the expectation that today's students will be lifelong learners" (p. 379). These views are similar to those by Benner, Sutphen, Leonard and Day (2010), who called for a radical transformation in the field of nursing education, emphasizing multiple ways of thinking.

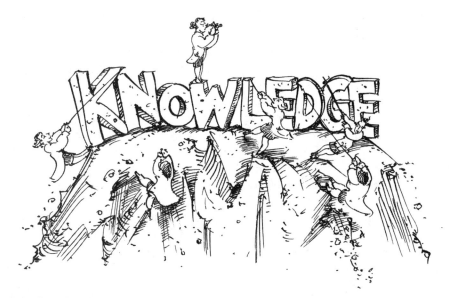

© Mark Steele. Reproduced by permission.

Minds for the Future

Howard Gardner had some interesting thoughts on what he called "five minds for the future." His contention was that the future will demand "capacities that until now have been mere options" (2006, p. 2). Those five minds are *disciplinary, synthesizing, creating, respectful,* and *ethical.* The disciplined mind has to do with mastery and continual honing of the skills of a profession or specialty. The synthesizing mind is particularly relevant to the health professions in that it is concerned with pulling together several sets of information and making an amalgam of that information. The creating mind is able to clarify and solve problems in innovative ways. The respectful mind appreciates the differences among people, and the ethical mind focuses on responsibility as citizens.

Gardner encouraged us to look at these minds relative to changes in today's world and how we educate future generations. He saw those without one or more disciplines as "being restricted to menial tasks," and those "without synthesizing capabilities . . . as overwhelmed by information and unable to make judicious decisions." Those without *creativity* "will be replaced by computers and will drive away those who have the creative spark." Those without respect "will poison the workplace," and those without ethics "will yield a world devoid of decent workers and responsible citizens" (2006, pp. 18–19).

Gardner's views are focused on needed changes in education, not just in formal settings, but in today's workplace:

> We should be concerned with how to nurture these minds in the younger generation, those who are being educated currently to become the leaders of

tomorrow. But we should be equally concerned with those in today's workplace: how best can we mobilize our skills—and those of our coworkers—so that all of us will remain current tomorrow and the day after tomorrow? (2006, p. 10)

As we anticipate changes in society, we must think of those changes as they are and will be mirrored in healthcare systems. Gardner's ideas are particularly relevant to helping health professionals learn differently than they have in the past and to focus on thinking. We need to reform nursing education, and we need a drastic change in our views of the workings of the mind. We're not sure what Gardner would say specifically about nursing education, but he had this to say about education in general: "current formal education still prepares students primarily for the world of the past, rather than for possible worlds of the future" (2006, p. 17). Perhaps closer to home for an applied science such as nursing is this comment: "We acknowledge the importance of science and technology but do not teach scientific ways of thinking, let alone how to develop individuals with the synthesizing and creative capacities essential for continual scientific and technological progress" (p. 17).

Although Gardner's labels—synthesizing in particular—are not identical, they are very similar to "integrative learning" advocated by the Association of American Colleges and Universities and the Carnegie Foundation for the Advancement of Teaching (2004), which had this to say:

Integrative learning comes in many varieties: connecting skills and knowledge from multiple sources and experiences; applying theory to practice in various settings; utilizing diverse and even contradictory points of view; and, understanding issues and positions contextually. Significant knowledge within individual disciplines serves as the foundation, but integrative learning goes beyond academic boundaries. Indeed, integrative experiences often occur as learners address real-world problems, unscripted and sufficiently broad to require multiple areas of knowledge and multiple modes of inquiry, offering multiple solutions and benefiting from multiple perspectives. (para. 2)

We think these descriptions sound very much like CT. Perhaps a change of labels, from *CT* to *integrative learning*, will help make the case that we must look closer at how we teach and learn thinking in nursing. Tanner made important links from integrative teaching to CT and nursing education. "*Integrative teaching and learning* may well become the buzz phrase for this decade, replacing the ubiquitous, yet conceptually fuzzy, emphasis on *critical thinking*" (2007, p. 531). Integrative teaching was also a focus of Benner et al., who advocated shifts in thinking and approaches to nursing education, one of which was the shift "from a focus on covering decontextualized knowledge to an emphasis on teaching for a sense of salience, situated cognition, and action in particular clinical situations" (2010, p. 89).

How change in teaching and learning will occur will not be easy. Frederic Moore Binder, former president of Hartwick College (Gaie's excellent alma mater), once cited this old adage: "Changing a college curriculum is like trying to move a cemetery" (2000, para. 5). Perhaps service-based educators have less buried patterns, but we'll bet you can relate. As educators who have struggled through curriculum changes, we can attest to the truth of that cemetery analogy.

We have a long tradition of teachers being authorities and all-knowing. Students come through an education system that largely uses this hierarchical model of teaching; they expect to be takers of information. When changes occur in practice, they are used to someone handing them new information. How, then, can nurse leaders and educators promote integrative or synthesis learning and knowledge-seeking behaviors? Myrick and Tamlyn (2007) dared educators to reflect critically on their teaching and to move to more enlightened approaches that promote student thinking. We are talking about a teaching and learning paradigm shift. That sounds like a big deal, and we'll discuss that shortly, but first let's focus on some easily overlooked but vital small things that can help us move to more enlightened teaching and learning.

Make Some Small Changes

Some students, probably more than we think, are affected by seemingly simple comments or actions. Look at **Box 4-3** for a list of such simple comments and nonverbal behaviors that can either promote or squelch CT.

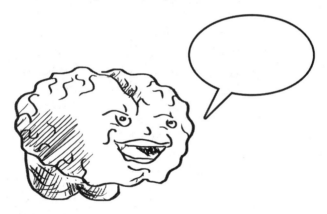

© Jesse Rubenfeld

Box 4-3 Comments and Behaviors That Promote or Squelch CT

COMMENTS AND BEHAVIORS THAT PROMOTE CT	COMMENTS AND BEHAVIORS THAT SQUELCH CT
■ That's an interesting question. ■ There's no such thing as a dumb question.	■ What a dumb question! ■ Don't you know that? ■ You should know that!

(continues)

Box 4-3 Comments and Behaviors That Promote or Squelch CT (continued)

COMMENTS AND BEHAVIORS THAT PROMOTE CT	COMMENTS AND BEHAVIORS THAT SQUELCH CT
■ Do you have a different idea how to do this?	■ We've always done it this way.
■ Let's explore this.	■ That's the wrong way to do that.
■ Let's think this through.	■ That'll never work here.
■ I'm not sure; can we figure this out?	■ Just do it this way.
■ Don't believe everything you read or hear.	■ Why do you have to make everything so complicated?
■ Show me how you came to that conclusion.	■ That will never fit in our budget.
■ Can we look at this from a different angle?	■ Just memorize it.
■ What do you think?	■ Stop with the questions, already!
■ Walk me through your thinking on this.	■ Because I said so, that's why!
■ Tell me about what you learned here.	■ If you're so sure of yourself, you figure it out.
■ Let's see what others have to say.	■ Mistakes are not tolerated here.
■ That's one option; let's see what other ways might also work.	■ Let's get moving; we don't have all day.
■ What are some possible outcomes of that approach?	■ I can't believe you don't know that by now.
■ That was a great example of how you used (insert the CT dimension used, such as *inquisitiveness*).	■ Come on, use your brain here!
■ That's a good idea; let's expand on it to make it even better.	■ It's too complicated to explain.
■ Use a neutral voice tone.	■ I can't believe you said/did that!
■ Use an enthusiastic voice tone.	■ Roll eyes.
■ Sit silently and patiently.	■ Smirk.
	■ Big sighs.
	■ Scowl.
	■ Foot-tapping or finger-tapping.
	■ Other nonverbal demonstrations of anger, frustration, irritation.
	■ Look at one's watch frequently.

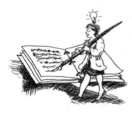

TACTICS 4-1: Promoting CT or Knowledge-Seeking Behavior

Clinicians

Using **Box 4-3**, reflect on your interactions with other staff over the past 2 days. How often have you made comments from the left column of the box, and how often from the right? Be honest! Think about how you feel when you hear comments from each side of that box.

Educators

Using Box 4-3, think about your teaching situation in the past 2 months. How often have you made comments from the left column of the box and how often from the right? Be honest! Alternatively, ask students to list what they think are the most and least productive teacher comments related to promoting knowledge-seeking behaviors. Use the responses as a self-inventory of the comments you make when teaching.

Discussion

You probably remember some of the CT-promoting and CT-squelching comments directed at you during your education. They stick in your mind, don't they? Especially the squelching ones. It's frightening to acknowledge the potential impact of our small comments, but it's healthy to contemplate how our behavior might help or hinder knowledge-seeking behavior.

Bigger Changes

Now, let's examine the bigger guns of teaching and learning approaches that will transform health professions' education in the 21st century. The philosopher John Dewey wrote *Democracy and Education* in 1916. Because his wisdom has withstood the test of time and because he links thinking and action, Dewey's ideas have particular relevance for teaching and learning in health care. Consider this gem from Dewey that should make you sit up and take note: "Information severed from thoughtful action is dead, a mind-crushing load" (1916/1966, p. 153). Think about that statement the next time you write exam items. Do you want a simple recall of information or a more cognitively sophisticated application item? For those of you who hunger for more of Dewey's thoughts on education and thinking, we've compiled some Dewey Diamonds in **Box 4-4**.

Box 4-4 Dewey Diamonds

(The first bold lines are our translations. Sorry, Dewey.)
Don't be too academic.
"Hence the first approach to any subject in school, if thought is to be aroused and not words acquired, should be as unscholastic as possible." (p. 154)
Both thinking without action and action without thinking get you nowhere.

(continues)

Box 4-4   Dewey Diamonds (continued)

"Thinking which is not connected with increase of efficiency in action, and with learning more about ourselves and the world in which we live, has something the matter with it just as thought. And skill obtained apart from thinking is not connected with any sense of the purposes for which it is to be used. It consequently leaves a man at the mercy of his routine habits and of the authoritative control of others." (p. 152)

Some people think you can improve thinking separately from what you do.

"Thinking is often regarded both in philosophic theory and in educational practice as something cut off from experience, and capable of being cultivated in isolation." (p. 153)

Teachers, don't make things too hard or too simple.

"A large part of the art of instruction lies in making the difficulty of new problems large enough to challenge thought, and small enough so that, in addition to the confusion naturally attending the novel elements, there shall be luminous familiar spots from which helpful suggestions may spring." (p. 157)

Education is all about thinking.

"The important thing is that thinking is the method of an educative experience. The essentials of method are therefore identical with the essentials of reflection." (p. 163)

Lectures on topics out of context are boring.

"Under the influence of the conception of the separation of mind and material, method tends to be reduced to a cut and dried routine, to following mechanically prescribed steps." (p. 169)

Some teachers think you're a troublemaker if you ask questions.

"Exorbitant desire for uniformity of procedure and for prompt external results are the chief foes which the open-minded attitude meets in school. The teacher who does not permit and encourage diversity of operation in dealing with questions is imposing intellectual blinders upon pupils—restricting their vision to the one path the teacher's mind happens to approve." (p. 175)

It's not all about quick answers.

"The zeal for 'answers' is the explanation of much of the zeal for rigid and mechanical methods." (p. 175)

Some people still want someone to just give them the answers.

"Men still want the crutch of dogma, of beliefs fixed by authority, to relieve them of the trouble of thinking and the responsibility of directing their activity by thought." (p. 339)

Source: Dewey, J. (1916). *Democracy and education*. New York, NY: Macmillan.

Dewey's ideas underpin the problem-based learning (PBL) movement, which was made popular by McMaster University in Ontario, Canada, and is in common use worldwide today (Kowalczyk, 2011; Oja, 2011; Rideout, 2001). This student-centered approach to learning links learning to action in that students are directed by relevant problems or issues rather than a set of topics defined by the teacher. Independent inquiry and *reflection* are important thinking components of this approach.

There are also many references to Dewey in Wiggins and McTighe's *Understanding by Design* (1998). They differentiated real understanding (that which uses learning in new ways) from knowledge that is "superficial, rote, out-of-context and easily tested" (p. 40). We want to promote real understanding, which Wiggins and McTighe viewed as having six facets: "When we truly understand, we can . . . explain . . . interpret . . . apply . . . have perspective . . . empathize . . . [and] have self-knowledge" (p. 44). Have you ever said the best way to learn something is to teach it? Look at those six facets and think about the last time you spent a lot of time and energy preparing a lesson. You probably drew on each of those six facets. A little later in this chapter, we're going to discuss the benefits of picturing yourself teaching something as a way of learning. We'll revisit the six facets then.

Another take on Dewey's ideals is Barr and Tagg's article (1995), which clearly identified the differences between teaching and learning. For example, teaching implies a hierarchy; learning is done in collaboration. Teaching implies covering material; learning implies performance outcomes. Teaching implies that "knowledge exists out there"; learning implies that "knowledge exists in each person's mind and is shaped by individual experience." Teaching implies that "knowledge comes in chunks and bits delivered by instructors"; learning implies that "knowledge is constructed, created, 'gotten'" (p. 17).

In today's healthcare world, where things change almost by the minute, we need to aim for competencies. Performance at competence level necessitates the kind of understanding that allows for transfer of information to fit new situations—what we call *transforming knowledge*. This is what Perry (1970) called "relativism," where knowledge is contextual and relative, and multiple perspectives fit into a big picture. This relativism is in contrast to "dualism," where there are right and wrong answers and the world is seen in absolute categories. In nursing, we are most familiar with the move from dualism to relativism in terms of ways of viewing situations and gaining knowledge from Benner's work (1984). Benner defined these differences as existing between novices and expert nurses. From her work, we have learned to do all we can to move nurses away from novice dualism to the relativistic or contextual thinking of experts.

Old dualistic teaching and learning methods just don't cut it. Clinicians cannot learn about new medications and procedures and expect that information to remain static; it will change, for example, as research reveals better procedures and as medications are shown to be valuable for off-label uses. Clinicians must be able to converse intelligently about new information with the healthcare team and with patients and families.

Educators shouldn't just test students for their recall of textbook information. Who cares what you know today if you won't be able to use that knowledge tomorrow when the context changes? We must help students process information and use it to define their own knowledge. We must move away from shoveling content at students and move toward learning partnerships focused on students discovering things for themselves. And we must develop new habits of the mind to help students do the same. "The development of understanding greatly depends on such attitudes and habits of mind as open-mindedness, self-discipline (autonomy), tolerance for ambiguity, and reflectiveness" (Wiggins & McTighe, 1998, p. 171).

On the academic side of nursing, any suggestion related to changing how content is taught generally sends seasoned faculty running, holding their lecture notes close to their hearts. We are too focused on teaching specific content, fearing that students will not learn content unless it is taught directly. Debates over content often get dichotomized because of the assumption that content and process are parallel and mutually exclusive. This leads to the idea that one must teach either process or content. For those teaching undergraduate students, one of the driving forces behind a rigid focus on content is that students must pass the National Council Licensure Examination. This kind of thinking presupposes that students will not learn content if it is not spoon-fed to them. Does that make any sense? No. We are caught in the providing-information paradigm.

So what needs to be done? Starting with simple steps, we need to redefine the process of acquiring knowledge and understanding. A teaching method is not the same as a learning process. Certainly, some teaching methods do seem to promote learning better than others, and we'll discuss some of those shortly. But learning is a whole other process, and it doesn't matter much what we teach and how we do it if no one learns.

We should also clarify what we mean by *content* and *process*: content is information, and process is what we do with that information. There's certainly a necessary marriage of the two in a practice discipline. However, that's too facile; we need to expand on the idea of content or knowledge. We need to distinguish between the acquisition of information and the process of true learning. True learning means internalizing information and transforming it into knowledge until it becomes part of the learner's ideas. Only then can the learner use that knowledge meaningfully (such as for patient care situations). In this context, Dewey's observations are helpful. He said that we don't convey ideas. Ideas form as we do something in our heads with the facts told to us. When facts are shared,

> the communication may stimulate that other person to realize the question for himself and to think out a like idea, or it may smother his intellectual interest and suppress his dawning effort at thought. But what he directly gets cannot be an idea. Only by wrestling with the conditions of the problem at first hand, seeking and finding his own way out, does he think. (1916/1966, pp. 159–160)

If that doesn't stimulate you to plan interactive teaching, nothing will! We'll bet that clinicians are nodding in agreement at this point, though educators may still be a bit skeptical. That's because clinicians are focused on using knowledge, not teaching it. Anyone who uses knowledge knows it's necessary to have it in idea form—what Wiggins and McTighe (1998) called "real understanding"—that can be used in a variety of ways. Ask clinicians how they learn best, and most will say by practicing or using something. In other words, they are thinking of ideas, not facts. They have done something with what they learned. They have internalized the information so they can use it. Educators need to take a lesson from clinicians and focus on what their students will be doing with the information they are receiving; then educators can adapt their teaching methods to the realities of healthcare practice. We have summarized some similarities and differences between teaching content and teaching process in **Box 4-5**.

Techniques to Promote Thinking and Knowledge Processing

Interestingly, nursing seems to be doing better than some other health professions in publishing reports of teaching methods that promote critical thinking, according to the systematic review conducted by Kowalczyk (2011), a radiation science educator. An athletic training educator, seeing the need to increase active learning strategies to promote critical thinking, looked to other sources, including nursing literature, to augment the limited research in her field (Walker, 2003). Popkess and McDaniel (2011) conducted a secondary analysis of data from a national survey of student engagement, comparing nursing students with two other groups: education and other health professions majors. The education majors exhibited higher scores in active and collaborative learning than the health professions and nursing majors. The authors emphasized the need to promote nursing students' active engagement in learning. "Educators in nursing and health professions continue to predominantly employ traditional, teacher-centered methods of instruction, such as lecture, that do not necessarily encourage the active and collaborative participation of students in class discussions and out-of-class activities" (p. 93).

Thankfully, there are many teaching method resources to promote thinking and processing knowledge for educators these days. Our favorite is what we call the "CAT" book (*Classroom Assessment Techniques*) by Angelo and Cross (1993). Even though it says "classroom," we think service educators will find it useful, too. Another helpful guide is by Billings and Halstead (2009). We have listed some of the techniques adapted from those sources in **Box 4-6**. Note that these are all interactive approaches.

In addition to the techniques identified a decade or so ago in Box 4-6, the literature has exploded with teaching strategies to enhance critical thinking. A brief summary of some current literature may whet your appetite to explore these teaching techniques:

- Distance education/Web-based classrooms: Stanley and Dougherty (2010) pointed out that many of today's students are nontraditional and "need a

Box 4-5 Similarities and Differences between Teaching Content and Teaching Process

	Role of Teacher	Role of Student	Example
Teaching content	Provide instruction on what to read. (May occur before or after class.)	Read the required materials in the text or course pack.	Course syllabus provides information on what reading is needed for the class on communication skills, what assignments are related to the communication content, and how student learning will be tested related to communication skills.
	Review content in class with classroom material, PowerPoint slides, lecture, group work to review key points of content.	Listen in class and take notes for later review and prep for exam.	The class content includes a PowerPoint presentation along with a handout. The instructor provides numerous examples of the different types of communication (e.g., verbal, nonverbal, written).
	Provide study sessions to prepare for exams.	Attend study sessions.	At the end of class the instructor uses the new clicker system to see if students have understood the key points of the class content.
	Design exams, usually with multiple-choice questions, that focus on recall of information with some items requiring application of knowledge.	Study for exams, take exam, and review exam afterward.	The examination items related to communication include several items in which students have to select the proper communication skill that is demonstrated (e.g., paraphrasing, summarizing, clarifying, etc.).
Teaching process	**Provide instruction on what information is necessary to read prior to class.**	Read required materials in text or course pack prior to class and then again after class as needed.	Course syllabus provides information on what reading is needed for the class on communication skills, what assignments are related to the communication content, and how student learning will be tested related to communication skills.
	Design classroom time to provide students with **opportunities to apply content** to case studies, problems, scenarios, real-life situations.	Listen in class, take notes, and participate in learning activities that require you to	Class time is divided into 15-minute segments in which groups of three students are each given roles to play with a given scenario. One student plays the nurse, one student plays the patient, and one student is the peer observer.

Design classroom time for dialogue, discussion, problem solving, and debriefing following activities.

Overtly discuss how content knowledge is transformed to customize nursing care in a patient-centered approach. Do not assume this transformation of knowledge just happens.

Design assessments of student learning outcomes that require a combination of recall, application, analysis, synthesis, and opportunities for students to demonstrate their ability to transform knowledge. This could be paper-and-pencil exams that moved beyond recall items, quizzes, written assignments, critical thinking vignettes.

engage many, if not all, of your 17 dimensions of critical thinking in nursing.

Complete student learning outcome assessments and discuss the results, providing rationales for your choices and selection of answers.

Both the nurse and patient play out their roles based on the scenario. The peer observer has a guideline sheet outlining the key communication skills covered in the readings and behaviors that tend to block communication.

The role playing lasts 10 minutes; then the peer observer provides feedback and allows for discussion. Roles are rotated every 15 minutes, with different scenarios provided by the teacher.

At the end of class, discussion with the whole group allows for identification of key strengths demonstrated and key areas for improvement.

Ideally students would be asked to summarize the key concepts related to communication skills, but if time does not permit, a handout or outline of the key concepts could be provided by the instructor.

The examination items related to communication include several items in which students have to select the proper communication skill that is demonstrated (e.g., paraphrasing, summarizing, clarifying, etc.), or students are required to fix a piece of communication and provide the rationale for the fix.

Box 4-6 Teaching Techniques to Promote Processing and Internalization of Knowledge

---

***Muddiest Point:** After presenting content, have students write on cards the muddiest point and hand in the cards anonymously; the teacher then discusses each of those points.

***One-Sentence Summary:** Have students sum up what they just learned in one sentence. Then, in groups, have students explain why they came up with that sentence.

***One-Word Summary:** A variation on the one-sentence summary, students choose one word and explain why that word summarizes the idea.

***Concept or Mind Maps:** Students map out ideas and the connections among them, questions, answers, and so on, in some way that is meaningful to them.

***Student-Generated Test Questions:** Students come up with test questions. These can be collected and used for tests and quizzes.

***Minute Paper:** At the end of the teaching session, students are asked to answer a question, such as, What was the most important thing you learned today? or What are you most curious to learn more about? Students are given a minute to write an answer.

***Empty Outline or Empty Mind Map:** The teacher gives students a partially completed outline or map; they need to fill in the blanks.

***Memory Matrix:** Students set up a grid with some ideas across the top and some down the side; they then fill in the squares to show relationships.

†**Algorithms:** Break tasks into yes/no steps to solve complex problems.

†**Argumentation/Debate:** This technique promotes *logical reasoning* and *open-mindedness* as students debate controversial issues. It works well when students have to argue the side opposite to their view.

†**Case Studies/Scenarios:** Use this technique to teach content; have students share cases with similar or different parts.

†**Collaborative Learning:** Form work groups for assignments or problem solving.

†**Newspaper Analysis:** Students analyze something written for the lay public, determine and critique sources of information, and discuss its relevance to nursing.

†**Reflection Projects/Logs:** Have students reflect on something, focusing specifically on their thinking.

Sources: Adapted from Angelo & Cross, *Classroom assessment techniques: A handbook for college teachers* (2nd ed.), pp. 28–29. Copyright (c) 1993 by Jossey-Bass. Reprinted with permission of John Wiley & Sons Inc.

This material was adapted from Teaching in Nursing, 3/e, Billings & Halstead, pp. 246–254. Copyright Elsevier 2009.

curriculum that supports their working lifestyle and that provides another venue for accessing higher learning education" (p. 379). Web-based approaches often promote more student involvement in learning.

- Team-based learning: Banfield, Fagan, and Janes (2012) used a problem-based group application of learned material. This three-phase approach focused on "pre-class preparation, readiness assurance tests, and application of course concepts" (p. 24). Both faculty and students saw this approach as an effective application of CT. The team-based learning model is referenced from Michaelsen, Knight, and Fink (2004).

- Problem-based learning (PBL): Kowalczyk (2011) did a systematic review and found that "of the 13 studies relating to PBL, 6 demonstrated significant differences in student critical thinking scores" (p. 130). Oja (2011) also conducted an evidence review of PBL relative to CT. Although there was support for positive relationships between the two, there were wide variations in the studies, especially in terms of how CT was measured and the teaching techniques related to PBL. Oja concluded that more rigorous studies were needed to find firm evidence that PBL improves CT.

- Reflection: Although *reflection* has been promoted for many years, there are limited data on its process and benefits. Bulman, Lathlean, and Gobbi (2012) used an ethnographic approach to study the perspectives of students and faculty on *reflection*, which was "perceived as intertwining cognitive, affective, as well as active elements" (p. e12). "It encourages an approach to nursing knowledge as requiring judgement in the context of experience, thus critically considering and using what comes from practice" (p. e12).

- Reflective writing or journaling: Kennison (2012) made a distinction between *reflection* via speech and *reflection* via writing, the latter containing more objectivity, as a way of promoting critical thinking and patterns of knowing. Marchigiano, Eduljee, and Harvey (2011), in a pilot study of CT skills in clinical assignments, found that journaling, as opposed to traditional care plan formats, provided students with greater *confidence* in their CT skills.

- Simulation: Simulation has become popular, and there are numerous reports touting its advantages and disadvantages. Sanford's review (2010) revealed advantages such as the nonthreatening simulation setting allowing for less stressful learning, promoting *reflection*, and possible substituting for clinical time. The disadvantages were the high cost of time and resources needed to purchase, prepare, run, and maintain the simulations, as well as the "lack of supporting theory and evidence-based research supporting the use of simulation" (p. 1010). Maneval et al. (2012) were unable to show a statistically significant relationship between high-fidelity patient simulation and improved critical thinking and clinical decision making.

- Debate: Hall (2011) reported on this method and noted the benefits. "Students reported the use of critical thinking skills in different ways, researching of controversial topics, learning how to organize thoughts, listening to both sides of an issue, learning new ways to communicate to colleagues and other professionals, and being able to analyze both sides of an issue" (p. 5). Walker (2003) also advocated debates of controversial issues. A variation of the debate approach was the development of "pro and con grids" (p. 265).

■ Case studies: Popil (2011) enumerated several benefits to case study methods of teaching. Often linked with PBL, and touted as an effective active learning strategy, case studies allow students to work individually or in groups to explore alternative solutions to patient problems and apply theory to practical situations. Not without limitations, case studies can be narrow in scope, "overly sterilized," and embedded with cultural biases.

■ Concept maps: Huang, Chen, Yeh, and Chung (2012) showed that case studies combined with concept maps improved CT skills and dispositions. Sinatra-Wilhelm (2012) also showed that some aspects of CT were improved when students used a concept map approach as opposed to traditional care plans. Taylor and Littleton-Kearney (2011) combined clinical rounds and concept mapping for advanced practice graduate nursing students to help them address the complexities of physiological and pathophysiological concepts. Although their report is anecdotal, these authors showed how this approach helps students integrate complex concepts.

■ Questioning: Lim (2011) presented what may seem simplistic, the notion that "a simple question to a single or group of students during the course of the clinical day will help enhance this interaction, improve clinical thinking, and promote the application of evidence-based practice" (p. 52). Some of these questions were as simple as, "What's the plan for this patient?" Walker (2003) suggested that "questions should be designed to promote evaluation and synthesis of facts and concepts" (p. 264). Practical suggestions were given: "Higher-level thinking questions should start or end with words or phrases such as, 'explain,' 'compare,' 'why,' 'which is a solution to the problem,' 'what is the best and why,' and 'do you agree or disagree with this statement?'" (pp. 264–265). Socratic questioning that promotes *inquisitiveness* and deep exploration of an issue was also advocated.

Many of these teaching techniques can also be used to assess CT competencies. If we view CT as just one of many competencies, then we need to be teaching so that students will be able to demonstrate their CT. We'll limit our discussion here to making sure that you link assessment with teaching and learning.

Teaching as Learning

One of our favorite questions to undergraduate nursing students is this: How would you explain that to a patient? Think about that. Inevitably, nurses have to impart most of their knowledge to patients. Remember our discussion of Wiggins and McTighe's (1998) six facets of true understanding—explain, interpret, apply, have perspective, empathize, have self-knowledge. If those ring true in your mind, you will agree that one of the best ways to learn something is to teach it to someone else. And having to teach someone who does not have your working vocabulary will make that an even more valuable learning experience, because now you have to translate the message, too. To do that, you really need to know it.

For our clinician readers, how often do you teach things to patients? Most of you will answer, continually. Each day, as you learn new things, think about how you would effectively explain these things to a patient. Paolo Freire said this beautifully: "Whoever teaches learns in the act of teaching, and whoever learns teaches in the act of learning" (1998, p. 31).

Learning in the Workplace

We'd like to sow the seeds for the learning environment. Carole Estabrooks, in her discussion of using research in practice, characterized nurses as generating knowledge within their "communities of practice" (2003, p. 60). People don't learn in isolation; they do it with others. Nurses produce knowledge, as well as use it, in their workplaces every day. We don't think Dewey would be surprised to read this, especially if he considered the huge amount of knowledge that nurses must learn and use daily.

Benner et al. (2010) enumerated integration of classroom and clinical teaching as one of their four shifts in nursing education. The idea of integrating learning and the practicalities of practice is not new: Carkhuff (1996) advocated reflective learning through the use of work and learning groups in the workplace. This approach is very helpful for service-based educators who want to move from the old goals of adaptive learning that focus on survival and maintenance, to a generative learning model based on *creativity* and continual learning (Watkins & Marsick, 1993). Carkhuff provided an excellent example of reflective group learning: While checking the competency of nurses to correctly identify and locate equipment on a crash cart, several nurses were unable to meet the criteria. Rather than reteach the crash cart criteria, the staff educator encouraged the group to reflect on and discuss why it was difficult to do this job without error. Together they came up with strategies to increase their competency. The keys to the success of this approach are that the learning was problem based, learner directed, contextual, and reflective.

Reflection in Practice

We'd like to talk more about the value of *reflection*, not just as a teaching and learning tool, but also as a way to increase clinicians' CT. A word to clinicians: in the past few pages, we've focused on educators, but it would be useful here for you to consider the thinking challenges you deal with daily. You probably do not practice as you once did because of the rapid pace of change in the healthcare arena. "Reflection in practice" is how Schon (1983) referred to this, a wonderful idea that is poignantly relevant today. Schon advocated that practitioners think about what they are doing and thinking while in the midst of action—to be "reflective practitioners" in response to changes in their professions. Although healthcare professionals were one of his intended audiences, he cited many professionals who have experienced a "crisis of confidence" because of "the mismatch of traditional patterns of practice and knowledge [and the] . . . complexity, uncertainty, instability, uniqueness, and value conflict" (p. 18) of the practice arena.

This complexity and uncertainty are especially found in what Schon called the "swampy lowland where situations are confusing 'messes' incapable of technical solution" (1983, p. 42). Whoa! Does that sound like a typical *when* and *where* for nurses? Schon also said that those who choose the swampy lowland "deliberately involve themselves in messy but crucially important problems and, when asked to describe their methods of inquiry, they speak of experience, trial and error, intuition, and muddling through" (p. 43). Can something be done to help clinicians "muddle through" better? Schon's answer is *reflection*.

How can clinicians use *reflection* to meet the goals that the IOM has advocated for practice? First and foremost, you must focus on thinking—not as a phenomenon separate from daily work, but as it is joined with action. Now, don't get the idea that nurses can ever practice without thinking. That is a scary thought. However, *reflection* in action is thinking about thinking and action as you are actively working. That *reflection* is necessary because of the changing nature of health care. What worked yesterday won't necessarily work today; what we did yesterday is not necessarily what we should be doing today. Thinking and acting are linked out of necessity; we don't have the luxury of sitting back and doing our thinking after the fact, nor would we be comfortable doing that. However, because it is so easy to concentrate on action rather than on thinking, we need reminders to think.

How Does *Reflection* in Action Work?

At the risk of being prescriptive, we've come up with a list of questions that clinicians should ask themselves as they reflect (see **Box 4-7**). As you see, they are essentially based on the CT habits of the mind and skills that we have already discussed. Now, would each clinician reflect on these things in a linear, checklist kind of way? Of course not. But it's helpful to have such a list to help us think about things fully.

TACTICS 4-2: *Reflection* in Action

Clinicians

Think about your most recent clinical day. Now think of a specific patient encounter or team meeting. Using the questions in Box 4-7, reflect on these events. Pay attention to how comfortable you are with *reflection*. Try to picture yourself in the midst of what was happening. Were you reflective at the time? As you recall the situation, do things occur to you now that you didn't consider while the event was happening?

Box 4-7   Suggestions for Clinicians' *Reflection* in Action

Am I...

reasonably sure of my thinking here?
taking into account the total context of this situation?
considering more creative, better approaches?
being too rigid? Too loose?
asking all the questions I should be asking?
using any preconceived notions that might be wrong?
going with my gut reactions or ignoring them?
closing my mind off to any possibilities?
sticking with this long enough, or is it time to just make a decision and get on with it?
breaking this down enough so I'm seeing all the pieces and how they fit together?
forgetting any important rules?
seeing the patterns and details?
missing anything?
making conclusions based on solid data?
able to predict where this is going?
adapting my knowledge to this situation?

Discussion

If the checklist idea seems a bit scripted to you, think about other ways to promote reflective practice. Perhaps this real-life situation will spark your *creativity*.

We asked our nurse practitioner colleague Jane Duerr, working in primary care, to describe her *reflection* in action. She talked about *where, when,* and *how* to reflect. (OK, so we prompted her with those words; nevertheless, this is what she said.)

> *I try to reflect with another clinician if I can because I think better when I can bounce ideas off someone else. I do that in several ways—both structured and informally. On the structured side, the nurse practitioners at my office get together for breakfast on a regular schedule to talk about practice issues. We make a point of not turning that into a complaining session about things we dislike, but, rather, we focus on things we've seen in practice that we're concerned with, new information we've found and so forth—real collaborative communication. The physicians and nurse practitioners also have a journal club where we reflect on our practice relative to the latest research findings. Less structured reflection occurs in the corridors and lunchroom; sometimes I call one of the docs or nurses to bounce ideas off them in the middle of the day.*

I also reflect with families and patients. Sometimes sitting down and going over things with them allows me to think aloud; we can think together and often come up with better actions than I would have come up with alone. It's very easy to forget that patients and families are there, too.

As to where I reflect, it's everywhere, especially places where I can find some solitude. I go into the lab, find an empty office, I do a lot of reflection in my car on the way home or to and from settings. I often take a longer route home so I can have more thinking time.

The challenge to clinicians is this: How are you managing *reflection* in practice? Do you do it enough? Where do you do it? Do you need to reflect on your *reflection*?

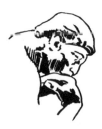

© Jesse Rubenfeld

PAUSE and Ponder

Think Ahead to Change

In this chapter, we've discussed *how* educators and clinicians need to grow to make sure that the competencies of providing patient-centered care, working in interdisciplinary teams, employing evidence-based practice, applying quality improvement, and using informatics become the norm of health care.

REFLECTION CUES

- The *how, when,* and *where* of CT for clinicians and educators are intrinsically interconnected: the *where* is healthcare practice and education; the *when* is today and tomorrow. What remains is to figure out the best *how.*
- The IOM has issued a challenge for health professions "to deliver patient-centered care as members of an interdisciplinary team, emphasizing evidence-based practice, quality improvement approaches, and informatics" and for healthcare educators to produce clinicians who can achieve this task (IOM, 2003, p. 3).
- Errors are inevitable. Blaming individuals is not the way to deal with those errors; errors need to be analyzed to determine ways to prevent them in the future.
- Meeting the IOM's challenge will require major changes in the practice and education of health professionals.
- Education must move away from the status quo of traditional teaching and start focusing on active learning rather than rote memorization.
- Thinking in education and practice requires us to expand our understanding of what Gardner (2006) referred to as the five minds of the future: disciplinary, synthesizing, creating, respectful, and ethical.
- Students must become finders of knowledge, not takers of information.

- Knowledge-seeking behavior can be affected by such simple things as casual comments and nonverbal behaviors directed toward learners.
- A primary goal must be to aim for understanding that allows for transfer of information in a variety of circumstances.
- Dewey's ideas on differences between providing knowledge and forming ideas are relevant to educators today.
- Various teaching techniques lend themselves to promoting knowledge processing.
- Encouraging students and clinicians to imagine themselves teaching patients to think and learn is helpful in developing new skills.
- Clinicians are encouraged to practice what Schon (1983) called "reflection in action" to promote thinking for today's ever-changing practice world.
- Reflecting on the differences between teaching and learning is helpful in gaining a new perspective on *how* to improve thinking.

REFERENCES

American Association of Colleges of Nursing. (2008). *The essentials of baccalaureate education for professional nursing practice*. Washington, DC: Author.

Angelo, T. A., & Cross, K. P. (1993). *Classroom assessment techniques: A handbook for college teachers* (2nd ed.). San Francisco, CA: Jossey-Bass.

Association of American Colleges and Universities & the Carnegie Foundation for the Advancement of Teaching. (2004). *A statement on integrative learning*. Retrieved from http://www.evergreen.edu /washingtoncenter/docs/intlearning/statementintlearning.pdf

Banfield, V., Fagan, B., & Janes, C. (2012). 2009–2010 Spacelabs innovation project award: Charting a new course in knowledge: Creating life-long critical care thinkers. *Dynamics, 23*(1), 24–28.

Bargagliotti, T., Luttrell, M., & Lenburg, C. (1999, September 30). Reducing threats to the implementation of a competency-based performance assessment system. *Online Journal of Issues in Nursing*. Retrieved from http://www.nursingworld.org/MainMenuCategories/ANAMarketplace /ANAPeriodicals/OJIN/TableofContents/Volume41999/No2Sep1999/ReducingThreatsto theImplementationofaCompetencyBasedPerformanceAssessmentSystem.html

Barr, R. B., & Tagg, J. (1995). From teaching to learning: A new paradigm for undergraduate education. *Change, 27*(6), 13–25.

Benner, P. (1984). *From novice to expert: Power and excellence in nursing practice*. Menlo Park, CA: Addison-Wesley.

Benner, P., Sutphen, M., Leonard, V., & Day, L. (2010). *Educating nurses: A call for radical transformation*. San Francisco, CA: Jossey-Bass.

Billings, D. M., & Halstead, J. A. (2009). *Teaching in nursing: A guide for faculty* (3rd ed.). Philadelphia, PA: Saunders Elsevier.

Binder, F. M. (2000). *So you want to be a college president?* Retrieved from http://www.cosmos-club.org /web/journals/2000/binder.html

Bulman, C., Lathlean, J., & Gobbi, M. (2012). The concept of reflection in nursing: Qualitative findings on student and teacher perspectives. *Nurse Education Today, 32*, e8–e13. doi: 10.1016/j.nedt.2011.10.007

Carkhuff, M. H. (1996). Reflective learning: Work groups as learning groups. *Journal of Continuing Education in Nursing, 27*, 209–214.

Dewey, J. (1966). *Democracy and education*. New York, NY: Free Press. (Original work published 1916)

Ellerbe, S., & Regen, D. (2012). Responding to health care reform by addressing the Institute of Medicine report on the future of nursing. *Nursing Administration Quarterly, 36*(3), 210–216. doi: 10.1097 /NAQ.0b013e318258bfa7

Estabrooks, C. A. (2003). Translating research into practice: Implications for organizations and administrators. *Canadian Journal of Nursing Research, 35*(3), 53–68.

Freire, P. (1998). *Pedagogy of freedom: Ethics, democracy, and civic courage* (P. Clarke, Trans.). Lanham, MD: Rowman & Littlefield.

Gardner, H. (2006). *Five minds for the future*. Boston, MA: Harvard Business School Press.

Giddens, J. F., & Brady, D. P. (2007). Rescuing nursing education from content saturation: The case for a concept-based curriculum. *Journal of Nursing Education, 46,* 65–69.

Hall, D. (2011). Debate: Innovative teaching to enhance critical thinking and communication skills in healthcare professionals. *Internet Journal of Allied Health Sciences and Practice, 9*(3). Retrieved from http://ijahsp.nova.edu/articles/Vol9Num3/pdf/Hall.pdf

Hassmiller, S. (2010). Nursing's role in healthcare reform. *American Nurse Today, 5*(9), 68–69. Retrieved from http://www.americannursetoday.com

Huang, Y.-C., Chen, H.-H., Yeh, M.-L., & Chung, Y.-C. (2012). Case studies combined with or without concept maps improve critical thinking in hospital-based nurses: A randomized-controlled trial. *International Journal of Nursing Studies, 49,* 747–754. doi: 10.1016/j.inurstu.2012.01.008

Hughes, R. G. (Ed.). (2008, April). *Patient safety and quality: An evidence-based handbook for nurses.* Rockville, MD: Agency for Healthcare Research and Quality. (AHRQ Publication No. 08-0043)

Institute of Medicine. (2000). *To err is human: Building a safer health system.* Washington, DC: National Academies Press.

Institute of Medicine. (2001). *Crossing the quality chasm: A new health system for the 21st century.* Washington, DC: National Academies Press.

Institute of Medicine. (2003). *Health professions education: A bridge to quality.* Washington, DC: National Academies Press.

Institute of Medicine. (2004a). *Keeping patients safe: Transforming the work environment of nurses.* Washington, DC: National Academies Press.

Institute of Medicine. (2004b). *Patient safety: Achieving a new standard for care.* Washington, DC: National Academies Press.

Institute of Medicine. (2011). *The future of nursing: Leading change, advancing health.* Washington, DC: National Academies Press.

Kennison, M. (2012). Developing reflective writing as effective pedagogy. *Nursing Education Perspectives, 33*(5), 306–311.

Kowalczyk, N. (2011). Review of teaching methods and critical thinking skills. *Radiologic Technology, 83*(2), 120–132.

Legislative Counsel. (2010). Patient Protection and Affordable Care Act: Health-related portions of the Health Care and Education Reconciliation Act of 2010. Retrieved from http://housedocs.house.gov/energycommerce/ppacacon.pdf

Lim, F. A. (2011). Questioning: A teaching strategy to foster clinical thinking and reasoning. *Nurse Educator, 36*(2), 52–53. doi: 10.1097/NNE.0b013e31820b4dd8

Maneval, R., Fowler, K. A., Kays, J. A., Boyd, T. M., Shuey, J., Harne-Britner, S., & Mastrine, C. (2012). The effect of high-fidelity patient simulation on the critical thinking and clinical decision-making skills of new graduate nurses. *Journal of Continuing Education in Nursing, 43*(3), 125–134. doi: 10.3928/00220124-20111101-02

Marchigiano, G., Eduljee, N., & Harvey, K. (2011). Developing critical thinking skills from clinical assignments: A pilot study on nursing students' self-reported perceptions. *Journal of Nursing Management, 19,* 143–152. doi: 10.1111/j.1365-2834.2010.01191.x

Michaelsen, L., Knight, A. B., & Fink, L. D. (2004). *Team-based learning: A transformative use of small groups in college teaching.* Sterling, VA: Stylus.

Myrick, F., & Tamlyn, D. (2007). Teaching can never be innocent: Fostering an enlightening educational experience. *Journal of Nursing Education, 46,* 299–303.

Oja, K. J. (2011). Using problem-based learning in the clinical setting to improve nursing students' critical thinking: An evidence review. *Journal of Nursing Education, 50*(3), 145–151. doi: 10.3928/01484834-20101230-10

Perry, W. G. (1970). *Forms of intellectual and ethical development in the college years*. New York, NY: Holt, Rinehart and Winston.

Popil, I. (2011). Promotion of critical thinking by using case studies as teaching method. *Nurse Education Today, 31*, 204–207. doi: 10.1016/j.nedt.2010.06.002

Popkess, A. M., & McDaniel, A. (2011). Are nursing students engaged in learning? A secondary analysis of data from the national survey of student engagement. *Nursing Education Perspectives, 32*(2), 89–94.

Rideout, W. (2001). *Transforming nursing education through problem-based learning*. Sudbury, MA: Jones and Bartlett.

Sanford, P. G. (2010). Simulation in nursing education: A review of the research. *The Qualitative Report, 15*(4), 1006–1111. Retrieved from http://www.nova.edu/ssss/QR/QR15-4/sanford.pdf

Scheffer, B. K., & Rubenfeld, M. G. (2006). Critical thinking: A tool in search of a job. *Journal of Nursing Education, 45*, 195–196.

Schon, D. A. (1983). *The reflective practitioner: How professionals think in action*. New York, NY: Basic Books.

Sinatra-Wilhelm, T. (2012). Nursing care plans versus concept maps in the enhancement of critical thinking skills in nursing students enrolled in a baccalaureate nursing program. *Creative Nursing, 18*(2), 78–84.

Stanley, M. J. C., & Dougherty, J. P. (2010). A paradigm shift in nursing education: A new model. *Nursing Education Perspectives, 31*(6), 378–380.

Tanner, C. A. (2007). Connecting the dots: What's all the buzz about integrative teaching? *Journal of Nursing Education, 46*, 531–532.

Taylor, L. A., & Littleton-Kearney, M. (2011). Concept mapping: A distinctive educational approach to foster critical thinking. *Nurse Educator, 36*(2), 84–88. doi: 10.1097/NNE.0b013e31820b5308

Walker, S. E. (2003). Active learning strategies to promote critical thinking. *Journal of Athletic Training, 38*(3), 263–267. Retrieved from www.journalofathletictraining.org

Watkins, K. E., & Marsick, V. J. (1993). *Sculpting the learning organization: Lessons in the art and science of systemic change*. San Francisco, CA: Jossey-Bass.

Wiggins, G., & McTighe, J. (1998). *Understanding by design*. Upper Saddle River, NJ: Merrill Prentice Hall.

CHAPTER 5

Critical Thinking, Quality Improvement, and Safety

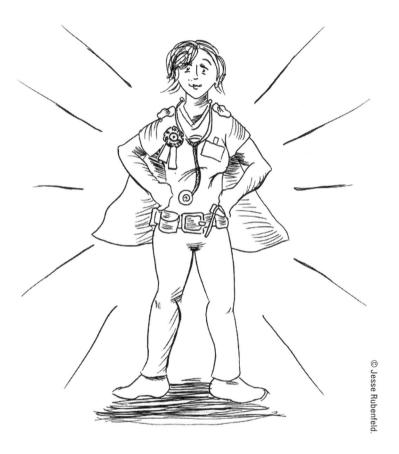

© Jesse Rubenfeld.

Quality improvement seems to be the one Institute of Medicine (IOM) competency toward which all others are aimed. We have, therefore, decided to start your thinking journey with this competency. Quality improvement and safety require all healthcare providers, including nurses, to change their thinking and their actions. To begin appreciating the impact of critical thinking (CT), or lack of CT, on patient quality and safety, read the following patient situation. You should wonder how this could happen in today's state-of-the-art healthcare system.

JW is a 76-year-old 170-pound woman in general good health but has significant immobility and pain secondary to degenerative joint disease in her left knee. She elected to have a knee replacement. Twenty-four hours after surgery to replace her left knee, during a transfer from her hospital bed to a wheelchair, her care providers dropped her to the floor, disrupting the surgical site. After her repair surgery and during her rehabilitation in extended care, she was fitted with a knee support brace in the wrong size. This was discovered after 3 weeks and resulted in another return to surgery to repair the improper and increasingly painful knee alignment. Infection set in after this third surgery, resulting in a long course of antibiotics. After the infections cleared, a fourth surgery fused her left knee, resulting in a permanently straight left leg. JW finally returned home after four surgeries and 5 months of inpatient and extended rehabilitation care. Her mobility is now less than presurgery.

Whether you are a beginning nursing student or have been practicing nursing for years, you can quickly identify the most obvious points at which CT *did not* occur in JW's care. Insufficient thinking contributed to healthcare worker errors (unsafe transferring practice and improper selection of equipment) and system errors (transfer policies and infection control), resulting in severely compromised patient care. Unacceptable outcomes such as those experienced by JW continue to trigger the need for nurses and other providers to engage all 17 dimensions of CT to achieve safe, quality health care.

The statistics on adverse events are alarming. The U.S. Office of Inspector General (2010) estimated that "13.5 percent of hospitalized Medicare beneficiaries experienced adverse events during their hospital stays" (p. i). Such an event contributed to death in 1.5% of Medicare beneficiaries. Forty-four percent of all events were deemed preventable and linked to "medical errors, substandard care, and lack of patient monitoring and assessment" (p. ii). The Joint Commission reviews adverse events each year and revises goals to improve safety. In their 2011 yearly review and update of patient safety goals (such as those related to patient identification, improved communication, medication safety, healthcare-associated infections, reduced falls, pressure ulcers, and risk assessment), The Joint Commission added a new goal for 2012 focused on catheter-associated urinary tract infection (The Joint Commission, 2013a).

To say that improving healthcare quality has become a priority for the U.S. government would be an understatement. Among the many seminal reports that emerge when one searches for quality-related policies are the 2011 report to Congress, *National Strategy for Quality Improvement in Health Care*, cited in the follow-up 2012 progress report (U.S. Department of Health and Human Services, 2012). That

2011 report described the need for better, affordable care, which became a reality in the Affordable Care Act (Legislative Counsel, 2010.) Three broad aims have been outlined: better care, healthy people and healthy communities, and affordable care.

This chapter examines the thinking that is essential to achieve safe, quality health care. We explore (1) definitions of quality and safety in health care and the stakeholders involved; (2) the scope of the healthcare quality–safety problem; (3) the relationships among quality, safety, and CT within a systems framework of structure, process, and outcomes; (4) the five IOM criteria guiding education and practice toward quality improvement and safe patient care; and (5) nurses as safety champions for enhancing quality and safety through thinking. Our goal is to make crystal clear how thinking is the key ingredient in all efforts to achieve safe, quality care for our patients, their families, and their communities.

Defining Quality and Safety in Health Care and Stakeholder Involvement

Definitions

Many groups have defined quality and safety in the past 2 decades. Such groups include the American Society for Quality, the American Medical Association, and The Joint Commission (Burhans, 2007). The American Nurses Association, the National Quality Forum (NQF), and the Agency for Healthcare Research and Quality (AHRQ) have also weighed in on the issue (Ridley, 2008). The AHRQ defined safety as "freedom from accidental injury or avoiding injuries or harm to patients from care that is intended to help them" (2003, p. 8).

The IOM defined quality as "the degree to which health services for individuals and populations increase the likelihood of desired health outcomes and are consistent with current professional knowledge" (1990, p. 4). We believe that they have retained this definition of quality over the years because it recognizes (1) the impact that health care has on quality of life for both patients and communities, (2) the probability of achieving better outcomes, and (3) the reliability of those outcomes stemming from sound information and CT.

Although there are varied definitions within and across disciplines, there are common themes in how we think about quality and safety. Those themes include "deficiency-free excellence; conformity and consistency with standards and current professional knowledge; stakeholder-specific subjectivity; and congruence with the structure-process-outcomes quality triad" (Burhans, 2007, p. 43). Thus, when defining quality and safety, we must think about error-free top-notch care, compliance with professional standards and evidence-based practice (EBP), appreciation of multiple points of view, and acknowledgment that thinking must focus on systems (structures, processes, and outcomes) and not simply individuals.

These four themes allow us to dissect the quality improvement issues and the thinking involved in each. The first theme identified by Burhans (2007), deficiency-free excellence, or error-free, top-notch care, is the overarching goal for all safety initiatives. However, we need to look at that goal realistically in today's world. The second theme is conformity and consistency with standards and professional knowledge. The third and fourth themes—stakeholders, and the structure, process, and outcomes of the system—are important areas for CT. We'll start with stakeholders because they are an ever-present influence on quality initiatives.

Stakeholders

Stakeholders are individuals or entities who participate in or experience the impact of some activity or event (Alexander, 2007; Burhans, 2007; Lundquist & Axelsson, 2007; Mastal, Joshi, & Schulke, 2007; Melichar, 2007; Needleman, Kurtzman, & Kizer, 2007). We are most concerned about the thinking employed by both individuals and organizations (entities) because thinking is the key if safety and quality care are the desired outcomes.

All stakeholders have a stake in the quality of care from the perspectives of cost and benefit or harm. In health care, there are four basic categories of stakeholders: those who pay for care, those who deliver care, those who receive care, and those who monitor the quality of care. The paying stakeholders include the national and state or provincial governments, insurance companies, and recipients of care who pay out-of-pocket costs. Those who deliver care include all healthcare disciplines and providers in health care. Those who receive care include individuals, families, and communities. Recipients of care have been joined by a whole cadre of public and private organizations and agencies whose goal is to improve quality and safety in health care. Examples of those who monitor quality are identified in **Box 5-1**.

Organizations concerned with quality explicitly or implicitly express the need for CT. Such organizations study and advocate for accurate information, emphasizing the need for collaborative thinking and discussion to find creative solutions. One organization, Quality and Safety Education for Nurses (QSEN), developed a website that invites ongoing critique and input to improve quality and safety strategies (Cronenwett et al., 2007). This group is specifically focused on enhancing prelicensure

---

Box 5-1 Groups and Organizations That Address Quality in Health Care

Institute of Medicine (IOM): http://www.iom.edu
Agency for Healthcare Research and Quality (AHRQ): http://www.ahrq.gov
The Joint Commission: http://www.jointcommission.org
National Quality Forum (NQF): http://www.qualityforum.org
IPRO Quality Improvement Organization: http://www.ipro.org
Quality and Safety Education for Nurses (QSEN): http://www.qsen.org

nursing education. QSEN has been further developed to identify competencies for nursing students at various levels (American Association of Colleges of Nursing [AACN] QSEN Education Consortium, 2012; Cronenwett et al., 2007; Forneris et al., 2012). See Box 5-1 for their website URL.

Nurse educators are also a group of stakeholders concerned about delivering quality and safety with patient care. The presidents of both nursing educational professional organizations, the National League for Nursing (NLN) and the AACN, cited the need for changes in the education of prenursing students regarding quality and safety (Bargagliotti & Lancaster, 2007). They described a gap between what nurse educators say they teach about quality and safety and how nursing graduates apply that teaching in the practice setting. The presidents recommended that faculty embrace "new ways of thinking, interacting and learning" (p. 156) to bridge the gap between education and practice of quality care. The AACN *Essentials of Baccalaureate Education for Professional Nursing Practice* includes an assumption that all baccalaureate graduates are prepared to "promote safe, quality patient care" (2008, p. 8)

The AACN (2006) also created a Patient Safety Task Force to emphasize the importance of quality and safety in the education and preparation of nurses. It is very important for nursing students and faculty to integrate the knowledge, skills, and attitudes of safe, quality care into all aspects of prelicensure education (Cronenwett et al., 2007)—in other words, integrate quality and safety thinking throughout nursing curricula.

Deficiency-Free Excellence: What Is the Scope of the Quality–Safety Problem?

We probably all agree that much of today's health care would not receive a 10 on a scale of 1–10, with 10 being the best. In contemplating goals for remediation, we first need to reflect on whether reaching 10 is possible. Attempting to achieve perfection in complex systems is not only unrealistic, but it also may make matters worse. Attempts at perfection have a tendency to increase the level of system complexity, which in turn potentially leads to more system failures. "Excellence is not perfection, excellence is striving. Perfection is the enemy of excellence" (E. Tagliareni, personal communication, July 30, 2008).

Given that we cannot score a 10 on healthcare quality and that achieving perfection is unrealistic, let's get a better handle on the scope of the problem to employ some thinking to resolve it. We start, of course, with the CT dimensions of *inquisitiveness, information seeking,* and *analysis. Information seeking* enables us to gather useful data about the current state of quality care. *Inquisitiveness* drives us to explore, to find out what is working and what is not working, and to wonder why. *Analysis* allows us to examine the parts of the problem in manageable segments so we can thoroughly define and frame the problem before using *logical reasoning* and *transforming knowledge* to find solutions. As you will see, discovering those solutions will require all the CT dimensions from a multitude of stakeholders, but particularly nurses, the safety champions.

A Bit of History

In the early 1990s, the IOM asked hard questions about healthcare quality and raised awareness of the overuse, misuse, and underuse of healthcare services in the United States. At that point, the IOM recommended switching to computer-based patient records as a way of monitoring healthcare issues (informatics enters the picture). Computerized data provided the means to find out how serious the problem with quality was (IOM, 2004a).

In 2000, the IOM issued *To Err Is Human: Building a Safer Health System*, and in 2001, *Crossing the Quality Chasm: A New Health System for the 21st Century*. Both reports revealed growing concerns about quality in health care. The data from the U.S. healthcare system revealed that on a yearly basis:

- 7% of patients suffer a medication error
- Every patient admitted to an intensive care unit suffers an adverse event
- 44,000 to 98,000 deaths [result from errors]
- $50 billion in total costs [result from errors] (Pronovost, 2004)

And to further help put this in perspective, "In the United States, the annual loss of life from medical errors approaches the loss of American combat deaths annually during World War II" (Bargagliotti & Lancaster, 2007, p. 156). These statistics should be a scary call to action.

Quality and Safety Lingo

Searching the literature to gain insight and data on safe, quality health care provided a plethora of articles that are growing exponentially. There are multiple concepts and terms closely associated with quality and safe care that should be acknowledged in our attempt to be good critical thinkers. **Box 5-2** includes many of the terms and phrases commonly used when discussing quality and safety. Time and space

---

Box 5-2 The Lingo of Quality

Active failures: Errors or harm as a result of direct actions or contact with a patient (Mitchell, 2008).

Adverse event: "An event that results in unintended harm to the patient by an act of commission or omission rather than by the underlying disease or condition of the patient" (IOM, 2004b, p. 201).

Continuous Quality Improvement: Also referred to as Total Quality Management. Focuses on the healthcare system and its overall structure versus individuals. Keys are measuring performance, making changes, and evaluating the effects of those changes (Newhouse & Poe, 2005).

Box 5-2   The Lingo of Quality (continued)

Culture of safety: A phrase describing an organization that acknowledges the following: (1) most errors are a result of systemic dysfunctional work processes, (2) blaming individuals is counterproductive, and (3) supporting a learning environment for both staff and the organization enhances safety (IOM, 2004a).

Failure to rescue: A situation resulting from delayed detection of changes in a patient's condition *and* slow responses to those changes (IOM, 2004a).

Latent failures: Errors or harm as a result of organizational policies, procedures, resources, or allocation of resources (Mitchell, 2008).

Near miss: "Acts of omission or commission that could have harmed the patient but did not cause harm as a result of chance, prevention or mitigation" (IOM, 2004b, p. 227).

Nurse dose: A concept with three equal parts: (1) the number or amount of care delivered by nurses (dose); (2) the educational preparation, expertise, and experience (of the nurse); and (3) the receptiveness of the organization or the patient (host response) (Brooten & Youngblut, 2006).

Nursing-sensitive databases: Standardized information on nursing quality and patient outcomes (Alexander, 2007).

Organizational system failures: Errors or harm as a result of management, organizational culture, processes, communication, or external resources (Mitchell, 2008).

Patient-centered outcome measures: Conditions experienced by the recipient of care after the care is provided.

Quality assurance: Terminology used to describe projects.

Quality improvement: Terminology used to describe moving from one level of care to a better level of care.

Risk management: Label for one department in an organization focused on minimizing both individual and system errors that could result not only in patient harm but also in monetary loss for the institution.

Sentinel event: "An unexpected occurrence involving death or serious physical or psychological injury, or the risk thereof. Serious injury specifically includes loss of limb or function. The phrase 'or the risk thereof' includes any process variation for which a recurrence would carry a significant chance of a serious adverse outcome" (The Joint Commission, 2013b, para 2).

Surveillance: A label in the Nursing Interventions Classification system and used to describe the equal role of the ongoing monitoring *and* interpretation of clinical information (Kelly & Vincent, 2010; Shever et al., 2008).

Technical failures: Errors or harm due to failure of facilities or resources (Mitchell, 2008).

Value-added care processes: Indicators that care has improved quality of life.

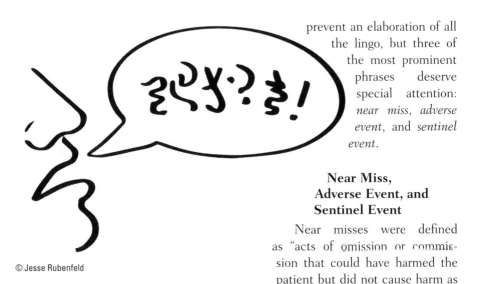

prevent an elaboration of all the lingo, but three of the most prominent phrases deserve special attention: *near miss*, *adverse event*, and *sentinel event*.

© Jesse Rubenfeld

Near Miss, Adverse Event, and Sentinel Event

Near misses were defined as "acts of omission or commission that could have harmed the patient but did not cause harm as a result of chance, prevention or mitigation" (IOM, 2004b, p. 227). An adverse event was defined as "an event that results in unintended harm to the patient by an act of commission or omission rather than by the underlying disease or condition of the patient" (p. 201). The most adverse event, or the sentinel event, was identified by The Joint Commission as "an unexpected occurrence involving death or serious physical or psychological injury, or the risk thereof. Serious injury specifically includes loss of limb or function. The phrase 'or the risk thereof' includes any process variation for which a recurrence would carry a significant chance of a serious adverse outcome" (2013b, para 2). These terms are discussed in more detail later in this chapter.

The Joint Commission publishes a *Sentinel Event Alert*, which includes a root cause analysis and contributing factors of one problem area at a time. These can be found on their website. Alert number 40, "Behaviors that Undermine a Culture of Safety," is particularly relevant to this chapter and will be discussed in more detail (The Joint Commission, 2008).

The 2004 IOM report, *Keeping Patients Safe: Transforming the Work Environment of Nurses*, added an additional dimension to the problem with quality in reference to the 44,000 to 98,000 deaths from errors: "This alarming number, which reflects only deaths occurring in hospital settings . . . does not reflect the many patients who survive, but sustain serious injuries" (2004a, p. 1). Thus, these data do not address most adverse events, and they do not address any near misses. It is important to recognize that quality and safety issues run the whole gamut of health care and nursing care. Although most of the focus has been on acute care settings, a growing body of literature is addressing quality and safety in long-term care, palliative care, physicians' offices, pharmacies, community clinics, and home care (Davies & Cripacc, 2008; Donaldson & Philip, 2004; Gruneir & Mor, 2008; Lynn et al., 2007; McBride-Henry & Foureur, 2007; Raterink, 2011; Whitson et al., 2008). Concern about quality care is not confined to the acute care setting, and CT cannot be, either.

So what is the role of nursing and thinking in all of this? It appears, from a study by Buerhaus and colleagues (2007), that there are very differing opinions. These researchers surveyed registered nurses (RNs), medical doctors (MDs), chief nursing officers (CNOs), and chief executive officers (CEOs) in health care to get an understanding of the impact of the nursing shortage on hospital patient care. One of their findings was very disturbing. When participants responded to the question, "Do you think the current [nursing] shortage will lead to lower-quality care for patients?" the "yes" responses were as follows (p. 859):

- 69% of the 142 CEOs said yes
- 71% of the 222 CNOs said yes
- 90% of the 657 RNs said yes
- 83% of the 445 MDs said yes

The above data represent a significant difference in the perceptions of nurses in administrative/executive roles (CNOs and CEOs) and the perceptions of nurses in practice roles. It is also noteworthy to compare all with the perceptions of the physicians (MDs) in the study, as they are our interprofessional parterns in patient care. *Inquisitiveness* and *perseverance* lead us to some challenging questions: How do these differing opinions make a difference in policies and procedures related to safe, quality patient care? How can nurses use their CT to enlighten policy makers about their role in safe, quality patient care? What impact do these perceptions have on staffing patterns? (What other questions do you have?)

Other studies have strongly acknowledged the significant role of nursing in both the thinking and the doing aspects of quality and patient safety. For example, Mitchell titled a chapter section "Nursing as the Key to Improving Quality Through Patient Safety" (2008, pp. 1–3). Numerous other authors support this perspective and the need for some good ol' CT (Kurtzman & Corrigan, 2007; Mastal et al., 2007; Miller & Chaboyer, 2006; Naylor, 2007; Needleman et al., 2007; Ridley, 2008; Schmalenberg & Kramer, 2008), providing more evidence that nurses are safety champions.

Reflection Pause

Now it's time for some *reflection* and *contextual perspective* to look back at the whole picture of the quality problem. A summary of the key points of this section will help us move on to examining the system that needs a good dose of CT to facilitate safe, quality healthcare outcomes:

- Perfection is not a realistic goal; in fact, attempts to achieve perfection will probably make matters worse.
- The volume of errors and deaths is enormous and unacceptable.
- Documented near misses, adverse events, and sentinel events provide concrete evidence of threats to patient safety and quality care.
- Quality and safety concerns and the CT that must accompany those concerns extend beyond acute care in all aspects of health care: long-term care, palliative care, home care, and so on.
- The perceptions of CNOs and CEOs regarding the role of nursing in patient safety (in one study) do not match the perceptions of nurses or physicians.

The Relationships among Quality, Safety, and Critical Thinking within a Systems Framework of Structure, Process, and Outcomes

Safe, quality health care can result from high-quality thinking and appreciating how systems function. **Figure 5-1** uses a medallion symbol, which represents the IOM competency of applying quality improvement. We selected this symbol because it generally represents a mark of excellence or an award for great work.

This more detailed illustration of the medallion acknowledges the overall health-care system. The center of the medallion represents the healthcare system triad of

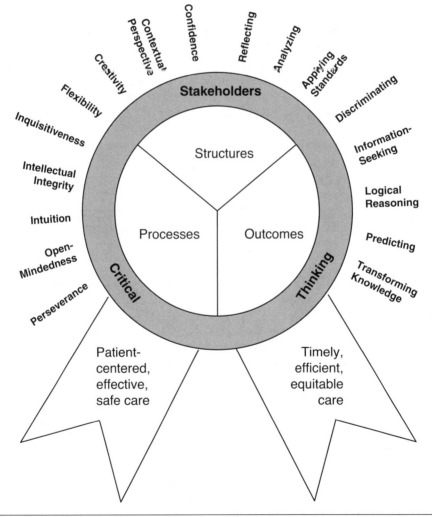

Figure 5-1 Medallion of safe, quality health care through critical thinking.

structure, process, and outcome. Thinking about how these components interact can guide decisions about quality and safety.

Surrounding the three system components is a ring that represents stakeholders' thinking. Beyond that ring are the 17 dimensions of CT used by all the stakeholders, especially the nurse (the safety champion), the interdisciplinary team, and the patient or family. The medallion ribbons represent the six IOM Aims for Quality Healthcare: patient centered, effective, safe, timely, efficient, and equitable. For the remainder of this chapter, when we refer to CT, remember that it represents both individual and interdisciplinary thinking. It is this collaborative thinking that ultimately changes the quality of patient care from good to better to best.

The Healthcare System and Safe, Quality Care

Attempts at quality improvement in health care have been addressed over the past several decades, beginning in the 1960s with Donabedian's work on quality assurance (Shortell, Bennett, & Byck, 1998). In a nutshell, Donabedian proposed a framework for quality assurance in health care using a systems perspective. Systems have three interacting components: structure, processes, and outcomes. Donabedian was ahead of his time in thinking about systems; unfortunately, the rest of the healthcare industry was not yet into systems thinking, and significant change did not occur. In the past few decades, numerous authors have developed models and tested those models, all based on Donabedian's systems approach to quality assurance (Burhans, 2007; Needleman et al., 2007). According to Leape, Berwick, and Bates, "the clear message of the IOM report, *To Err Is Human*, is that safety is primarily a systems problem" (2002, p. 504). Today, as we embrace that awareness and appreciate the complexity of those systems, we move to new levels of thinking.

Healthcare systems have moved well beyond complicated and into the realm of complex. Complex systems are not like machines; they are more like conscious entities (Wheatley, 1994) or living organisms. As such, healthcare systems are constantly adaptive (Plsek, 2003). In other words, people, responsibilities, and workloads do not stay in their nice little boxes on organizational charts. Systems (the inner circle on the medallion in Figure 5-1) are dynamic and constantly changing. All aspects of systems (structures, processes, and outcomes) must be actively addressed when looking for solutions to problems of inadequate quality in health care.

Thinking in systems is another level of thinking. Einstein said, "We cannot solve our problems with the same thinking we used when we created them" (BrainyQuote, 2013). We will let you imagine the kinds of thinking that created the problems of quality in health care, but we are certain it will take a concerted interdisciplinary team effort, using all 17 CT dimensions, to deal with the current level of complexity.

But for now, we need to artificially break down the healthcare system to explore the CT needed to examine the structure, process, and outcomes of healthcare systems as they relate to quality and safety, and thinking. By now, you should be able to automatically say, "Aha, we need some *analyzing*, some *open-mindedness*, and some *reflection* here!" And that's just for starters! Let's use some *analysis* to examine the three major components of a system (structure, process, outcome—the inner circle of our medallion) in health care.

Structure

Structure was a system component addressed in the IOM publication *To Err Is Human* (2000). Newhouse and Poe described structure as "having the right things" (2005, p. 61). Structure includes healthcare system resources and infrastructure such as information, the organization itself, physical aspects, human aspects, and fiscal aspects (Handler, Issel, & Turnock, 2001). When using *reflection* and *inquisitiveness*, think about how the following very simplistic example has an impact on safety related to infection control:

> **Information:** What data are available, and how reliable are they for making decisions about a recent rise in staphylococcal infections?
>
> **Organization:** Who in the organization has authority and responsibility to monitor infection rates? Are there any policies and procedures to guide infection control?
>
> **Physical:** Do the staff have the necessary equipment, such as sterile dressing kits, and antiseptic hand-washing liquid, in convenient locations? Are there sinks in every room?
>
> **Human:** Are there adequate numbers of nurses and ancillary staff to manage the acuity of the patient load with infections? Are the staff adequately prepared for their role in infection control? Are patients and family members, nursing and medical students, and the interdisciplinary members taught how to avoid contamination?
>
> **Fiscal:** Is there money in the budget to install hand-washing sinks in each patient room? Which is more cost-effective, paper gowns or cloth gowns for isolation units? What is the cost of iatrogenic infections if these other factors are not addressed?

What dimensions of thinking help us to understand all these structure resources? An obvious one is *contextual perspective*, or looking at the big picture. It is far too easy to blame someone for a mistake but forget the structural constraints that may have contributed to it. *Discriminating* is vital when you are trying to determine which policies and procedures are working and which aren't. *Logical reasoning* is necessary to ensure that the inferences you draw are based on all the facts.

As broad as the structural components are, they are at least somewhat tangible; they can generally be seen, touched, and even measured in some manner. But the next part of the system, process, is a bit harder to capture, let alone measure.

Process

If structure is having the right things, then process is what is done with those things. Processes are actions. Processes in health care are not new to nursing students, nurses, or nurse educators. Beginning nursing students consider processes to be the steps or activities taken to achieve a task, such as inserting a urinary catheter. However, when students move from the learning laboratory to the real world of patient care, they soon realize (we hope!) that those process steps described in textbooks have limited value without the use of CT. For example, one needs to use *flexibility* and *transforming knowledge* to insert a catheter in a patient with cerebral palsy and severe hip contractures.

Examples of other processes that are used daily and that require constant CT are the nursing process, therapeutic communication, teaching, and working in interdisciplinary teams. A related, influential, and somewhat elusive process relevant to this quality discussion is the functioning of the organizational culture. An organization's culture has a powerful influence on quality and safety because it embodies our values, attitudes, and thinking about quality, safety, and care. In short, it affects every process. Later in this chapter, we elaborate on the organizational culture in relation to thinking and errors and, more specifically, the culture of safety, the goal for our safety champion nurses.

Look back to JW's story at the beginning of this chapter. What are the processes that you can identify? Obviously the nursing process stands out; the parts of that process—assessing, planning, implementing, and evaluating care—may well have been problematic. It is quite possible that JW did not receive proper teaching or that communication went awry. Certainly, there seems to have been a breakdown in the interdisciplinary team interactions. Now, consider how difficult it might be to measure the quality of those processes. In contrast to the tangible qualities of structure, the processes can easily become elusive, taken-on-faith actions.

Outcomes

The third portion of the systems triad (the inner circle of the medallion) is outcomes. Outcomes are results brought on by processes. They are often predetermined as goals toward which providers aim their interventions. Outcomes, specifically patient outcomes, became a major focus over the past decade as healthcare providers and quality monitoring organizations began looking at the value-added aspects and outcomes of health care (Kurtzman & Corrigan, 2007).

It would be hard to imagine anyone in nursing, even a nursing student, who does not recognize the phrase *outcome measures*. Typically, outcomes or outcome measures are the part of nursing care plans that we think about ahead of time to later determine if our interventions had the planned effect and the patient achieved a goal. That same terminology is used to think about quality. What are we looking for? Alexander (2007) identified three characteristics of outcomes related to quality: (1) measurable, (2) verifiable, and (3) cost-effective. *Measurable* requires something quantitative, such as shorter length of stay, fewer falls, or no postoperative infections; *verifiable* means that more than one person agrees with the outcome; and *cost-effective* refers to both time and money.

Perhaps because outcomes are concrete and measurable, they have become a hot topic. Much has been written about outcomes, and the language to describe them has expanded. There is a wide variety in what is called an *outcome*. Some outcomes are clearly within the purview of nursing, while others cross over disciplinary lines. The AHRQ patient safety indicators (PSI) were used by Zrelak and colleagues (2012) to target nursing quality improvement processes. Five PSIs were linked with nursing opportunities for improving outcomes: central line–related blood stream infection, postoperative deep vein thrombosis or pulmonary embolus, postoperative sepsis, postoperative respiratory failure, and pressure ulcer. The authors identified several nursing opportunities for improvement of each of these PSIs, finding common trends to be "lack of documentation of an accurate and timely patient assessment, lack of adherence to national standards of care related to prophylaxis or prevention, and delays in recognition and intervention" (pp. 103–104).

Open-mindedness, along with other CT dimensions, is important to a consideration of outcomes. *Applying standards* is a necessity. Standards come in many forms: professional, institutional, personal, and ethical, to name a few. Just what should our standards for outcomes be? This is a question on the minds of many nurses and nursing administrators who are *analyzing* outcomes and *applying standards* (Mitty, 2007; Wise, 2007). Although this is hardly a topic that can be dealt with in one paragraph, the need for ethical standards cannot be overemphasized. We encourage those interested to explore documents from the Hastings Center and the report titled "The Ethics of Using QI Methods to Improve Health Care Quality and Safety" from their project (Mitty, 2007).

Going back to our example of JW, most of you can probably identify which outcomes were missing. What went wrong? Was it the projected outcome that was amiss, or were the processes and structures the biggest contributing factors to this disaster? We know that reasonable outcomes were not reached. Perhaps you can see that even though outcomes have received lots of attention lately, looking at outcomes alone would not be adequate in figuring out what went wrong in JW's case. We need to remember that outcomes are only one-third of the systems triad. If we want to make a difference in safety and quality, we must engage our thinking to examine all three components—structures, processes, and outcomes—of the whole system (Burhans, 2007).

Five IOM Criteria Guiding Education and Practice Toward Quality Improvement and Safe Patient Care

Luckily the IOM (2003) established five criteria for the educational changes necessary to improve quality in health care. As you read these five criteria in **Box 5-3**, think about what needs to change in healthcare practice, education, and thinking patterns to move in those directions. Our new level of thinking requires clinicians and educators to engage as many of the 17 CT dimensions as possible and as often as possible.

Although all 17 CT dimensions are necessary to achieve the five IOM criteria, only some will be used in our examples, for the sake of time and also so you can discover the others on your own. Each criterion and its necessary CT will be discussed separately for the remainder of the chapter.

Box 5-3 IOM Five Criteria for Achieving Quality

---

1. Continually understand and measure quality of care in terms of structure . . . process . . . and outcomes . . . in relation to patient and community needs.
2. Assess current practices and compare them with relevant better practices elsewhere as a means of identifying opportunities for improvement.
3. Design and test interventions to change the process of care, with the objective of improving quality.
4. Identify errors and hazards in care; understand and implement basic safety design principles.
5. Both act as an effective member of an IDT [interdisciplinary team] and improve the quality of one's own performance through self-assessment and personal change.

Source: Reproduced with permission from *Health Professions Education: A Bridge to Quality,* 2003 by the National Academy of Sciences, Courtesy of the National Academies Press, Washington, D.C.

IOM Criterion #1

#1—Continually understand and measure quality of care in terms of "structure," or the inputs into the system, such as patients, staff, and environments; "process," or the interactions between clinicians and patients; and "outcomes," or evidence about changes in patients' health status in relation to patient and community needs. (IOM, 2003, p. 59)

This criterion addresses the quality improvement concepts of structure, process, and outcomes that we have just discussed. Structure, process, and outcomes are valuable concepts in health care but are more valuable when all three are looked at as a whole. Remember the saying, "The whole is greater than the sum of its parts." Basically, this means we have to recognize the whole as its own conscious entity in addition to the contributions of its parts.

To illustrate how these three concepts work together as a system, and the thinking that is involved, complete **TACTICS 5-1**, which uses **Scenario 5-1**.

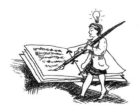

TACTICS 5-1: Thinking for Criterion #1

1. Read Scenario 5-1. Notice that we have inserted some of the CT used by the nurses.
2. Identify any additional CT dimensions we have not cited.

3. Identify the aspects of this situation that represent structure, process, and outcomes.
4. Think about some other possible solutions that the staff did not consider.

Scenario 5-1: Thinking for Criterion #1

The community health nurses working in the well-baby clinic noticed that fewer and fewer new mothers were bringing in their babies for immunizations over the past 6 months. They were concerned about the potential for increasing the incidence of measles during the coming months when measles generally peaks among infants. They wanted to understand both patient and community needs. (**Predicting**)

They want to find out what is happening that may have precipitated this change in behavior and begin to ask the mothers who come if they have any ideas. They also consult the Centers for Disease Control and Prevention (CDC) website to see if this is a national or regional occurrence or if it is unique to their clinic. They consult pediatricians' offices as well. (**Information seeking**)

The mothers who visit the clinic have no idea what the problem could be; they are very pleased with the service they receive. The CDC website has no indication that this is a widespread problem; local pediatricians' offices have not experienced the problem either. The nurses, however, are not about to give up. They meet with the other clinic staff and try to brainstorm ideas. Are they doing something to discourage the return of certain patients? Are they missing some culturally sensitive information, considering that they serve a population of rural migrant workers? Maybe the parents have been listening to the news reports about mercury in the immunizations causing autism and are afraid of immunizing their children. (**Perseverance, open-mindedness, intellectual integrity**)

The nurses decide to try to contact the new mothers directly and ask them what is happening. Because few of the mothers have phones, the nurses make several home visits and ask about the missed appointments. They get only vague excuses about not having time or forgetting.

While driving to a final home visit, a nurse begins to think about one forgotten piece of the whole process of immunizations: access to service. She notices that all the bus stops that used to be in this part of the county are no longer there. When she arrives at a home, she asks the mother about the missed appointments, gets the same vague answer, and then asks about the missing bus stops. (**Contextual perspective**)

With some encouragement, the mother admits that she does not have enough money for a taxi to bring her daughter to the clinic for her immunizations. The *nurse compares the dates of the decline in immunization appointments with the date that the busses stopped servicing some areas of the county and found a match. She and the rest of the clinic team know that declining immunizations puts the children and the community at risk. They combine their thinking and discuss how to approach this situation using the structure-process-outcomes framework recommended by the IOM. (**Analysis, logical reasoning**)*

Discussion

What other CT dimensions did you identify? What did you see as structure, process, and outcomes? Initially the staff thought that the lack of culturally sensitive interventions for immunizations might be a process problem. It turned out to be a structural problem: transportation. What started as an observation by an inquisitive nurse (declining immunization appointments in a well-baby clinic) became a broader system issue that required CT as the nurses and others examined the structure, process, and outcomes.

The thinking about *structure* included perspectives from the parents of the under-immunized children, from transportation authorities who make bus routes, from city officials who provide tax money to the transportation authority, and from volunteer agencies that provide free transportation. Thinking about *process* included collaboration with all parties to examine causes as well as solutions—for example, considering if the staff were culturally sensitive to this population's needs. Thinking about outcomes ultimately focused on the rates of immunization and led to an increase in the quality of health of the children and the community.

If the staff in the clinic had gone even further in their thinking, they would have reflected on the overall system and how immunization outcomes could be more assured. They might have identified ways to use what they learned to deal with other current and future problems. They might have begun to think about how to create a system of mobile satellite clinics that would provide families in outlying areas access to a full range of healthcare services. And they might have thought about how to seek grant money to fund the project.

IOM Criteria #2 and #3

#2—Assess current practices and compare them with relevant better practices elsewhere as a means of identifying opportunities for improvement.
#3—Design and test interventions to change the process of care, with the objective of improving quality. (IOM, 2003, p. 59)

These criteria are being discussed together because they both deal with EBP. Criterion #2 implies the use of evidence-based guidelines that would be the relevant better practices as comparisons with current practice. Comparisons require *information seeking* to locate the best practice guidelines and *applying standards* to select the best fit.

Criterion #3 then pushes for implementation of best practices and testing how the change in practice makes things better. As a quick prelude, consider *flexibility, creativity, transforming knowledge,* and *contextual perspective. Flexibility* helps clinicians adjust practices as better evidence emerges. *Creativity* is particularly necessary for finding ways to implement evidence-based guidelines. *Transforming knowledge* is used to find evidence and translate it into practice. And *contextual perspective* helps customize best practices to the individual patient.

Criteria #2 and #3 and the incorporation of EBP ultimately lead to safe, effective, and efficient care. The IOM addressed six attributes for quality health care systems: "(1) safe, (2) effective, (3) patient centered, (4) timely, (5) efficient, and (6) equitable" (2000, pp. 41–42). Of those six attributes, effective and efficient, timely care fit well with criteria #2 and #3 and are discussed next. Safe care is discussed with IOM criterion #4.

Effective Care

Effective care refers to providing the right type and amount of care to specifically address the problem at hand. The right type of care should be what is recommended by solid evidence. We use CT, specifically *logical reasoning,* to accurately match data and conclusions drawn from those data sets with interventions.

Matching the data with conclusions, matching the right provider to patient needs, and matching appropriate tests and procedures to patient conditions are essential aspects of effective care. This can be a delicate balancing act. Providers need to avoid overdoing things, such as ordering unnecessary tests or procedures. Not everyone with neck pain needs magnetic resonance imaging. Antibiotics are not proper treatment for viral infections. Patients with back pain do not necessarily need orthopedic surgery; many will do much better with treatment from a physical therapist who specializes in back pain.

Overuse is wasteful, and underuse can lead to errors and death. For example, for a patient with a brain tumor who complains of headaches and is diagnosed and treated for migraines, care is not effective. The best CT along with the best evidence makes the difference between effective-quality and ineffective-quality health care.

Effectiveness has implications for CT in teaching as well, whether it is in the academic classroom or practice setting. **Scenario 5-2** illustrates the problems that ensue when quality thinking impacts teaching and quality care.

Scenario 5-2: Earl's Staff Development Teaching Effectiveness

Earl is a staff development instructor for a 30-bed step-down unit in an urban hospital. It is time to do his annual in-service on care of central lines to meet The Joint Commission standards. He has done this several times over the last few years and pulls out his file with lecture notes, grabs the video off the shelf, runs to make copies of the quiz he designed when he first prepared the material, and heads off to the conference room.

During his presentation, two nurses seemed to be napping, but they scored fine on the quiz, so he decides not to say anything. The one new staff member, Jill, did not score well, however. Earl decides he'd better meet with her and review some of the material. When he talks with Jill, she tells him she learned to do central line dressings differently in school and that's why she answered the way she did. Earl says he will check that out.

Later that week at the weekly staff meeting, the new unit manager shares some data she has been collecting on quality and notices the increasing frequency of infections for patients on this unit who have central lines.

Earl looks surprised and says, "I don't know how that can be. I've been doing in-services on central lines consistently for the last few years and everyone attends and passes the post-quiz. I hope we aren't getting another strain of staph on the unit."

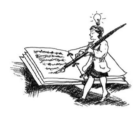

TACTICS 5-2: Thinking and Effectiveness

After reading Scenario 5-2, identify the CT skills and habits of the mind that were not used.

Discussion

The obvious missing CT dimensions are these:

- No *information seeking* on Earl's part to update his information.
- No *reflection* on Earl's part to consider examining his information, teaching style, or measurement instrument before or after his teaching.
- No evidence of *inquisitiveness* to find out about changes in central line care since he first prepared his teaching material and to ask why Jill has different information.
- No *intellectual integrity* on Earl's part to explore the possibility that he might not be teaching accurate information.

A significant area of improvement would be for Earl to use EBP. Earl could have done a literature review or gone to the Internet (the CDC website would have been a good place to start) to look up the latest practice guidelines for central lines. This would have provided him with a better match for the problem—central line care and the proper interventions—thus promoting effective care, as opposed to outdated practice. This behavior requires using at least the listed CT dimensions, plus most other dimensions. Give yourself some stars for additional ones that we did not list, and if you see Earl, tell him about EBP.

Efficient Care

Criteria #2 and #3 also expect efficient care. "Efficiency . . . calls for conducting production activities in as cost-effective and time-efficient a manner as possible" (IOM, 2004a, p. 114). Again, balance is important. Excessive cost-cutting measures without attention to quality frequently lead to decreased staffing, less equipment, and fewer opportunities for catching errors. An example of useful efficiency measures would be to analyze a procedure that has 50 steps, look at all its parts, and see how it could be simplified (by using *logical reasoning*) to determine what could be safely eliminated. If that procedure could be reduced to 35 steps without sacrificing safety, then time, money, and energy would be saved. **Scenario 5-3** illustrates the problems with efficiency in pain management.

Scenario 5-3: Efficient Pain Control Care

Mr. Cashin, a 63-year-old man with lung cancer metastasized to his thoracic and lumbar spine, was scheduled for his initial assessment prior to receiving radiation. However, his health status was too poor to start the treatment. He was hospitalized with severe back pain. Among his many comorbidities were obesity (5 feet 10 inches and 335 pounds), right- and left-sided heart failure, hypertension, 4+ edema of his lower extremities, and 3+ edema up to the T9 area of his back. He had very limited range of motion. He was very sensitive to narcotics, and in the past, it seemed that half a Vicodin knocked him out. He was prescribed a fentanyl patch. When the nurse practitioner (NP) came to his room to identify the specific point of pain area and prepare him for focused radiation, she found him in pain, with no fentanyl patch. Upon questioning the patient's wife, she discovered that Mrs. Cashin had removed the patch, thinking that it was a Band-Aid left behind from an earlier procedure. She said her husband kept calling the nurse during the night because he was in so much pain. The patient was unable to identify an area of the back that was causing the pain, stating that it was all over and radiated down his legs. The frustrated NP went to look at his chart and found these entries in the nursing notes: "3 AM: Patient reported pain at level 4 to nursing assistant." "4 AM: When assessed by the nurse, patient reported a pain level of 7/8. Two Vicodin given. Patient continued to use call light every half hour through the night." Wanting to check the specific time of the pain medication administration, the NP looked at the drug-dispensing computer record and found it was 3:40 when the medication was given. When discussing the matter with the nurse, she found the nurse surprised that it had taken 40 minutes for her to give the medication. She reported that the night had been very busy and said, "I'm doing my best; I've been juggling things all night." The NP returned to the radiation oncology department, stating that radiation would be delayed until a full assessment could be completed.

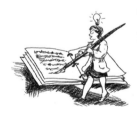

TACTICS 5-3: Thinking and Efficiency for Mr. Cashin

1. After reading Scenario 5-3, how would you describe the efficiency of the night nurse? The NP?
2. Identify what thinking skills and habits of the mind could have been used to make the care more efficient for Mr. Cashin.

Discussion

This situation may be all too familiar to harried nurses trying to do their jobs with too few staff and too many demands. Many of you may immediately become defensive of the harried night nurse because you've been in similar situations. If you could set that defensiveness aside and try to think of efficiency issues, what would you come up with? In terms of efficiency, the delay in pain medication administration created a cascade of events that made both the night nurse and the NP inefficient. Some *contextual perspective* was needed; the nurse needed to realize that the assistant was not equipped to assess pain thoroughly and that, considering the patient's history, she should have assessed pain herself at specific points during the night. If the pain had been controlled, the NP would have been able to accomplish her job of getting the patient ready for radiation. Some *discriminating* by the nurse could have helped her delegate other tasks, not pain assessment, to the nursing assistant. The NP might have been able to be more *discriminating* and assured that the staff knew specifically what the patient needed. *Applying standards* of care would have ensured that the patient's wife was taught about the fentanyl patch. It may be that both the nurse and the NP needed some *confidence* in their thinking so they could articulate the system problems that led to this patient's pain being ill-controlled.

IOM Criterion #4

#4—Identify errors and hazards in care; understand and implement basic safety design principles, such as standardization and simplification and human factors training. (IOM, 2003, p. 59)

Criterion #4 is aimed at safe care. Safety is the gold standard for quality these days. Safety is also something that is very amenable to thinking. *Analysis, logical reasoning, inquisitiveness, predicting,* and *intellectual integrity* are 5 of the 17 CT dimensions necessary to prevent errors and hazards.

Because there is a lot of material in this section, we have provided a road map to help you stay on track. We start with **TACTICS 5-4** to examine a safety issue, error identification, in health care. From there, we (1) discuss errors and hazards that hinder safety and how they are categorized, (2) explore how the current organizational culture influences error identification, and (3) identify solutions for better safety.

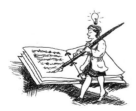

TACTICS 5-4: CT for Assessing Safety

1. Read **Scenario 5-4**.
2. Find the dimensions of thinking that are used and those that are missing.
3. Determine what kinds of errors, if any, are present in this situation.

Scenario 5-4: Safety with Medications

Mr. Davis is being discharged today and has a list of medications he needs to take at home. He has been taking Celexa during his hospital stay. His nurse, Betty, who is staffing five patients today because someone called in sick, is in a rush to give blood and doesn't notice the order for Celebrex instead of Celexa. She asks Sara, who just came on, to help out and finish the discharge teaching for Mr. Davis.

Sara is new to this unit; she examines the discharge meds before going in to teach Mr. Davis. She doesn't recognize the name of one drug on the list, Celebrex, but notices from the chart that it looks like what Mr. Davis has been taking. Sara looks for the drug book to check it out but can't find it. She sees Mr. Davis's doctor rushing off the unit and doesn't want to bother him. She calls the pharmacy, but the line is busy, and just then, Mrs. Davis arrives at the nurses' station.

Mrs. Davis says she has the dog in the car and it's hot outside; she has Mr. Davis all set in the wheelchair and is ready to go. Sara escorts Mr. Davis to the hospital entrance, reminding him to get his prescriptions filled as soon as possible and to call if he has any questions. Mr. Davis goes home with a prescription for Celebrex instead of Celexa.

Discussion

What do you think is the likelihood of this happening? We hope it is not common, but considering the national and international nursing shortage, its potential is rising. Did you find some use of CT dimensions? We came up with these missing CT dimensions. Compare our list with yours, and for all additional dimensions you thought of, give yourself an extra star (or if you're lucky enough to be slim, have chocolate!). If you're not so slim, have the chocolate anyway, but take a break from reading and go for a walk.

Missing Thinking:

■ Insufficient *discrimination* of the different medications by Betty and Sara.
■ Insufficient *applying standards* relative to medication administration by Sara.
■ Beginning *perseverance*, but not enough, by Sara in identifying the medication discrepancy.
■ No *confidence* in her reasoning, as seen when Sara does not pursue her concerns.

As part of our CT, we would look to the system for ways to protect Mr. Davis and other patients from taking the wrong medication. Many groups, such as The Joint Commission and the U.S. Food and Drug Administration, recommend attention to look-alike/sound-alike drugs—that is, medications with similar names, medications with similar packaging, medications that are not commonly used, and commonly used medications that trigger allergic reactions. Attention also should be given to drugs that require close monitoring. Mr. Davis would have benefited from his nurses' CT and attention to medications with similar names.

Also, think about who needs to participate in team thinking about how to decrease medication errors. How could those participants create system strategies to alert staff to commonly misread medication names? What should they think about besides assigning blame to individuals? Hold that thought; we'll talk more about a culture of safety shortly.

Hazards and Errors

The first words in IOM criterion #4 are "Identify errors and hazards in care." We must engage our thinking dimensions to (1) identify and diminish hazards, and (2) minimize errors. Health care is so complex these days that it is foolish to think that things won't go wrong. Once we accept that, we can constructively use *information seeking* and *inquisitiveness* to hunt for hazards and errors and realistically seek to improve safety for patients. Or, as Dr. John Banja, Center for Ethics at Emory University in Atlanta, Georgia, encouraged nurses at the 2008 Michigan nursing summit, "We must accept that the more we are required to make judgments in a complex system, the higher the probability of errors, and the more we need to find ways to close the holes in the Swiss cheese of the healthcare system" (J. Banja, personal communication, July 31, 2008).

Again, we need to examine the concepts. What are hazards? A hazard is an error waiting to happen. Ideally, we will use *predicting* to anticipate hazards and prevent potential errors. And as we examine errors that have occurred with *intellectual integrity* and *logical reasoning*, we can then use *analysis* and *transforming knowledge* to diminish and decrease the probability of future errors.

What is an error? Some prefer the term *complication* because it helps to move away the culture of blaming and redirects us to focus more on thinking about what in the system needs fixing. In general, an error or complication can be collecting insufficient data, making the wrong diagnoses, giving the wrong medications, or providing the wrong treatments by the wrong providers. All of this and more can result in patient outcomes ranging from discomfort, to increased length of stay, to permanent disability, to death. By initially employing *logical reasoning* and *analysis*, critically thinking nurses are key players in identifying the causes of errors. A lot of *reflection* is also useful for this task.

Reason (2000) used the term *failure* to address underlying causes of errors. He identified two types of failure, or causes of errors: *active failure* (acts of commission or omission that have an immediate effect on a patient), or what we typically consider an error; and *latent failure* (aspects of care that may lie dormant initially but lead to errors). Examples of these latent failures are poor communication among all members of the interdisciplinary team, ineffective management and leadership styles, stressful work environments, short staffing, and poorly designed organizational changes (Currie & Watterson, 2007). Additional latent failures have been identified in long-term care settings. Examples of these include high turnover of staff, adversarial regulatory requirements, and a pervasive system of punishment for errors (Gruneir & Mor, 2008).

Root causes of errors also have been addressed by the NQF as (1) latent failures (related to organizational policies, procedures, and resources); (2) active failures (related to actions when directly interacting with patients); (3) organizational system failures (related to management, organizational culture, and communication); and (4) technical failures (related to facilities and external resources) (Mitchell, 2008). Errors have also been labeled as adverse events and near misses.

We like to focus on thinking-related issues that have to do with errors. Cimiotti, Aiken, Sloane, and Wu (2012) studied the relationship among nurse staffing, burnout, and healthcare-associated infection, finding significant relationships between patient-to-nurse staffing ratios, burnout, and patient urinary tract and surgical site infections. Of particular interest was their hypothesis that burnout was associated with "cognitive detachment" in nurses (p. 488). Problems with "cognitive load" and "working memory" were described by Cornell and Riordan (2011, p. 407) in their study of workflow interruptions and task switching among nurses. Studying the work of nurses on a medical–surgical unit and a pediatric oncology unit, these researchers confirmed the complexity of nurses' work flow; "these data imply that nurses continually load and unload patient and procedural data in their working memory" (p. 411). The task switching contributes to a task orientation in work but not to the cognitive processes necessary to good nursing. Cornell and Riordan concluded, "If they wish staff to be more engaged in critical thinking, nurse leaders must institute changes to alter these circumstances" (p. 414).

The dangers of interruptions were also noted by Lewis, Smith, and Williams-Jones (2012), along with factors for staff to think about when contemplating interrupting a nurse: situation (context of what the nurse is doing), significance (how necessary is the interruption), frequency (how often has that nurse been interrupted), timing (medication administration should not be interrupted), and urgency (how important the interruption is). Barriers and enhancers to CT in long-term care were the focus of a survey by Raterink (2011) of staff nurses in three nursing homes. The results of this survey supported earlier studies where nurses identified teamwork and staff support as enhancers or barriers to CT, depending if those factors were present or lacking in the environment.

Adverse Events and Near Misses

We defined *adverse events* and *near misses* at the beginning of this chapter, but we'll repeat them here to refresh your memory as we elaborate on the concepts. An adverse event is "an event that results in unintended harm to the patient by an act of commission or omission rather than by the underlying disease or condition of the patient" (IOM, 2004b, p. 201).

These events (errors) are frequently attributed to the poor design, communication patterns, and organization of the healthcare delivery system, not individuals. Such errors generally lead to incident reports and, if the errors lead to death or permanent injury, a sentinel event report. Nurses and others need "not only the knowledge to recognize an error, but also the *confidence* and communication skills to address the issue with appropriate personnel" (Henneman & Gawlinski, 2004, p. 200). That requires both *confidence* (in reasoning) and *intellectual integrity*.

Near misses are defined as "acts of omission or commission that could have harmed the patient but did not cause harm as a result of chance, prevention or mitigation" (IOM, 2004b, p. 227). Near misses occur frequently, as much as 100 times more often than adverse events. Depending on the organizational culture, near-miss data may or may not be reported. *Perseverance* is important in paying attention to patterns and consistently collecting data that are needed to document those patterns and make changes.

Organizational Culture Influences on Thinking and Error Identification

Changing how we think about hazards and errors is a matter of changing our individual thinking. We have to consider the whole of the healthcare system and, in particular, the culture of the organizational system. Organizations are not inanimate objects; they are groups of people who relate, interact, think, and work together for many hours each day. Organizations, therefore, have all the characteristics of any group of people, including a culture. Cultures have values, beliefs, and attitudes that influence behaviors, such as identifying errors.

Look at your organizational culture. What are the values, beliefs, and attitudes that might be promoting errors? When something goes wrong, do people quickly find someone to blame, or does the thinking go further to other possible factors? Does anyone look for a quick fix? All these factors stifle cognitive inquiry and quality in healthcare organizations. Thinking through errors and their prevention requires thinking together with one's team. (That's a cue to appreciate interdisciplinary teams.)

Although healthcare cultures vary, historically, all have had two traditional beliefs: (1) avoiding all errors is possible, and (2) finding the one or more persons who are to blame for an error is a goal (IOM, 2004a). We must transform our thinking about the myth that we can avoid all errors because it is counterproductive to developing a new culture of safety. Old beliefs and attitudes about perfection and avoiding errors severely limit our ability to collect accurate data for research and decisions on system changes.

We must also move beyond blaming individuals. According to Benner (2001), a culture of blame and shame actually discourages the reporting of errors for fear of punishment and being singled out for responsibility. Organizational cultures that retain values of blaming and pretending that all errors can be avoided ultimately have a much more difficult job of improving quality (Henneman & Gawlinski, 2004). A more effective approach is to move our thinking to a culture of safety.

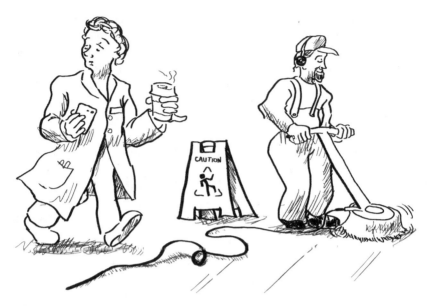

© Jesse Rubenfeld

Culture of Safety and Thinking

Healthcare providers must be open and attentive to finding their errors, errors of others, and errors in the system, and not be overtly or covertly punished in the process. If the current culture hinders that openness and attentiveness, the obvious solution is to change the culture. The question is, change it to what, and how?

A culture of safety is complex. In an attempt to clarify the complexities of a culture of safety, Sammer, Lykens, Singh, Mains, and Lackan (2010) enumerated seven subcultures: leadership, teamwork, evidence based, communication, learning, just, and patient safety. These categories are helpful to address the many aspects of an organization that might be contributing to or hindering their culture of safety. To move an organization toward this complex culture of safety necessitates an equally complex set of thinking dimensions (such as all 17 of the dimensions we've been discussing). All players in the culture have to be involved in that thinking process.

Benner had two suggestions for changing the healthcare culture to a focus on safety. One is to accept the fact that "practice is broader and more flexible than the science and technology that support practice" (2001, p. 283). Clinicians who accept that and educators who teach that will be promoting a culture of safety, one that acknowledges the need for *flexibility* and *contextual perspective* in the CT of providers. Benner's second suggestion was to focus on self-improvement, which requires *reflection*. Both *self-reflection* and *reflection* on the organizational system are essential to changing a culture. We'll discuss this issue of *reflection* in more detail with criterion #5.

Affonso and Doran (2002) also addressed solutions for changing the healthcare culture. Their version calls for revolutionary thinking to develop a science of safety by encouraging creative thinking. Their conceptual framework focuses on patient safety through research, education, and practice by creating conditions for critical thinking, ethical practice, and opportunities for learning.

The IOM's *Keeping Patients Safe: Transforming the Work Environment of Nurses* (2004a) confirms the need for more opportunities for thinking to sustain a culture of safety. An entire chapter of the report ("Creating and Sustaining a Culture of Safety") addressed issues of (1) empowering employees with decision-making rights, (2) encouraging staff to question orders with *confidence*, (3) using *creativity* to think of ways to improve procedures, (4) developing staff members' *prediction* abilities to anticipate adverse events, and (5) being able to use *discrimination* abilities to make decisions and select the best practice interventions. The italics are ours (by now you should know why we added them).

The first two of these issues were echoed in Sayre, McNeese-Smith, Leach, and Phillips' 2012 quasi-experimental study of an educational intervention with nurses that was effective in increasing nurses' speaking-up behaviors. Empowered nurses is also a message in the 2011 IOM report, *The Future of Nursing: Leading Change, Advancing Health*, which stated that nurses should be equal partners in healthcare redesign to promote quality. Empowered, thinking nurses are key players in the quest for improved safety.

Nurses' work schedule characteristics and staffing were the focus of the Trinkoff and colleagues (2011) study of patient mortality in relation to these factors. Long hours and insufficient time off were noted schedule characteristics that contributed to fatigue, and, ultimately, to lapses in patient safety and quality. These researchers recommended offering alternative scheduling to 12-hour shifts. "In addition, nurses need to be able to take breaks (completely relieved breaks) combined with the opportunity to take strategically placed naps because these can improve vigilance and alertness" (p. 7). Tired nurses do not think well!

Nurses' level of education has also been linked to patient outcomes. Blegen, Goode, Park, Vaughn, and Spetz (2013), in a survey using data from 21 hospitals, found that those hospitals with a higher percentage of baccalaureate-prepared nurses had better outcomes, and not just in terms of decreased mortality rates, which have already been associated with higher education. Other outcomes associated with higher education were lower congestive heart failure mortality; fewer decubitus ulcers, incidents of failure to rescue, and postoperative deep vein thrombosis or pulmonary embolism; and shorter length of stay. These researchers noted that their results supported the IOM (2011) recommendation that the percentage of baccalaureate-prepared RNs should increase from 50% to 80% by 2020. Aiken and colleagues (2011), in addition to finding repeated patient quality support for an increased percentage of baccalaureate-prepared nurses, also found that improving work environments made a significant difference to quality.

CT is also essential for transformational leadership and evidence-based management. The IOM (2004a) emphasized the need for top management to "provide time for thinking, learning and training . . . [;] employees must have sufficient time for reflection and analysis . . . Only if top management explicitly frees up employee time for this purpose does learning occur with any regularity" (p. 130). With all this focus on thinking, *reflection*, and *analysis*, it makes us wonder if all 17 of our dimensions could be found if we scrutinized that report.

The AHRQ published *Patient Safety and Quality: An Evidence-Based Handbook for Nurses*. In this document, the authors focused an entire chapter (chapter 6) on the paradigm shift needed to "enable nurses to think more critically . . . to ultimately achieve high-quality care in every care setting and for all patients" (Hughes, 2008, p. vi).

Effective communication among nurses, members of the interdisciplinary team, and the patient and family is essential for this cultural paradigm shift (Bartlett, Blais, Tamblyn, Clermont, & MacGibbon, 2008; Currie & Watterson, 2007; Sherwood & Drenkard, 2007; Whitson et al., 2008). Communication was at issue in *Seminal Event Alert* number 40 (July 9, 2008), which addressed the "Behaviors that Undermine a Culture of Safety" (The Joint Commission, 2008).

So what is the relationship between communication and thinking, and quality care? That is a subject for another book, but let's focus for a minute on the primary thinking dimension needed here, *confidence*. Remember, *confidence* is focused on your reasoning abilities, not simply being able to do something. Nurses who are *confident* in their reasoning know they have *sought information*; they have used *analysis*, along with *contextual perspective*, *predicting*, and even some *transforming knowledge*, to draw some inferences with *logical reasoning*. Nurses who have *confidence* in their reasoning are more likely to share their thinking with the interdisciplinary team and *persevere* in being heard by using appropriate communication skills to achieve quality care outcomes.

Processes for Collecting, Monitoring, and Analyzing Errors

Organizations that are conscious entities operate as living organisms that need to be fed (Wheatley, 1994). Information is their food, informatics is the grocery store, and CT is the digestive system for the organization, allowing the information to be transformed into usable knowledge. To extend our analogy, we need to look at the grocery carts, or devices used to collect the information we want to transform.

Some devices used by the experts to collect data include *root cause analysis*, *near-miss analysis*, and *adverse-events analysis* (IOM, 2004b). After data are collected, CT is used to determine what to monitor and how to analyze the errors that lead to safety gaps.

Root cause analysis is an earlier error identification strategy. This analysis searches for underlying causes or system failures that contribute to errors. The major problem with root cause analysis is that it is done after the fact and is considered too subjective. There is little evidence of its value in actually reducing errors (AHRQ, 1999), yet the analysis continues to be used for tracking errors.

Near-miss analysis examines data about situations in which potential errors were caught before they occurred. The IOM identified three goals for near-miss analysis: (1) modeling (gaining qualitative insight into these types of errors), (2) trending (gaining quantitative insight into the patterns of errors), and (3) mindfulness (maintaining a high level of alertness to dangers). Unfortunately, near-miss analysis data are not routinely collected throughout the United States (IOM, 2004b).

The purposes of adverse-event analysis are to define events that need investigating, to design ways to detect the events, and to determine what data should be collected. Adverse-event analyses help identify events labeled as iatrogenic injuries. The major problem associated with adverse-event analysis is that most events are not reported. The IOM (2004b) recommended three areas for improvement: (1) automated surveillance systems to capture the data, (2) more research to determine the effectiveness of the monitoring, and (3) integration of the data collection systems with patient care standards.

We have designed an adverse-event analysis guideline to emphasize the thinking that is useful in *analyzing* errors. See **Box 5-4** for the guidelines needed to complete **TACTICS 5-5**.

Box 5-4   Guidelines for *Analyzing* CT in an Event

Directions: Circle the number that best represents your conclusion.

	2 Yes, 1 Maybe, 0 No
1. Was the nurse confident in his or her reasoning?	2 1 0
2. Was the whole situation (relationships, background, environment) taken into consideration?	2 1 0
3. Was there adequate consideration of alternatives, even those that were nontraditional or creative?	2 1 0
4. Was the nurse flexible enough?	2 1 0
5. Was the nurse engaged enough to really want to understand fully?	2 1 0
6. Were decisions based on usual practice or bias, or was the truth sought even if it went contrary to usual practice?	2 1 0
7. Were there any intuitive signs of this happening?	2 1 0
8. Were all views considered? (The field was not narrowed too quickly.)	2 1 0
9. Did the nurse keep trying to solve the problem? (The nurse didn't give up too quickly.)	2 1 0

(continues)

Box 5-4 Guidelines for *Analyzing* CT in an Event (continued)

---

10. Was there evidence of anyone standing back and reflecting on what was happening?   2   1   0

11. Was there evidence of the nurse breaking the situation down to better understand what was happening?   2   1   0

12. Were applicable standards upheld?   2   1   0

13. Were similarities or differences among parts of the issue distinguished carefully?   2   1   0

14. Was all possible information gathered?   2   1   0

15. Was there adequate evidence to support the conclusions drawn?   2   1   0

16. Was there evidence that this incident could have been predicted?   2   1   0

17. Was knowledge applied well in this situation?   2   1   0

Total Score: _____

INTERPRET SCORE

0–15:   Deficient CT probably contributed to event.
16–25:   Insufficient CT possibly contributed to event.
26–30:   CT may be insufficient, but consider additional contributing factors.
31–34:   CT was good; consider other contributing factors.

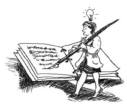

TACTICS 5-5: Thinking through an Adverse Event

Clinicians and Educators

1. Ask nurses or students to record the details of a patient safety incident, paying particular attention to what they were thinking. To maintain anonymity, if that is desired, have those reports typed without names. Even better, have the event voice recorded so verbal nuances can be heard.

2. Give the incident to other nurses to analyze in terms of the CT dimensions.

3. Use the guidelines in Box 5-4 to help with that analysis. If several nurses analyze the same event, the total scores can be compared.

4. Discuss the how and why of each score.

Discussion

How did you and your colleagues do? Were you consistent in your scoring? In the recorded event, which CT dimensions were strong and which could be enhanced? Consider how you could modify this guideline to fit your practice setting or course content. How can you use this to help emphasize the CT needed to improve safe care?

There is an interesting new process for collecting, monitoring, and *analyzing* errors that has addressed a frequently cited problem with nursing-related safety outcomes—that is, the lack of consistent and nursing-specific data gathering and analysis. The State of Ohio Board of Nursing recently instituted a system that responds to that issue: "The time is right for nursing organizations, employers and regulators to more closely collaborate for patient safety" (2010, p. 3).

The Ohio Board of Nursing's work takes up the challenge presented by the National Council of State Boards of Nursing (NCSBN), as reported by Benner and colleagues (2006), to create a national database on nursing errors. A Taxonomy of Error, Root Cause Analysis and Practice Responsibility (TERCAP) was developed that could help classify nursing practice breakdowns in the following categories: safe administration of medication, documentation, attentiveness and surveillance, clinical reasoning, prevention, intervention, interpretation of authorized providers' orders, and professional responsibility (Benner et al., 2006). The Ohio initiative was also based on the principles of just culture as outlined by Griffith (2009).

Taking what at first might seem a simplistic approach to determining quality from a process prospective, McHugh and Stimpfel asked nurses about their perceptions of quality and found that a "10% increment in the proportion of nurses reporting excellent quality of care was associated with lower odds of mortality and failure to rescue; greater patient satisfaction; and higher composite process of care scores for acute myocardial infarction, pneumonia, and surgical patients" (2012, p. 566). McHugh and Stimpfel postulated that, because nurses spent extended time with patients and could directly observe that care, their perceptions were a valid answer to the obstacles to measuring healthcare quality. They posed one simple question to nurses: "How would you describe the quality of nursing care delivered to patients in your unit?" (p. 567) They then used discharge databases of 396 hospitals in a four-state region to look at the patient outcomes in relation to nurses' perceptions of quality.

Their findings were consistent with those found by Aiken and colleagues (2011), who also asked nurses questions about quality.

Safety Goals

Part of IOM criterion #4 recommended implementing basic safety design principles. The IOM (2004b) began the process by designing safety goals. The Joint Commission established and updated yearly patient safety goals for various healthcare settings, including hospitals (2013a).

These patient safety goals require informatics to collect (*information seeking*), monitor, and interpret the aggregate data (*analysis* and *logical reasoning*), think about underlying system problems (*reflection* and *inquisitiveness*), and develop strategies to achieve safety goals (*flexibility, creativity, transforming knowledge, intuition, contextual perspective, perseverance,* and so forth). You get the picture?

IOM Criterion #5

#5—Both act as an effective member of the interdisciplinary team and improve the quality of one's own performance through self assessment and personal change. (IOM, 2003, p. 59)

This last criterion addresses CT directly; it refers to self-assessment or *reflection*, which is one of the 10 CT habits of the mind and has been defined as "contemplation upon a subject, especially one's assumptions, and thinking for the purposes of deeper understanding and self evaluation" (Scheffer & Rubenfeld, 2000, p. 358).

The standard version of self-assessment (*reflection*) is typically done independently. *Reflection* encourages us to look back at our actions, behaviors, biases, and faulty reasoning. *Reflection* helps us find things we missed, consider things we want to work on differently, see patterns that we did not recognize initially, wonder about solutions we did not consider at the time, and, yes, even celebrate when our thinking was brilliant!

But self-assessment is enhanced when it is validated by thinking and input from other perspectives. Brookfield (1995) identified four lenses, or sources of feedback for *reflection*: autobiography, theory, students, and colleagues. Each lens is considered to have equal value during *reflection*. Each lens provides the educator or clinician with another point of view from which he or she can make comparisons and see patterns that confirm or discount what one or more of the other lenses reflects.

Self-Assessment for Educators and Clinicians

Brookfield's (1995) four lenses of *reflection* can easily be used by educators or clinicians. **Scenario 5-5** describes a shortened version of a clinician's use of the four lenses.

Scenario 5-5: Using Four Lenses for Reflection

Carol has been the nurse manager on an inpatient 24-bed psychiatric unit for the past 3 months. She has been trying to implement changes in interdisciplinary teamwork and wonders why the staff show little interest or do not follow through on plans after each staff meeting. She decides to do some reflection to better understand what is happening. Over the course of the next few weeks, she uses all four lenses.

Autobiographical lens: Carol considered herself a facilitative leader and promoter of collaboration. She took a continuing education course in leadership last year and went back to her notes to check off all the things the course recommended. She was doing them. From her perspective, she was doing all the right things.

Patient/staff lens: Carol asked some staff members what they thought about her leadership. They told her she was doing a great job. It appeared the staff thought she was doing well, but she wondered if they were just being nice. She didn't ask patients.

Theoretical lens: Carol decided she would get on the Internet. She obtained more updated information on management and leadership. She found others who were having similar problems with getting changes made. Carol found extensive information about management and about interdisciplinary teams. She read the management material, tried to schedule meetings more conveniently, and gave the staff copies of everything she downloaded about interdisciplinary teams.

The results were the same. The staff were not following through.

Colleague's lens: Carol remembered she had one more lens to use. She asked a colleague to sit in on the next few meetings and give her feedback. After the third meeting, the colleague's feedback included, "Have you ever noticed how often you interrupt your staff with your own ideas?" The colleague also suggested how Carol might assign staff to search out reasons why interdisciplinary teamwork such as this would encourage their more active participation. Her colleague reminded her about the discovery learning workshop they had attended.

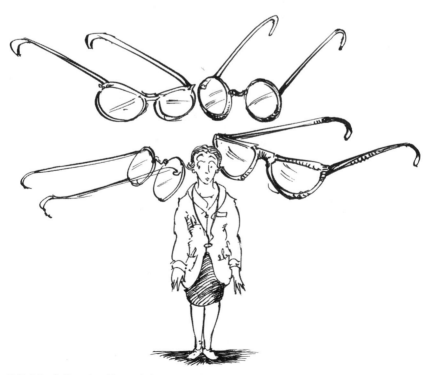

Self-reflection's multiple lenses allow clinicians and educators to examine and think about their practice and teach more effectively and accurately. We must, however, consciously and actively create opportunities to combine our thinking with the thinking of colleagues, patients, and students, and use the best available evidence to achieve the level of self-assessment that will more accurately lead to quality improvement. Again, we believe the IOM would endorse this kind of *reflection* for clinicians as well as educators.

Summary of the Five IOM Criteria for Quality Improvement

Our journey of thinking through the five IOM criteria for quality improvement has only begun. (And you thought this was the end!) To achieve quality through safe, effective, and efficient care, we need to continually reflect on these criteria and use all dimensions of our CT to make them a reality in practice. Educators must incorporate these criteria into curricula if future practitioners are to effectively apply quality improvement strategies.

We have one last TACTIC to illustrate how CT, the five IOM criteria for achieving quality improvement, and the five IOM competencies all come together.

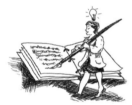

TACTICS 5-6: Quality Care through CT

Read the following questions and answer them as you read and reflect on **Scenario 5-6**.

1. Which of the 17 thinking dimensions were demonstrated in the scenario?
2. How did Jeff achieve the five IOM criteria for quality improvement?
3. Which of the five IOM competencies (patient-centered care, interdisciplinary care, EBP, informatics, and quality improvement; see Box 5-3) were demonstrated in the scenario? How could you have improved on them?

Scenario 5-6: Quality Care through Individual and Team Thinking

Jeff is a rural parish nurse. His clinic, 200 miles from the nearest hospital, includes a team of nurses, social workers, an NP, and physical therapists. Contact with the hospital is by phone, email, and fax. Jeff was scheduled to visit Mr. Youngblood, a 60-year-old single farmer, on his first day home from the hospital, where he'd had a bowel resection for diverticulitis. He has a temporary colostomy.

Faxed orders for an initial home visit were for colostomy care. It had been some time since Jeff had done colostomy care, so he got on the Internet to check for

EBP guidelines and called the Wound, Ostomy and Continence Nurses Society for help. Based on the information he found and feedback from the team, he questioned the frequency of the ordered bowel irrigations. He contacted the doctor and explained his concerns, and the order was changed.

The social worker knew Mr. Youngblood and provided information about his healthcare beliefs and how much he valued his privacy. The team would meet again after Jeff's first visit to modify and adjust care planning.

Mr. Youngblood lived about 50 miles from the clinic. He had no phone, but Jeff left a message at the hospital before discharge to tell him the visit would be in the afternoon of his day of discharge.

Based on past experiences with patients in rural areas, Jeff stocked his truck with a variety of items just in case there were some unexpected circumstances. He knew that not all homes had all the amenities needed for standard healthcare procedures. He made sure his cell phone was fully charged even though he would be able to use it only when he was on the tops of the mountain ridges.

When Jeff arrived, he found Mr. Youngblood sitting on his porch. He was sleeping in his rocking chair and needed physical contact to be aroused. With permission, Jeff began his assessment with vital signs. Although Mr. Youngblood was still weak from surgery, the assessment indicated that all systems were within normal limits, with the exception of elimination and possibly his hearing. Assessment of the home environment revealed no indoor plumbing, and water was brought to the house daily from a nearby stream. The home itself was neat and clean, and he had adequate food supplies. Mr. Youngblood still drove. His nearest neighbor was 2 miles away.

Mr. Youngblood convinced his physician to discharge him early because he believed he would heal more quickly at home, with the fresh air and peace and quiet that did not exist in the hospital. Besides, he did not believe it was good to have young female nurses doing what needed to be done. Mr. Youngblood was also adamant that he couldn't be bothered by doing "all this colostomy stuff more than once a day" because he needed to be in the fields all day long. Jeff did not remind him that work in the fields was probably going to have to wait until his strength returned.

Encouraging Mr. Youngblood to help with the problem solving, they worked out a plan for colostomy care that respected Mr. Youngblood's dignity, personal prefer- ences, and need for quality colostomy care. The plan included Jeff filling empty gallon milk containers with spring water and bringing them to the house to use for irrigation. Because of inadequate lighting in the house, they worked out a plan to do the irrigations and dressing changes by the window that received the best morning light, using an old bucket from the barn for the irrigation waste.

Disposing of the waste in the bucket was a concern. Mr. Youngblood told him not to worry. Jeff had a feeling that Mr. Youngblood, who had been very independent all his life, would try to solve this on his own. Jeff returned to the barn and found an old wagon that still worked. Until his strength returned, Mr. Young-blood agreed to use the bucket in the house, take it outside to the wagon at the end of the porch, and pull it to the outhouse to be dumped. Suspecting that Mr. Youngblood might still try to carry the bucket on his own, Jeff asked him to promise to use the wagon for at least the first few weeks. He reluctantly agreed. Extra gallon water jugs were left by the outhouse for rinsing the bucket.

After returning to the office, Jeff realized that he had misread Mr. Youngblood's antibiotic prescription. He had read "iii" on the Rx as "ii" because of the fuzziness of the fax. He visited the next day to correct his error and notified the physician. Jeff told the team to pay close attention to faxed information in all future orders.

Mr. Youngblood's strength gradually returned; he did use the wagon for a week until he was stronger and able to carry the bucket. He continued to do safe colos-tomy care with no complications and take the correct dosage of his antibiotic. His second surgery to reconnect his bowel was successful. Jeff continued to visit to monitor progress, working with the healthcare team and following Mr. Young-blood's preferences. Further assessment revealed that Mr. Youngblood was losing his hearing, but he refused suggestions for a hearing test. The team respected his wishes in spite of the increased risk to his safety while living alone.

Discussion

Thinking Used:

Transforming knowledge was demonstrated when Jeff had to adapt what he knew were normal procedures for colostomy care in a hospital to a rural environment with fewer resources.

Confidence was demonstrated in challenging the physician's order for frequency of bowel irrigations.

Contextual perspective was demonstrated when Jeff assessed the home environment and Mr. Youngblood's healthcare beliefs and incorporated the input from the social worker.

Creativity was demonstrated when Jeff and Mr. Youngblood came up with several plans for using the available resources to achieve safe care.

Predicting was demonstrated when Jeff thought about the extra supplies he might need in a rural setting.

Intuition was demonstrated when Jeff suspected that Mr. Youngblood would try to be too independent before his strength returned.

Five IOM Criteria for Achieving Quality Improvement

#1—Jeff considered structure by taking into consideration Mr. Youngblood's preferences and his environment. He paid attention to process in his interactions with Mr. Youngblood and the other healthcare providers. He monitored outcomes in the form of Mr. Youngblood's tolerance for the medications, his ability to stay infection free, and his ability to maintain a quality of life that he preferred.

#2—Jeff assessed current practice and searched for better practice when he used the Internet and conferred with his colleagues for the best approaches.

#3—Jeff very creatively designed and monitored his interventions for effectiveness.

#4—Jeff identified his error and the defect in the fax system. He took steps to avoid this adverse event in the future.

#5—Jeff's scenario does not highlight *reflection*, but we will assume he did so when he realized the medication error.

IOM Competencies Addressed

Patient-centered care was demonstrated when Jeff worked to meet Mr. Youngblood's desire to be home during his recovery, and Jeff did not push Mr. Youngblood to follow up on his hearing loss after it was clear that he preferred not to.

Interdisciplinary teamwork was demonstrated when Jeff consulted with the nursing team, the physician, and the social worker, and together they created a plan.

EBP was demonstrated when Jeff searched the Internet for current guidelines for colostomy care.

Informatics utilization was demonstrated when Jeff used the Internet and the fax machine for information.

Applying quality improvement was demonstrated when Jeff provided safe, effective, and efficient care in Mr. Youngblood's home environment. He also applied quality improvement by recognizing a medication error, fixing the error, and addressing the system problem that created it.

Nurses Are Safety Champions for Enhancing Quality and Safety Through Thinking

Look back to the first page of this chapter and put your face in the safety champion picture! You—the nursing student, the practicing nurse, the nurse educator, the education coordinator—are a safety champion. You are developing, or have, the CT skills to keep patients safe and provide the best quality care possible. The nursing literature is beginning to use the term *champion* in relationship to nursing's role in promoting quality care (Mastal et al., 2007; Miller & Chaboyer, 2006). As Miller and Chaboyer stated, "Nurses cannot afford to remain on the periphery of the patient safety movement but must actively engage with it at personal, institutional and professional levels" (p. 266). You are not alone in this mission, but you will need to continually use your CT to facilitate interdisciplinary thinking and systems thinking to make this work. The following are some recommendations to consider along with our thinking:

■ Expand research to address issues of quality and safety beyond the acute care setting. It must include home care, long-term care, outpatient settings, and palliative care. Better measures are needed to address nursing-sensitive outcomes and positive versus negative outcomes.

■ Consider whole systems, including structure and process, not just the outcomes.

■ Recognize that measuring processes is challenging, but we must find a way.

■ Help CEOs and CNOs recognize and appreciate the impact that nurses and the nursing shortage have on quality and safety.

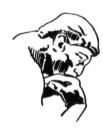

© Jesse Rubenfeld

PAUSE and Ponder

Safety Champions of Quality Improvement

Well, here we are at the end of the chapter. Because safe, quality care is the ultimate outcome we seek, it's important to make it the first chapter in our study about the thinking required for the five IOM competencies. If we know what we are aiming for, we are more likely to know when we have achieved it! The current healthcare situation regarding the number of deaths resulting from errors is not tolerable. Engaging thinking to achieve quality and safe patient care is mandatory. What will the future of quality improvement hold? How are you and other providers going to take up the challenge and become the safety champions of quality improvement and safe patient care? You are the providers who will take care of us and our families (and your families) and educate future providers, so we have a vested interest in cultivating all your CT skills and habits of mind to achieve the quality outcomes we want. We believe you are up to the challenge of being a safety champion.

REFLECTION CUES

■ "Quality is the degree to which health services for individuals and populations increase the likelihood of desired health outcomes and are consistent with current professional knowledge" (IOM, 1990, p. 4).

■ Errors in health care have led to as many as 98,000 deaths a year.

■ Structure, process, and outcomes remain valuable concepts in health care but are more valuable when all three are looked at as a whole.

- When we accept that errors will occur, we can constructively look for errors and hazards and realistically seek to improve safety for patients.
- *Near misses* and *adverse events* are frequently attributed to the poor design, communication patterns, and organization of the healthcare delivery system, not individuals.
- *Root cause analysis, near-miss analysis,* and *adverse-event analysis* are three strategies for collecting the data necessary to improve systems to decrease errors.
- Refocusing our thinking toward prevention of errors and identifying system problems, as opposed to blaming individuals, is essential.
- Changing the organizational culture to a culture of safety requires thinking from individuals, administration, and the interdisciplinary team to change values, attitudes, and beliefs about errors.
- Thinking remains the key to applying quality improvement in health care to achieve patient-centered, effective, safe, timely, efficient, and equitable care.
- Matching the data with conclusions, matching the right provider to patient needs, and matching appropriate tests and procedures to patient conditions are essential aspects of effective care.
- Old beliefs and attitudes about perfection and avoiding errors severely limit our ability to collect accurate data for research and for making decisions about system changes.
- Improvements in quality require nurses to be safety champions who (1) use all 17 dimensions of CT in both practice and education, (2) focus on the five IOM criteria for achieving quality, and (3) address the six IOM aims for high-quality healthcare systems.

REFERENCES

Affonso, D. D., & Doran, D. (2002). Cultivating discoveries in patient safety research: A framework. *International Nursing Perspectives, 2*(1), 33–47.

Agency for Healthcare Research and Quality. (1999). *Making healthcare safer: A critical analysis of patient safety practices.* Rockville, MD: Author.

Agency for Healthcare Research and Quality. (2003). *AHRQ quality indicators.* Retrieved from www .qualityindicators.ahrq.gov/downloads/modules/psi/v32/psi_technical_specs_v32.pdf

Aiken, L. H., Cimiotti, J. P., Sloane, D. M., Smith, H. L., Flynn, L., & Neff, D. F. (2011). Effects of nurse staffing and nurse education on patient deaths in hospitals with different nurse work environments. *Medical Care, 49,* 1047–1053.

Alexander, G. R. (2007). Nursing sensitive databases: Their existence, challenges, and importance. *Medical Care Research and Review, 64*(44), 44S–63S. doi:10.1177/1077558707299244

American Association of Colleges of Nursing. (2006). Hallmarks of quality and patient safety: Recommended baccalaureate competencies and curricular guidelines to ensure high quality and safe patient care. *Journal of Professional Nursing, 22,* 329–330.

American Association of Colleges of Nursing. (2008). *The essentials of baccalaureate education for professional nursing practice.* Washington, DC: Author.

American Association of Colleges of Nursing QSEN Education Consortium. (2012, September 24). *Graduate-level QSEN competencies: Knowledge, skills and attitudes.* Retrieved from www.aacn.nche .edu/faculty/qsen/competencies.pdf

Bargagliotti, L. A., & Lancaster, J. (2007). Quality and safety education in nursing: More than new wine in old skins. *Nursing Outlook, 55,* 156–158.

Bartlett, G., Blais, R., Tamblyn, R., Clermont, R. J., & MacGibbon, B. (2008). Impact of patient communication problems on the risk of preventable adverse events in acute care settings. *Canadian Medical Association Journal, 178,* 1555–1562.

Benner, P. (2001). Creating a culture of safety and improvement: A key to reducing medical error. *American Journal of Critical Care, 10,* 281–284.

Benner, P., Malloch, K., Sheets, V., Bitz, K., Emrich, L., Thomas, M. B., . . . Farrell, M. (2006). TERCAP: Creating a national database on nursing errors. *Harvard Health Policy Review, 7*(1), 28–43.

Blegen, M. A., Goode, C. J., Park, S. H., Vaughn, T., & Spetz, J. (2013). Baccalaureate education in nursing and patient outcomes. *The Journal of Nursing Administration, 43*(2), 89–94. doi: 10.1097 /NNA.0b013e31827f2028

BrainyQuote. (2013). *Curiosity quotes.* Retrieved from http://www.brainyquote.com/quotes/keywords /curiosity.html

Brookfield, S. D. (1995). *Becoming a critically reflective teacher.* San Francisco, CA: Jossey-Bass.

Brooten, D., & Youngblut, J. M. (2006). Nurse dose as a concept. *Journal of Nursing Scholarship, 38,* 94–99.

Buerhaus, P. I., Donelan, K., Ulrich, B. T., Norman, L., DesRoches, C., & Dittus, R. (2007). Impact of the nurse shortage on hospital patient care: Comparative perspectives. *Health Affairs, 26,* 853–862. doi:10.1377/hlthaff.26.3.853

Burhans, L. D. (2007). What is quality? Do we agree, and does it matter? *Journal of Healthcare Quality, 29,* 39–54.

Cimiotti, J. P., Aiken, L. H., Sloane, D. M., & Wu, E. S. (2012). Nurse staffing, burnout, and health care-associated infection. *American Journal of Infection Control, 40,* 486–490. doi: 10.1016/j.ajic.2012.02.029

Cornell, P., & Riordan, M. (2011). Barriers to critical thinking: Workflow interruptions and task switching among nurses. *The Journal of Nursing Administration, 41*(10), 407–414. doi: 10.1097/ NNA.0b013e31822edd42

Cronenwett, L., Sherwood, G., Barnsteiner, J., Disch, J., Johnson, J., Mitchell, P., . . . Warren, J. (2007). Quality and Safety Education for Nurses. *Nursing Outlook, 55,* 122–131.

Currie, L., & Watterson, L. (2007). Challenges in delivering safe patient care: A commentary on a quality improvement initiative. *Journal of Nursing Management, 15,* 162–168.

Davies, S., & Cripacc, D. G. (2008). Supporting quality improvement in care homes for older people: The contribution of primary care nurses. *Journal of Nursing Management, 16,* 115–120.

Donaldson, L., & Philip, P. (2004). Patient safety—a global priority. *Bulletin of the World Health Organization, 82,* 892–893.

Forneris, S. G., Crownover, J. G., Dorsey, L., Leahy, N., Maas, N. A., Wong, L., . . . Zavertnik, J. E. (2012). Integrating QSEN and ACES: An NLN simulation leader project. *Nursing Education Perspectives, 33*(3), 184–187.

Griffith, K. S. (2009). Column: The growth of a just culture. *The Joint Commission Perspectives on Patient Safety, 9*(12), 26–27. Retrieved from http://legacy.justculture.org/media/Joint_Commission -Just_Culture.pdf

Gruneir, A., & Mor, V. (2008). Nursing home safety: Current issues and barriers to improvement. *Annual Review of Public Health, 29,* 369–382.

Handler, A., Issel, M., & Turnock, B. (2001). A conceptual framework to measure performance of the public health system. *American Journal of Public Health, 92,* 1235–1239.

Henneman, E. A., & Gawlinski, A. (2004). A "near-miss" model for describing the nurse's role in the recovery of medical errors. *Journal of Professional Nursing, 20,* 196–201.

Hughes, R. G. (2008, April). *Patient safety and quality: An evidence-based handbook for nurses.* Rockville, MD: Agency for Healthcare Research and Quality. (AHRQ Publication No. 08-0043)

Institute of Medicine. (1990). *Medicare: A strategy for quality assurance: Executive summary IOM committee to design a strategy for quality review and assurance in Medicare.* Washington, DC: National Academies Press.

Institute of Medicine. (2000). *To err is human: Building a safer health system.* Washington, DC: National Academies Press.

Institute of Medicine. (2001). *Crossing the quality chasm: A new health system for the 21st century.* Washington, DC: National Academies Press.

Institute of Medicine. (2003). *Health professions education: A bridge to quality.* Washington, DC: National Academies Press.

Institute of Medicine. (2004a). *Keeping patients safe: Transforming the work environment of nurses.* Washington, DC: National Academies Press.

Institute of Medicine. (2004b). *Patient safety: Achieving a new standard for care.* Washington, DC: National Academies Press.

Institute of Medicine. (2011). *The future of nursing: Leading change, advancing health.* Washington, DC: National Academies Press.

The Joint Commission. (2008). Behaviors that undermine a culture of safety. *Joint Commission Sentinel Event Alert, 40.* Retrieved from http://www.jointcommission.org /sentinel_event_alert_issue_40_behaviors_that_undermine_a_culture_of_safety/

The Joint Commission. (2013a). *National patient safety goals.* Retrieved from hhttp://www.jointcommission. org/standards_information/npsgs.aspx

The Joint Commission. (2013b). *Sentinel event.* Retrieved from http://www.jointcommission.org/sentinel_ event.aspx

Kelly, L., & Vincent, D. (2010). The dimensions of nursing surveillance: A concept analysis. *Journal of Advanced Nursing, 67*(3), 652–661. doi: 10.1111/j.1365-2648.2010.05525.x

Kurtzman, E. T., & Corrigan, J. M. (2007). Measuring the contribution of nursing to quality, patient safety, and health care outcomes. *Policy, Politics, & Nursing Practice, 8*(20), 20–36. doi: 10.1177/1527154407302115

Leape, L. L., Berwick, D. M., & Bates, D. W. (2002). What practices will most improve safety? Evidence-based medicine meets patient safety. *Journal of the American Medical Association, 288,* 501–507.

Legislative Counsel. (2010). Patient Protection and Affordable Care Act: Health-related portions of the Health Care and Education Reconciliation Act of 2010. Retrieved from http://housedocs.house.gov /energycommerce/ppacacon.pdf

Lewis, T. P., Smith, C. B., & Williams-Jones, P. (2012). Tips to reduce dangerous interruptions by healthcare staff. *Nursing 2012, 42*(11), 65–67. doi: 10.1097/01.NURSE.0000421387.36112.e0

Lundquist, M. J., & Axelsson, A. (2007). Nurses' perceptions of quality assurance. *Journal of Nursing Management, 15,* 51–58.

Lynn, J., West, J., Hausmann, S., Gifford, D., Nelson, R., McGann, P., . . . Ryan, J. A. (2007). Collaborative clinical quality improvement for pressure ulcers in nursing homes. *Journal of the American Geriatric Society, 55,* 1663–1669.

Mastal, M. G., Joshi, M., & Schulke, K. (2007). Nursing leadership: Championing quality and patient safety in the boardroom. *Nursing Economics, 25,* 323–330.

McBride-Henry, K., & Foureur, M. (2007). A secondary care nursing perspective on medication administration safety. *Journal of Advanced Nursing, 60,* 58–66.

McHugh, M. D., & Stimpfel, A. W. (2012). Nurse reported quality of care: A measure of hospital quality. *Research in Nursing and Health, 35,* 566–575. doi: 10.1002/nur.21503

Melichar, L. (2007). Introduction: Improving health care in America through nursing quality measurement research. *Medical Care Research and Review, 64*(3), 3S–9S. doi:10.1177/1077558707299673

Miller, A., & Chaboyer, W. (2006). Captain and champion: Nurses' role in patient safety. *British Association of Critical Care Nurses, Nursing in Critical Care, 11,* 265–266.

Mitchell, P. H. (2008). Defining patient safety and quality care. In R. G. Hughes (Ed.), *Patient safety and quality: An evidence-based handbook for nurses* (Vol. 1, pp. 1-1–1-5, Publication No. 08-0043). Rockville, MD: Agency for Healthcare Research and Quality.

Mitty, E. (2007). Hastings Center special report: The ethics of using QI methods to improve health care quality and safety. *Journal of Nursing Care Quality, 22,* 97–101.

Naylor, M. D. (2007). Advancing the science in the measurement of health care quality influenced by nurses. *Medical Care Research and Review, 64*(144), 144S–169S. doi: 10.1177/1077558707299257

Needleman, J., Kurtzman, E. T., & Kizer, K. W. (2007). Performance measurement of nursing care: State of the science and the current consensus. *Medical Care Research and Review, 64*(10), 10S–43S. doi:10.1177/1077558707299260

Newhouse, R., & Poe, S. (Eds.). (2005). *Measuring patient safety.* Sudbury, MA: Jones and Bartlett.

Office of Inspector General. (2010, November). *Adverse events in hospitals: National incidence among Medicare beneficiaries.* (OEI-06-09-00090). Washington, DC: U.S. Department of Health and Human Services. Retrieved from https://oig.hhs.gov/oei/reports/oei-06-09-00090.pdf

Ohio Board of Nursing. (2010). *Patient safety initiative: Creating a culture of safety and accountability.* Retrieved from http://www.nursing.ohio.gov/PDFS/Discipline/PatientSafety/PSI-Booklet01212011.pdf

Plsek, P. (2003, January). *Complexity and the adoptions of innovation in healthcare.* Paper presented at the National Institute for Healthcare Management Foundation and National Committee for Quality Healthcare conference, Accelerating Quality Improvement in Healthcare Strategies to Speed the Diffusion of Evidence-Based Innovations, Washington, DC.

Pronovost, P. J. (2004, March). *Healthcare safety and quality revolution.* Presentation at the American Association of Colleges of Nursing spring annual meeting, Washington, DC.

Raterink, G. (2011). Critical thinking: Reported enhancers and barriers by nurses in long-term care: Implications for staff development. *Journal for Nurses in Staff Development, 27*(3), 136–142. doi: 10.1097/NND.0b013e318217b3f3

Reason, J. (2000). Human error: Models and management. *British Medical Journal, 320,* 768–770.

Ridley, R. T. (2008). The relationship between nurse education level and patient safety: An integrative review. *Journal of Nursing Education, 47,* 149–156.

Sammer, C. E., Lykens, K., Singh, K. P., Mains, D. A., & Lackan, N. A. (2010). What is patient safety culture? A review of the literature. *Journal of Nursing Scholarship, 42*(2), 156–165. doi: 10.1111/j.1547-5069.2009.01330.x

Sayre, M. M., McNeese-Smith, D., Leach, L. S., & Phillips, L. R. (2012). An educational intervention to increase "speaking-up" behaviors in nurses and improve patient safety. *Journal of Nursing Care Quality, 27*(2), 154–160. doi: 10.1097/NCQ.0b013e318241d9ff

Scheffer, B. K., & Rubenfeld, M. G. (2000). A consensus statement on critical thinking in nursing. *Journal of Nursing Education, 39,* 352–359.

Schmalenberg, C., & Kramer, M. (2008). Essentials of a productive nurse work environment. *Nursing Research, 57,* 2–13.

Sherwood, G., & Drenkard, K. (2007). Quality and safety curricula in nursing education: Matching practice realities. *Nursing Outlook, 55,* 151–155.

Shever, L. L., Titler, M. G., Kerr, P., Qin, R., Taikyoung, K., & Picone, D. M. (2008). The effect of high nursing surveillance on hospital cost. *Journal of Nursing Scholarship, 40,* 161–169.

Shortell, S. M., Bennett, C. L., & Byck, G. R. (1998). Assessing the impact of continuous quality improvement on clinical practice: What it will take to accelerate progress. *The Milbank Quarterly, 76,* 755–757.

Trinkoff, A. M., Johantgen, M., Storr, C. L., Gurses, A. P., Liang, Y., & Han, K. (2011). Nurses' work schedule characteristics, nurse staffing, and patient mortality. *Nursing Research, 60*(1), 1–8. doi: 10.1097/NNR.0b013e3181fff15d

U.S. Department of Health and Human Services. (2012, April). 2012 annual progress report to Congress: National strategy for quality improvement in health care. Retrieved from http://www.ahrq.gov/workingforquality/nqs/nqs2012annlrpt.pdf

Wheatley, M. J. (1994). *Leadership and the new science: Learning about organization from an orderly universe.* San Francisco, CA: Berrett-Koehler.

Whitson, H. E., Hastings, S. N., Lekan, D. A., Sloane, R., White, H. K., & McConnell, E. S. (2008). A quality improvement program to enhance after-hours telephone communication between nurses and physicians in a long-term care facility. *Journal of the American Geriatric Society, 56,* 1080–1086.

Wise, L. C. (2007). Ethical issues surrounding quality improvement activities. *Journal of Nursing Administration, 37,* 272–278.

Zrelak, P. A., Utter, G. H., Sadeghi, B., Cuny, J., Baron, R., & Romano, P. S. (2012). Using the Agency for Healthcare Research and Quality patient safety indicators for targeting nursing quality improvement. *Journal of Nursing Care Quality, 27*(2), 99–108. doi: 10.1097/NCQ.0b013e318237e0e3

CHAPTER 6

Critical Thinking and Patient-Centered Care

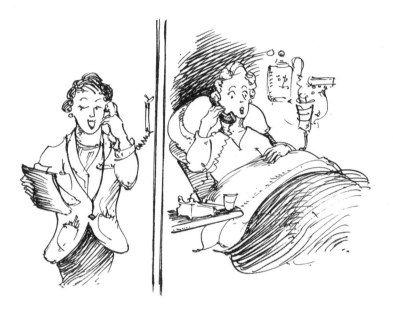

'OH... MS. McGREGOR LOOKS GOOD. HER BLOOD PRESSURE IS DOWN AND SHE'LL BE DISCHARGED IN A DAY OR TWO!'

Perhaps you heard the joke that went around before strict patient privacy laws were instituted. It goes something like this: One night the nurse on the 600 unit gets a phone call from somebody asking about Mary McGregor. The nurse grabs the chart and says, "Oh, Ms. McGregor looks good. Her blood pressure is down and she'll be discharged in a day or two!" The caller replies with obvious glee, "Oh, thank you." The nurse asks, "Are you a relative?" to which the caller replies, "No, I'm Mary McGregor and I haven't been able to get anyone to tell me anything about how I'm doing." Funny as it is, if the Institute of Medicine (IOM) gets its way, no one will be able to relate to that joke because it will be so preposterous.

Providing patient-centered care has been defined by the IOM (2003) as being able to

> identify, respect, and care about patients' differences, values, preferences, and expressed needs; relieve pain and suffering; coordinate continuous care; listen to, clearly inform, communicate with, and educate patients; *share decision making* [italics added] and management; and continuously advocate disease prevention, wellness, and promotion of healthy lifestyles, including a focus on population health. (p. 4)

The italicized words highlight how nurses' critical thinking (CT) interfaces with patients' CT. In this chapter, we focus on the thinking involved in patient-centered care. But first, let's consider circumstances that probably instigated our joke. And we'll look at the state of patient–provider relationships and why this IOM competency is so important. (It is important, you know, not just for being nice, but to improve patient satisfaction and outcomes.) For providers who have not yet made this paradigm shift, patient-centered care will require a drastic modification in their thinking about the relationship between patients and providers.

Changing Patient–Provider Relationships

Let's take a look at that traditional patient–provider relationship. As a patient, what decisions have you made about your health issues? Have you ever had a health provider dismiss you when you offered what you thought was a reasonable solution to your health problem? Worse yet, have you had a provider remind you that he or she knows better and that you should do what you're told? How did you feel? Angry? Stupid? Inept? Devalued? All of the above? These situations exemplify the all-powerful and disrespectful healthcare provider. And, until confronted about their behavior, most healthcare providers who behave this way are usually oblivious to other options for patient–provider relationships.

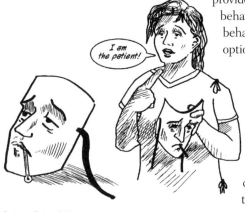

When the IOM vision becomes a reality, healthcare professionals and patients will work in partnerships. In this new relationship, they will respect each other for having different, but valuable, knowledge. In the IOM version of patient-centered care, patients will no longer tolerate the traditional relationship. They will expect care tailored to their

© Jesse Rubenfeld

individual needs. Providers, in turn, will expect patients to do sophisticated research on the Internet, think through their health situations, and come up with conclusions and questions that they will expect to have considered. Gone will be the days when health providers are viewed as all-knowing.

Patient-centered care is not just an IOM concept, nor is it a new one. Some of you, especially those practicing in mental health, will remember the tenets of Hildegard Peplau (the mother of psychiatric nursing) regarding the collaborative relationship required between patient and nurse to achieve what we now call patient-centered care (Peplau, 1952). These days the literature is full of a mixture of terminology describing what the IOM calls patient-centered care. See **Box 6-1** for the lingo related to this concept.

Box 6-1 Lingo Related to Patient-Centered Care

Lingo/Terminology	*Sources*
Client centered	Brown, McWilliam, & Ward-Griffin, 2006; deWitte, Schoot, & Proot, 2006
Consumer specialist	Calabretta, 2002
Informative relations	Benbassat, Pilpel, & Tidhar, 1998
Partnerships	Enehaug, 2000; Lee, 2007
Patient-centered care	Campinha-Bacote, 2011; Disch, 2012; Epstein & Street, 2011; Fiester, 2012; Fights, 2012; Fredericks et al., 2012; Van Mossel, Alford, & Watson, 2011
Patient-centered healthcare	Stichler, 2011
Patient engagement	Barello, Graffigna, & Vegni, 2012
Patient-, family- and population-centered interprofessional care	Cipriano, 2012
Patient-focused care	McCauley & Irwin, 2006; Medina, 2006
Person-centered care	Crandall, White, Schuldheis, & Talerico, 2007; Landers & McCarthy, 2007; McCormack, 2004; McCormack & McCance, 2006; Pope, 2012; Rosemond, Hanson, Ennett, Schenck, & Weiner, 2012
Person centeredness	McCance, McCormack, & Dewing, 2011; Saha, Beach, & Cooper, 2008
Person-centered framework	McGilton et al., 2012
Relationship-based care	Cropley, 2012; Woolley et al., 2012
Relationship-centered care	Nolan, Davies, Brown, Keady, & Nolan, 2004
Service partnership	Buch & Edgren, 2001

Under a variety of other terms, this movement has been studied from moral and ethical perspectives (Hewitt-Taylor, 2003), with a consumer specialist focus (Calabretta, 2002), and as a service partnership (Buch & Edgren, 2001). McCauley and Irwin called it "care we would want for our own family members" (2006, p. 1573). In spite of the differences in nomenclature and focus, the underlying messages and descriptions are quite similar. In **Box 6-2**, we've compiled some examples of patient-centered care descriptors we've found. Although there are many more phrases, these should give you a snapshot of what patient-centered care looks like.

Where does your experience fit in terms of the descriptors shown in the box? Are you more familiar with the old-fashioned paternalistic provider relationships, or are these examples part of your experience? If it's the latter, you recognize the wisdom of the IOM's vision. We hope that by now, patient-centered care is becoming more common; unfortunately, Redman might be right—patient-centered care is still "an

---

Box 6-2   Examples of Descriptors of Patient-Centered Care

- Balance of power between provider and patient
- Empowered patients
- Focus on interpersonal relationships
- Shared decision making
- Understanding others' perspectives
- Collaboration and partnership
- Common goals
- Patient autonomy promoted
- Mutual respect for each other's expertise
- Negotiation
- Acknowledgment of provider as not having all the knowledge
- Discussions of uncertainty OK
- Patient responsibility for health behaviors
- Open communication and information exchange
- Consumer control over information
- Connectedness
- Truthfulness and honesty
- Cultural sensitivity
- Culture of caring
- Mutuality
- Customized, individualized care

Sources: Buch & Edgren, 2001; Calabretta, 2002; Campinha-Bacote, 2011; Carter et al., 2008; Crandall et al., 2007; Enehaug, 2000; Fiester, 2012; Hewitt-Taylor, 2003; Knoerl, Esper, & Hasenau, 2011; McCormack, 2004; Nolan et al., 2004; O'Donovan, 2007; Sidani, 2008; Slater, 2006.

aspiration, not a reality" (2008, p. 5). One thing we know for sure is this: this alternative to traditional approaches will affect and be affected by the thinking of both providers and patients.

Patient-Centered Care and Critical Thinking

Patient-centered care acknowledges and celebrates patients as critical thinkers. This may be a shift in perception for many. Nurses and other providers need to consider not just their CT, but how their thinking interfaces with patients' CT. Because most patients have one or more family members and significant others who actively participate in their healthcare decision making, the actual group of affected thinkers can get fairly large. In the IOM's ideal healthcare delivery world, everyone's thinking would merge to find resolutions to the issues at hand. **Figure 6-1** depicts this model of thinking through a patient's healthcare issue.

Those thinking clouds should merge naturally, but in fact, this doesn't happen automatically. We have a long history of viewing health providers as experts to whom patients must defer; the expert model gives power to the provider, with an implication of compliance for the patient (Brown et al., 2006). Many older patients, especially, have that deferential attitude. However, that patient–provider relationship is changing rapidly. Patients of all generations can access vast amounts of health information today. With the implementation of patient-centered care, providers will be more likely to acknowledge and value patients' knowledge and collaborate with them in addressing health issues. However, providers cannot yet assume that patients have the necessary level of knowledge even though so much information is out there.

Patient thinking has been studied by several authors. Anderson (2007) found that couples' decision making for genetic issues could be enumerated into nine types of thinking: analytical, ethical, moral, reflective, practical, hypothetical, judgmental, scary, and second sight. People can access other patients' experiences online, and this becomes an important part of their decision making relative to newly acquired conditions (Ziebland & Herxheimer, 2008). Consumer health informatics is a burgeoning field, but it is not without drawbacks—not the least of which is the often undependable quality of knowledge that is now available (Eysenbach & Jadad, 2001). Therefore, providers will need to assess patients' knowledge much more critically in the future (Coulter, Entwistle, & Gilbert, 1999).

Our challenge for now is fourfold. We must (1) address the patient's health literacy, (2) assess the patient's readiness, willingness, and ability to participate in the healthcare thinking process, (3) facilitate patients' actual process of thinking about their own health care, and (4) merge our thinking and the patient's thinking to create a mutually satisfying and functional process that leads to quality outcomes. According to the IOM, "in many cases, the best window on the safety and quality of care is through the eyes of the patient" (2001, p. 45).

Health Literacy Effects on Patient-Centered Care

Health literacy is a huge and important issue, one that must be approached from a CT perspective. Without a basic understanding of their health issues, patients cannot begin to think critically about their health care (Clancy, 2008). Without understanding and thinking input, patient-centered care becomes an empty descriptor. Nielsen-Bohlman, Panzer, and Kindig, of the IOM, focused on health literacy, citing that "nearly half of all American adults—90 million people—have difficulty understanding and acting upon health information" (2004, p. 1).

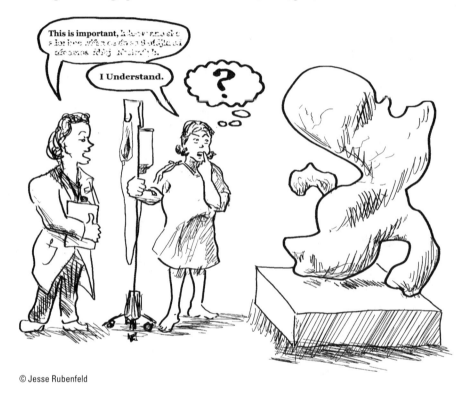

© Jesse Rubenfeld

Health literacy is addressed in multiple forums these days. It is a frequently stated priority in U.S. government agencies. For example, health communication and health information technology are part of the goals of *Healthy People 2020* (U.S. Department of Health and Human Services [DHHS], 2010a), and the DHHS devised an action plan to improve health literacy (2010b). The Plain Writing Act (2010), signed into law by President Obama, specified that all federal documents be written clearly and concisely. Hopefully, these prescriptive edicts will meet their desired goals.

Speros, touting health literacy promotion as a nursing imperative, cited that "nearly 9 out of 10 adults in the United States experience difficulty understanding and using basic health information provided to them in hospitals, clinics, and physicians' offices, or through media outlets such as television and the web" (2011, p. 321). Speros provided a comprehensive set of strategies to promote health literacy in five categories: creating a shame-free environment; using clear, purposeful communication; communicating in a patient-centered manner; reinforcing the spoken word; and verifying understanding.

In spite of what seems logical in response to the need for nursing to be involved in health literacy, Sand-Jecklin, Murray, Summers, and Watson (2010) noted that nursing education has failed to identify a standard approach to health literacy in schools of nursing. Nurses are ill-prepared to deal with this healthcare need. A few years ago we started teaching an elective course for registered nurse (RN)-to-Bachelors of Science in Nursing (BSN) students on health literacy; at the start of each class, we asked who had received health literacy education in their basic nursing program. Very rarely did a student say yes.

Low patient levels of health literacy are often not identified by healthcare providers who may be afraid to assess literacy for fear of patients being ashamed (Townsend, 2011; Wolf et al., 2007). However, there are abundant resources available to assess health literacy without shaming patients. For example, the National Institutes of Health has set up a helpful website at http://www.nih.gov/clearcommunication/healthliteracy.htm. A dated but very relevant, helpful resource that students have used in our health literacy course was written by Doak, Doak, and Root (1996), which the Harvard School of Public Health has made available online. The school's website (http://www.hsph.harvard.edu/healthliteracy/resources/) lists many other resources that nurses would find helpful. Other helpful resources are the PRISM tool kit by Ridpath, Greene, and Wiese (2007) and the quick assessment of health literacy offered by Weiss et al. (2005) and supported by Vangeest, Welch, and Weiner (2010). The Weiss instrument used a sample food label to assess a person's ability to read and understand basic nutritional information. We have had our students use this instrument, and it has been very helpful as an opening into discussions of patients' health literacy. Those discussions were very eye opening to students who had glossed over patient health literacy issues without much thought.

Assessing health literacy is the starting point for patient engagement in the process of providing health care. Ask yourself if your patient is engaged in the thinking necessary for patient-centered care. If not, why? Could it be that the patient has little understanding of what is being said?

Assessing Patient Readiness, Willingness, and Ability to Participate in Critical Thinking and Patient-Centered Care

After the patient's level of health literacy has been established, other factors that contribute to patient engagement must be assessed. Patient engagement involves more factors than just health literacy. It has been identified as multifaceted but poorly defined (Barello et al., 2012). We are addressing it here as readiness, willingness, and ability to participate in CT and patient-centered care. It is all too easy to skip to tasks at hand without checking to see if the patient is engaged. Nurses can get mired by the many checklists they are required to follow. Fights (2012) cautioned against scripted patient interactions. When a nurse follows a script, neither the nurse nor the patient may be engaged in thinking.

Perhaps 50 years from now patients will be more engaged in their health care because they will be accustomed to accessing information (and the standards to judge its quality) and self-diagnostic kits. But we're not there yet. Some patients might be uncomfortable with what they see as the extra burden of being full participants in healthcare decision making; others might be dissatisfied that they are not included in the thinking process. For now, we need some way to estimate how engaged a patient is, or wants to be, and to track potential growth in that engagement. For that, we can look at CT habits of the mind.

Remembering that habits of the mind are dynamic states that reflect one's penchant for CT, we could use a checklist to rate patients' thinking tendencies. Assessing habits of the mind is different than assessing the patient's actual skills at thinking (which we will address later); habits of the mind focus more on readiness and willingness. Before rating a patient's thinking tendencies, however, engage a bit of *contextual perspective* in your thinking. Look at yourself (*reflection*) and consider how your habits of the mind will correlate with the patient's habits. Remember, partnership in care decisions is at the core of patient-centered care, not simply out of respect, which is important, but to achieve quality outcomes.

Now, move to the patient's context. First, the basics: Can the patient speak and understand English? (Nailon, 2007). What is the status of the patient's senses; can he or she see and hear adequately to be a partner in decision making? Second, consider the magnitude of the physical and emotional stress experienced in the current health situation. Pain and anxiety can powerfully override natural thinking habits of the mind. Third, there may be cognitive deficits that are caused by developmental factors, neurological disease, and conditions such as dementia and delirium. Although it is not considered a cognitive deficit, the patient's educational level may affect thinking. In these cases, don't forget the patients' significant others as thinking team members; complete the checklist with them in mind. Fourth, cultural or generational issues might cause a patient to think it is disrespectful to openly participate in health-issue thinking. In these cases, it is our responsibility to let those people know that it is not only OK, but desirable to think along with us.

After you have considered the contextual issues, look at the checklist in **Box 6-3** and think about how you might use such a checklist in your practice. Even if you don't specifically rate patients' thinking habits of the mind, asking yourself these questions about each patient will help you focus on the patient as a thinking person and not some blank slate on which you and the team do things.

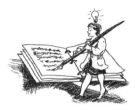

TACTICS 6-1: Reflect on Your Patients' Habits of the Mind

Clinicians and Educators

Think back to a patient encounter you (or, for educators, your student) had recently. Use the checklist in Box 6-3 to rate that patient. How did it feel to rate the patient? Can you see how such a rating might be valuable? How did it help you consider your patient in a different light?

Discussion

If you have patients who rate very low on this scale, what were the possible reasons? To what can you attribute higher scores? How did you use *contextual perspective* to find these contributing factors? Are any of those factors changeable? If so, how?

Box 6-3 CT Habits of the Mind Patient-Rating Checklist

Insert the patient's name in the blank for each item. Rate each habit of the mind as 1 (no), 2 (maybe), or 3 (yes) and mark the rating on the line. Remember that circumstances can change these scores, so use this information to assess where the patient is today. If the patient scores between 10 and 15, he or she is probably less likely to be an active team thinker; between 16 and 21, he or she is probably a moderately active team thinker; between 22 and 30, he or she is a very active team thinker.

___ *Confidence:* Does ___ seem sure of himself or herself in thinking through this situation?

___ *Contextual perspective:* Is ___ thinking of the whole picture?

___ *Creativity:* Is ___ likely to adapt to the situation with plans that are not immediately obvious to us?

___ *Flexibility:* Is ___ able to adapt his or her thinking to this health situation?

___ *Inquisitiveness:* Will ___ seek out information on his or her own?

___ *Intellectual integrity:* Will ___ consider the truth about this situation even if it goes against his or her hopes and wishes?

___ *Intuition:* Is ___ likely to respond at a gut level?

___ *Open-mindedness:* Will ___ choose the best path toward health, even if it means changing his or her behavior?

___ *Perseverance:* Will ___ hang in there and work this through?

___ *Reflection:* Is ___ someone who stops to think back on things?

_____**Total Score**

Facilitating Patients' Critical Thinking Skills

Once we have a feel for patients' CT tendencies, we can better gauge how much encouragement, if any, they need to exercise their thinking skills alongside ours. In other words, for patients and significant others, we need to determine what's in those thinking clouds shown in Figure 6-1. To help you focus on their thinking, let's look at each of the seven CT skills, explore how patients use those skills, and consider what we can do to promote them. We have addressed the skills in alphabetical order, but this does not imply any ranking of their importance.

Analyzing

Separating or breaking a whole into parts to discover their nature, function, and relationships. Can you imagine patients breaking down options for their care, such as for treatment of diabetes? Of course you can. Studying the pros and cons of insulin therapy and oral hypoglycemics is an analytical process. Helping patients *analyze* the complexities of a diabetic diet helps them follow recommendations. It's not enough to hand dietary guidelines to patients; they need to break that down into something that translates into their breakfast, lunch, dinner, snacks, grocery lists, restaurant options, vacation diets, sick days, and so on. Coulter et al. (1999), using focus groups, found that patients were dissatisfied with the information they got from healthcare providers. They wanted a full range of treatment options and to learn the pros and cons of each. They wanted materials to help them feel knowledgeable enough to participate equally in decision making. They didn't want simplistic conclusions; they wanted empowerment through knowledge. If providers and patients analyze situations together—break things down to essential information—they will better understand which options are appropriate and make more informed decisions. Patients will then be more likely to adhere to treatments such as dietary changes because those treatments will be tailored to their lifestyle.

Applying Standards

Judging according to established personal, professional, or social rules or criteria. This is an interesting cognitive skill. It is closely aligned with what one values. In a recent class exercise, we asked RN and BSN students to share personal standards they applied in their practices. Here are some of their answers:

- "I always check to see if my patients need pain medication right at the end of my shift, and I remind them that staff will be in transition for the next hour. I don't want them sitting there waiting for pain medication."
- "I always talk about what I'm doing while I'm doing tasks in patients' rooms."
- "I try to teach something every time I'm in the room."
- "I always ask patients, 'How can I help you today?'"

Aren't those wonderful standards?

Now, let's think about patients' standards. How often do we ask patients what they expect of us? What is their definition of standard of care, and might their definitions be in conflict with ours? Healthcare providers are apt to forget that patients don't know the usual routines that are taken for granted in health care. Patients might expect every nurse to ask about pain medication at the end of the shift, as the nurse just mentioned did. If the nurse on the next shift doesn't, patients are apt to think that she isn't doing her job.

Think about the patient who is constantly pressing his call light for seemingly trivial reasons. Might that patient think this is the expected standard of nursing care on an evening shift on a medical floor? People often think of nurses as being like waiters—you just call them when you want something. Rather than getting frustrated with patients like this, we can try to educate them about the norms and standards of care and ask them what they expect as routines.

A common example of conflicting standards is the patient who is angry at having to wait in the office for 45 minutes for his or her physician or nurse practitioner (NP). These patients obviously have an expectation that a 3 p.m. appointment means that they'll be seen within 5 minutes or so—as at the hairdresser, for example. Sometimes a straightforward explanation of what life is like in a medical office—people have unexpected needs that disrupt schedules—is enough to help a patient develop a more realistic standard and expectation of care. Patients and providers must have a full knowledge of how the system works for a true partnership to exist (Enehaug, 2000).

Another consideration concerning *applying standards* is linked to patient access to information. Patients not only read about healthcare issues in magazines, but also, for example, they can go online and retrieve the same guidelines for diabetes management that their health provider is using. In line with this diabetes management example, the National Institutes of Health and the Centers for Disease Control and Prevention have a practice transformation website (http://ndep.nih.gov/hcp-businesses-and-schools/practice-transformation/) that cites several dimensions of patient-centered care, including respect, information and communication, and coordination and integration of care (National Diabetes Education Program, n.d.). This site promotes a true partnership between patients with diabetes and their providers. Patients who use the thinking skill of *applying standards* will keep us on our toes. If we focus only on our application of standards without considering the patients' application of those same standards, we will create conflict, waste time, and diminish patient-centered care.

One final word and a bit of caution when *applying standards*: standards change, such as acceptable measures for blood pressure and blood glucose. Some standards are also culturally biased. For example, most height and weight charts for children are normalized for Caucasians. An Asian-Pacific colleague has to keep that in mind when her pediatrician's records show her son as consistently in the lower percentile for height. The lesson is that we need CT, even with standards, to customize patient-centered care.

Discriminating

Recognizing differences and similarities among things or situations and distinguishing carefully as to category or rank. We might not think of this as a cognitive skill that we readily identify from patients' perspectives. After all, we see distinguishing the finer points in healthcare situations as requiring our expert eyes, ears, and *intuition.* However, when we consider patients' abilities to make fine distinctions about their bodies, we can appreciate their ability to discriminate.

Pain assessment, for example, requires patient *discrimination.* Consider the question, On a scale of 0 to 10, with 10 being your worst pain, what number do you rank your pain at now? The answer requires mighty powers of *discrimination,* with potentially dire consequences (often unrealized by patients). Nurses decide between Tylenol and Vicodin based on those numbers! Should we pay more attention to how well patients are able to *discriminate* when we ask that question? And we must not let our own biases invade. Imagine the scenario going through this nurse's mind as she asks a patient to rate pain: This patient ranks her pain at a 3 on the 1–10 scale. She is a woman, so the worst pain she's had is probably childbirth. I had a baby so I have a good idea of what her 3 would be. OK, so she's in reasonable pain. But what if this woman suffers from migraine or cluster headaches? She may be using that pain as her standard.

The point is, the number is minimally relevant unless we can relate it to a baseline. The number allows for accurate *discrimination* only when the patient shares what the pain compares with. We must ask about that comparison to find out how the patient is making the distinction between, say, 5 and 3. Patient-centered care depends on understanding the patient's unique perspective, thinking, and *discriminating* skills.

Calabretta (2002) went so far as to call patients "consumer specialists" because of this acute self-discriminating ability relative to their health. "Because patients can afford to focus narrowly on their own concerns, learning only about their condition, they have the possibility of ultimately becoming 'consumer specialists.' In addition, all patients have the inherent knowledge of their own symptoms and the experience of living with a disease that physicians lack" (p. 33).

Information Seeking

Searching for evidence, facts, or knowledge by identifying relevant sources and gathering objective, subjective, historical, and current data from those sources. In today's world of easy access to information, patients can and will access information with or without our help. They can, for example, go to the American Diabetes Association website, pull up the section for healthcare professionals, and read the recommendations for care. Increasingly, we find patients doing just that. They read self-help books and magazine articles and view TV shows, all of which provide information. Whereas some patients are able to do extensive research on their health issues on their own, others could and might do so if healthcare providers guided them by identifying resources such as websites, patient-information libraries, and self-help books.

Providers must coach patients to be seekers of information. We must help them evaluate which sources of information are legitimate. We are well past the days when our role in patients' *information seeking* is simply to hand them brochures. We now need to be partners in seeking information. We must listen to and value what our patients find and respond not in a dismissive manner but collegially in deciding together the value of that information. Sharing and valuing each other's information promotes patient-centered care.

The issue of judging information, especially that found on the Internet, is still problematic. Some organizations are working diligently to improve this situation and develop instruments to judge the quality of website information. Unfortunately, we have a long way to go before these instruments are consistently validated. Gagliardi and Jadad (2002) found 51 new website rating instruments; only 5 had information allowing them to be evaluated, and none of those had been validated. They questioned the value of these incompletely developed instruments, asking, "Is it desirable or necessary to assess the quality of health information on the internet? If so, is it an achievable goal given that quality is a construct for which we have no gold standard?" (p. 571). Until these questions are answered, we must use our CT, and help patients use their CT, to choose the best sources of information and evaluate the quality of that information. The folks at Vanderbilt University had an interesting system to help patients get the best information. Their medical center and Eskind Biomedical Library have developed the Patient Informatics Consult Service, which gives patients "information prescriptions" they can take to librarians who then collect the information and create a report that is delivered to the clinician and patient (Williams, Gish, Giuse, Sathe, & Carrell, 2001). Now that's CT *creativity* at work!

Logical Reasoning

Drawing inferences or conclusions that are supported in or justified by evidence. This cognitive skill is used by everyone to some degree. Most patients today will not accept pat answers that aren't supported by the evidence of their symptoms. They will, and should, question these answers. On the other hand, we can also point out to patients that there is much we still don't know—that we don't have evidence for some things. "Healthcare professionals should acknowledge that they do not possess complete and irrefutable knowledge . . . [and] enter into discussions with patients in which uncertainties and conflicting views can be explored openly" (Hewitt-Taylor, 2003, p. 1327). Working together with patients and using available information, however incomplete it might be, we can help patients draw conclusions that are easier to accept because they can see the logic behind them.

Consider this case study: Mrs. Jones is 75 years old. She has a diagnosis of diverticulosis and colonic stricture; she has been suffering from diarrhea since finishing one course of antibiotics for a recent urinary tract infection. Based on her physical exam findings, she was placed on metronidazole to cover both clostridium difficile colitis and diverticulitis. When Mrs. Jones sees her NP on a follow-up visit, she states that she has stopped taking the metronidazole because it made her nauseated and she didn't like the taste it left in her mouth. When the NP said she needed a referral to a gastroenterologist and an abdominal scan, Mrs. Jones replied, "I don't like that doctor and I'm not having another scan." Continuing to ask for something to help stop the diarrhea but refusing all suggestions, the patient was a challenge to the NP, who was struggling alone with *logical reasoning*. Totally frustrated, the NP finally laid all the facts in front of the patient, including ways to disguise the taste of the pill, and said, "Here are the only conclusions I can make with these facts. Do you see a different conclusion here?" The patient replied, "Oh, I thought there were other things I could do, but I see that these are my choices."

Initially, this passive patient wanted the nurse to draw all the conclusions and make the decisions. Ultimately, however, when presented with the facts and given the option to draw her own conclusion, the patient engaged her *logical reasoning* and drew inferences based on the available evidence. (By the way, the patient reported that metronidazole and peanut butter taste great!) This situation is not unusual. Patients who see health providers as all-knowing don't engage in the decision making, but wait passively until a conclusion is passed down. Patients often can state what they don't want without knowing all the possible choices. When faced with making decisions themselves or in partnership with providers, they can see the logic used by the provider and add their own *logical reasoning*.

Predicting

Envisioning a plan and its consequences. Patients may be better at the cognitive skill of *predicting* than healthcare providers are; they can see how their lives will change by the health issue at hand. A good question to help patients use this skill, for example, is, Knowing that diabetes is a progressive condition (meaning that you will likely need more medications over time), how do you see yourself dealing with this over the next few years? This question helps patients think about the future and increases the chances that they will recognize the consequences of their decisions. It is important for providers to help patients see alternative right answers. There may be good, better, and best options, or even three betters and two bests.

Helping patients with *predictive* thinking is valuable because patients know themselves and the circumstances of their daily lives best. *Predicting* is especially important when patients are first faced with a chronic illness that will change their lifestyle. The process of *predicting* helps them internalize their new health situation and accept their realities. *Predicting* consequences may not come naturally to some and can be based on culture and be dependent on cognitive and developmental skills. Our job as providers is to facilitate opportunities for patients to use this skill to promote patient-centered care.

Predictive thinking, so important in dealing with chronic illness, is a driving force behind the shift away from provider-centered care, a paradigm for acute illness management (National Diabetes Education Program, n.d.). In the case of an acute illness, the provider takes more control; with chronic illness management, once the patient is out the hospital or office door, he or she is the one in control. Predictive thinking about what's outside that door must be the result of a partnership between patients and providers.

Transforming Knowledge

Patients probably have to transform knowledge (*change or convert the condition, nature, form, or function of concepts among contexts*) more than their providers do. Patients with this skill use information to take control of new health situations. Consider patient education: you know that you need to impart medical knowledge in a way that patients can understand. Among the most successful *knowledge transformation* examples are consumer self-help groups, which allow patients with similar conditions to talk to each other, teach each other, and translate medical lingo into something they can learn from.

It behooves healthcare providers to think about how they can learn from consumer groups. Some primary care settings have done this by having group appointments for patients with similar conditions, such as diabetes or pregnancy. The provider saves time by not having to repeat things, and patients benefit by receiving information from both the provider and others in similar situations. Group interactions are great facilitators for *transforming knowledge*. Transforming the provider's knowledge into the patient's reality, and vice versa, provides increased opportunities for patient-centered care.

How to Merge Our Thinking with Patient Thinking

With this perspective of how patients can and do use their thinking skills, what can educators and clinicians do to make this collaborative thinking the norm? Kleiman would say that we need to revitalize "the humanistic imperative in nursing practice" (2007, p. 209). Eldh, Ekman, and Ehnfors (2006), while studying patients' participation in health care, found that two conditions were necessary for true participation—recognition of each patient's unique knowledge, and respect for the patient. Even though it seems like a ludicrous statement, it is easy to forget the patient, a human being deserving of our respect and honesty, as we go along our way as healthcare providers.

The first job, then, is to remember the patient and acknowledge his or her "natural standpoint" (Anderson, 2007, p. 15). The second is to validate, validate, validate our conclusions with the patient. The third job is to coax and coach patient thinking.

Remember the Patient

In our nursing classes, when we get to the part about drawing conclusions—such as nursing diagnoses—we often ask our students, Now that you've concluded that there is a problem needing nursing care, what will your next step be? The typical response (based on the students' familiarity with the assessing, planning, implementing, and evaluating phases of the nursing process) is start planning. The answer we are looking for, however, is validate that conclusion with the patient. In all our years of teaching, neither of us has ever gotten that response without prompting. And that's even with teaching patient-centered care from the get-go. Why is it so easy to forget the patient when we keep saying that we value patient-centered care?

Here's an example. A student caring for a patient whose wife had died 4 months earlier made a nursing diagnosis of dysfunctional grieving based on evidence that the patient could not speak of his wife without crying. That student, with the teacher's prompting, sought the patient's validation of that conclusion by asking, "Mr. Jones, based on my assessment, I'm thinking that my nursing diagnosis is dysfunctional grieving. What do you think?" Mr. Jones was quick to put the student in her place. "I am grieving, but there's nothing dysfunctional about crying over my wonderful wife who left me only 4 months ago!" In response, this student, with the help of Mr. Jones, changed her diagnosis to incomplete grieving, even though the NANDA classification (NANDA International, 2012) had no such label (and still doesn't— it has only "grieving," "complicated grieving," and "risk for complicated grieving"). There wasn't a problem—just a conclusion, based on facts, made jointly with the patient. In this example, the patient's *logical reasoning* was better than the student's. She was more focused, initially, on following context-free rules—a common occurrence with novice-level thinking. But she was able, with the patient's partnership, to demonstrate *logical reasoning* and *transforming knowledge.*

Validate, Validate, Validate

The process of validation cannot be overemphasized. Think about your practice; how often do you solicit patients' validation to see if your thinking is on track? How often do you validate with yourself that you are valuing the patient's part in the thinking process? See **Box 6-4** for examples of remarks that support both kinds of validation.

TACTICS 6-2: Reflect on Your Validation Remarks

Clinicians

Carry a copy of the validation remarks in Box 6-4 in your pocket for a few days as you work with patients. Periodically, pull it out and check off which comments you've made. At the end of each day, look at how many comments you've made.

Educators

Distribute a copy of Box 6-4 to your students and ask them to track how many times they make such remarks over the course of a day or two when working with patients.

Box 6-4   Validation Remarks to Promote Patient Participation in Decisions

---

- Here's what I think; do you agree?
- What would you say is going on here?
- How is all of this affecting you?
- Does it seem that way to you? It does to me, but I want your opinion.
- Let's think about this together for a minute.
- Only you know your daily living situation.
- Can we find a way through this together?
- Let me explain my thinking to you.
- What do you think?
- How does this feel?
- Do you agree with this?
- This is what I'm thinking; what do you think?
- I'm interested in your take on all of this.
- If you could change this, what would be different?
- If you had a magic wand, what would you have it do?

You might also think about how many of these comments you use with students to validate your thinking with them.

Discussion

These remarks may seem simple, but many important things we do as nurses are simple. Remember the old adage, For want of a nail the shoe is lost, for want of a shoe the horse is lost, for want of a horse the rider is lost. There's a lot of truth to that; don't forget the simple things; they have huge consequences. Simple can be powerful.

Buch and Edgren suggested that patients be interviewed soon after admission to the hospital to "explore expectations, needs and demands" (2001, p. 69). Doing that would set the stage for thinking partnerships at the outset of the patient–provider encounter. The patient would expect to be a partner in decision making, either as a direct participant or by validating conclusions.

Coaxing and Coaching Patient Thinking

Most patients respect healthcare providers; they don't want to step on their toes or take up their time. They are also reluctant to push for collaborative thinking if their providers don't indicate that this is desirable. Using the validation remarks listed in Box 6-4 might help providers encourage patient participation, but there's more to it than that. We must do more than just verbally validate our thinking with them; we have to personify openness to their thinking and show them that we value them as people, not only as patients. That's a tough one to put in a box—it's linked to our personal interaction styles and requires subtle nonverbal communication. We asked some nurses how they show patients that they are open to sitting down and thinking together. **Box 6-5** lists ideas that those nurses shared. Add your unique ideas to this list.

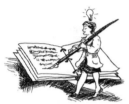

TACTICS 6-3: Whose Critical Thinking Provided the Best Guidance for George's Care?

Scenario 6-3: George

George is a 75-year-old male living at home with his significant other. After recovery from a stroke 2 years ago, he was recently diagnosed with metastatic renal carcinoma and has been admitted to hospice care at home. He might be labeled by some as an old curmudgeon who is not particularly verbal. He is being seen for the first time by the hospice nurse for an intake interview. The nurse initially meets with him privately.

Read the following interaction in the left column. Write your thinking impressions in the column on the right. Answer the following questions for each interaction: (1) What do you think about this portion of the interaction?;

Box 6-5 Strategies to Help Healthcare Providers Encourage Patient Participation in the Thinking Process

- Stay in the room; don't talk to them from the doorway.
- Pay attention to your body language and to theirs.
- Sit down so you're at eye level with them.
- Use open questions and comments, such as, Tell me about, instead of closed questions, which imply that you expect a short answer.
- Touch them, but be respectful of their space and cultural norms.
- Use collaborative thinking language such as, We should think this through, Let's look at some possible conclusions, and Can we analyze this together?
- Use phrases that let them know their situation is not so unusual that they can't discuss it; for example, Some people feel anxious when . . .
- Address them respectfully; find out if they prefer Mr. or Mrs. or Professor, Reverend, and so on.
- Don't look at your watch, no matter how busy you are.
- Be direct and honest; for example, tell them when the schedule is backed up and why.
- If you feel like avoiding a patient, reflect on why you feel that way.

(2) What critical thinking dimensions were being used, or should have been used, and by whom? Along with your comments, identify which of the 17 dimensions you believe were being used, or should have been used, by either the nurse or the significant other.

Interaction	Your Thinking Impressions
Nurse (while completing the intake assessment form): "Are you ever feeling down or depressed?" George: "Yes."	1.
Nurse: "How often do you feel this way?" George: "All the time."	2.
After assessing George, the nurse talks with his significant other. That conversation includes the following:	1.
"I think we should consider adding an antidepressant to his medications. I'll have the nurse practitioner call in a prescription. What pharmacy do you use?"	2.
Significant other: "Why do you think he needs an antidepressant medication?"	1.
	2.
Nurse: "He says he is depressed all the time." Significant other: "Let's go check this out with him."	1.
	2.
Significant other: "George, did you tell the nurse you were depressed?" George: "Yes."	1.
Significant other: "What do you think is making you depressed?" George: "I can't have sex anymore!"	2.

Discussion

What happened to the assessment process being used by the nurse? What pieces of CT could the nurse have used to avoid jumping to a premature conclusion (e.g., *intellectual integrity, inquisitiveness, information seeking, contextual perspective*)? What would have happened if the significant other had not used her CT skills to seek out more information?

Are There Negatives to Patient-Centered Care?

Clearly, we value patient-centered care, but are there negatives to this? Certainly. Two of the biggest are time and power. It takes more time to practice true patient-centered care—or so it would seem on the face of it. As providers, we have to give up power and share it with patients, and, if we consider it honestly, that makes us feel vulnerable. It's hard to admit that we don't have all the control or all the answers.

Time

Let's look at time. Say you have a passive patient who doesn't push to get involved in decisions. What do you do? You probably answer, Get the patient involved, of course. Now, picture yourself on a particularly busy medical unit and ask yourself what you'd do. If you're like most, you'd be happy that the patient is not slowing you down, asking questions, or expressing opinions on how things should be done. This is our reality; we're busy people, and practicing patient-centered care can be very time consuming. That's probably the real reason why it's not the norm.

We ask you to reconsider this assumption. Does patient-centered care really take more time in the long run, or does it seem that way in the short run? How much time do we spend doing things that we decide are best for the patients, only to find that those patients have no investment in our ideas because they weren't involved in the decisions? How many extra trips down the hall do we have to make because our patients feel isolated and at the mercy of all those providers who are making decisions for them? What is the price of making our patients feel powerless?

Power

Now, let's look at power—ours and patients'. According to the IOM, "the patient is the source of control" (2003, p. 47), and providers must "allow patients to have unfettered access to the information contained in their medical records" (p. 52).

Don't you wonder why, in the not so distant past (or perhaps still today), we kept patients' health information secret from them? Did it help us keep a sense of power as the experts? Were we trying to protect patients from something scary? Were we afraid of litigation (a fairly legitimate concern in the litigious-minded United States)? Were we just fulfilling a rescuer model of nursing care? Were we trying to keep our distance from serious or life-threatening conditions that we just did not want to deal with? The answer could be any or all of the above, but it was and is not the way to provide quality patient-centered care.

Our job as nurses and healthcare providers is not to protect patients and their families from the truth, but to work together and think together to deal with their healthcare issues. And if you are still worried about the litigation potential, consider the finding of a 2002 study by Hickson and colleagues: "patients who saw physicians with the highest numbers of lawsuits were more likely to complain that their physicians would not listen or return telephone calls, were rude, and did not show respect" (p. 2955). If we respect patients, respect their right to information about their health condition, and respect their thinking, then we are truly providing patient-centered care.

But let's back up a bit and look at some of the foundation needed for respecting patients and providing patient-centered care. Who else do we need to respect for patient-centered care to permeate your healthcare environment? How about each other? Tellis-Nayak (2007) concluded that a person-centered workplace would turn workers into person-centered caregivers. Although caring about people is considered a natural characteristic of nurses, unfortunately, it doesn't always carry over to those with whom we work. The old, very sad adage that we eat our young is still in play, and it isn't always focused on our young. Lateral violence, professional bullying, or whatever else you choose to call it does occur and significantly impedes thinking, let alone patient-centered care. For more information on this topic see Clark (2012) and Jenkins, Kerber, and Woith (2013), who studied civility among nursing students. It's time for a marvelous example of how nurses in one large healthcare organization are clearly capturing the essence of patient-centered care.

A Patient-Centered Care Story

From Kari Szczechowski, RN, BSN, PCCN, Relationship Oriented Care Program Coordinator
Oakwood Healthcare System, Michigan

Nurses at the Oakwood Healthcare System in Michigan have been using a patient- and family-centered care approach to positively impact the patient experience. Since 2007, Oakwood has been using Relationship Oriented Care (ROC) as the means of care delivery based on their Professional Practice Model, Patient and Family Centered Care. ROC is a way of providing exceptional, personalized care that focuses on incorporating patients and their families in their healthcare plan. Hearing "you ROC" throughout the organization has become a way of acknowledging those staff members who are living the organization's credo, patients come first.

The ROC program was developed as a version of Ruth Hansten's model, Relation-ship and Results-Oriented Healthcare. This model emphasizes developing fundamental relationships, using critical thinking and high-impact team practices to create positive healthcare outcomes (Hansten, 2005). At its inception, over 3,000 employees, including nurses and ancillary staff, were introduced to ROC by attending one of the 300 in-service programs provided throughout the organization. In addition, more than 150 nurses participated in further training through Hansten Healthcare and were recognized as Relationship and Results-Oriented Health Care Level 1 Specialists.

While ROC became a way for nurses to provide care, it was felt that this program should be extended to the nursing support staff, who are a crucial part of the healthcare team providing quality patient care. In 2010, the Oakwood Healthcare System's ROC Ambassador Program was developed by Diane DiFiore, RN, MSA, the then director of Nurse Recruitment & Retention; Janet Johnson, RN, BSN, nurse educator; and Sandra Schmitt, RN, BSN, manager of Nursing Development. The program's purpose was and is to raise awareness and attention around ROC values, educate participants regarding overcoming barriers to obtain and maintain ROC on their units, and assist and support the participants to become ROC role models in their area. The program has had over 100 nursing support staff participants and continues to be offered twice a year.

The foundation for patient- and family-centered care was created by providing educational sessions for nurses and nursing support staff that focused on the three main elements driving practice: developing fundamental relationships, constant and effective communication, and teamwork. Direct care staff members incorporate these key concepts of ROC into their daily practice by performing bedside reports, conducting patient-focused interviews, documenting on patient Care Boards, conducting hourly rounding, and utilizing delegation skills to complete required tasks.

The introduction of ROC to Oakwood's care delivery practice changed the healthcare team's thought process from, What tasks do I have to do for my patients today? to How are we going to work together, with the patients, to meet their needs for today? The thought process for the patients has also changed. In the past, patients were accustomed to coming into a hospital setting and being at the mercy of the healthcare team. Now they are being asked what they want to accomplish for the day or what time frame works for them to complete daily care needs. This is reinforced by performing patient-focused interviews not only at the beginning of a shift, but also throughout the course of the patient's stay.

The nurses and nursing support team spend time introducing themselves while at the same time establishing a relationship with patients and their support systems. Patients are asked, What is your goal for today? Many times the initial response is, To feel better, or To go home; however, this response changes as the patient and the family become accustomed to this process. Their goals change to, I want to get out of bed for each of my meals, or I want to walk farther than I did yesterday. These goals are placed on the Patient Care Board. In addition, there is a spot on the board for placing the patient's name, the healthcare team members' names, and patient and family communication.

There is an interesting story about the interview and care board. When a nurse asked one patient, Aloysius, what name he wanted to be called, he thought for awhile and then said, "Al." His daughter looked up and said, "Dad, since when have you wanted to be called Al?" He replied, "All my life but nobody ever asked." Nurses consistently say they are listening to their patients, but have they really been doing that? Patients know and appreciate when we are truly listening to them; it builds trust.

The initiation of bedside reporting was at first an uncomfortable task for the staff to embrace. Talking in front of the patients and their family members about the patient's care was something new. Report had always taken place in a report room and took the staff away from the patients for at least 30 minutes during this time. With education and support from nurse leaders, some units saw their report time decrease by 50%. In addition, patient satisfaction increased significantly. Bedside reporting not only improves patient satisfaction; it improves patient safety and staff accountability as well. For example, potential falls can be prevented, and nurses are held more accountable for the way they are leaving a patient care area with this process.

As ROC continues to grow at Oakwood, nurses are thinking ahead about how to improve the patient experience. Nurses and nursing assistants are working together to keep one another informed about patients, while at the same time updating the patient and family on a regular basis. Hourly rounds are being conducted to assess our patients so that their personal needs are met and their safety is maintained. Nurses are working with physicians, social workers, physical therapists, and other disciplines to begin discharge planning for patients, from the time they are admitted so we can provide them with the resources they will need after leaving our facility. The culture is changing; the thought process to approaching patient care is changing. The increased focus on ROC has positively impacted patients' experiences at Oakwood!

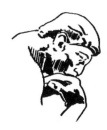

© Jesse Rubenfeld

PAUSE and Ponder

Where Is the Balance?

What else can educators and clinicians do? We will leave this question for you to ponder. Keep in mind that there are no easy answers to these complex issues. We'll bet that every reader can think of a patient who was so controlling that the only solution seemed to be to say, "Could you just listen to me and do as I ask?" Such negative situations always seem to stand out more than the positive ones. We've also had many patients who reached wonderful aha points after collaborative problem solving. There will, of course, always be extremes that challenge our commitment to patient-centered care.

One useful guideline to remember is balance. Ideal patient-centered care is a balance of patient thinking and provider thinking within the realities of each situation. Many factors—knowledge, access to knowledge, overt and covert permission to think, cultural beliefs about roles, habits of the mind and thinking skills, power and control—affect thinking and patient-centered care. Our job is to keep thinking in spite of time constraints, taking advantage of our CT and that of our patients.

REFLECTION CUES

- Patient-centered care, as envisioned by the IOM, must include a focus on patient and provider thinking.
- Traditional patient–provider relationships were hierarchical, with the provider doing the thinking for the patient.
- Patient-centered care must start with a collaborative nurse–patient relationship.
- Patients, significant others, and the team of healthcare providers must work to merge their thinking toward one end: a safe, high-quality healthcare issue outcome.
- Challenges for providers who want to think with patients are threefold. We must assess the patient's readiness, willingness, and ability to participate in the healthcare thinking process; help patients with the actual process of thinking about their own health care; and merge our thinking and the patient's thinking to create a mutually satisfying and functional process.
- Assessing health literacy is especially important to promoting patient engagement.
- Assessing readiness, willingness, and ability to participate in collaborative thinking can be done by considering patients' CT habits of the mind and taking into account contextual factors that might affect those habits of the mind.
- Helping patients with their thinking processes can be done by focusing on each of seven CT cognitive skills.
- Patients can be encouraged to *analyze*, breaking issues down into manageable parts.
- Providers can determine patients' expectations of standards of care and share with patients their *application of standards*.
- Patients are often able to *discriminate* the nuances of their responses as well as, or better than, providers.
- Sharing *logical reasoning* processes with patients can help them see how we come to conclusions, enabling them to draw their own conclusions.
- *Predictive* thinking helps patients see the reality ahead and may help them through a grief process brought on by a change in health.
- *Transforming knowledge* is crucial to effective patient teaching; consumer groups often do very well at transforming medical knowledge into a usable form for consumers.
- Merging provider and patient thinking means remembering to engage patients' thinking and validating conclusions with them.
- Negative aspects of patient-centered care can be seen as time and power issues.
- Although patient-centered care may seem time consuming, in the long run, it may save time.
- Giving up the power of the traditional hierarchical provider–patient relationship can make us feel vulnerable.

■ One nurse describes her institution's success with relationship-centered care: it can be done.

■ The best patient-centered care occurs when providers also care about each other and work together.

REFERENCES

Anderson, G. (2007). Patient decision-making for clinical genetics. *Nursing Inquiry, 14*(1), 13–22.

Barello, S., Graffigna, G., & Vegni, E. (2012). Patient engagement as an emerging challenge for healthcare services: Mapping the literature. *Nursing Research and Practice,* Article ID 905934, 7 pages. doi: 10.1155/2012/905934

Benbassat, J., Pilpel, D., & Tidhar, M. (1998). Patients' preferences for participation in clinical decision making: A review of published surveys. *Behavioral Medicine, 24*(2), 81–88.

Brown, D., McWilliam, C., & Ward-Griffin, C. (2006). Client-centered empowering partnering in nursing. *Journal of Advanced Nursing, 53,* 160–168.

Buch, T., & Edgren, L. (2001). Patients as partners in intensive care units: A conceptual analysis of the literature. *Nursing in Critical Care, 6,* 64–70.

Calabretta, N. (2002). Consumer-driven, patient-centered health care in the age of electronic information. *Journal of the Medical Library Association, 90,* 32–37.

Campinha-Bacote, J. (2011). Delivering patient-centered care in the midst of a cultural conflict: The role of cultural competence. *OJIN: The Online Journal of Issues in Nursing, 16*(2), Manuscript 5. doi: 10.3912/OJIN.Vol16No02Man05

Carter, L. C., Nelson, J. L., Sievers, B. A., Dukek, S. L., Pipe, T. B., & Holland, D. E. (2008). Exploring a culture of caring. *Nursing Administration Quarterly, 32*(1), 57–63.

Cipriano, P. (2012). American Academy of Nursing on policy: The imperative for patient-, family-, and population centered interprofessional approaches to care coordination and transitional care: A policy brief by the American Academy of Nursing's Care Coordination Task Force, *Nursing Outlook, 60,* 330–333. doi: 10.1016/j.outlook.2012.06.021

Clancy, C. (2008, May). *What is your health literacy score? Navigating the health care system: Advice columns from Dr. Carolyn Clancy.* Rockville, MD: Agency for Healthcare Research and Quality. Retrieved from http://www.ahrq.gov/consumer/cc/cc052008.htm

Clark, C. (2012). *Creating and sustaining civility in nursing education.* Indianapolis, IN: Sigma Theta Tau International.

Coulter, A., Entwistle, V., & Gilbert, D. (1999). Sharing decisions with patients: Is the information good enough? *British Medical Journal, 318,* 318–322.

Crandall, L. G., White, D. L., Schuldheis, S., & Talerico, K. A. (2007). Initiating person-centered care practices in long-term care facilities. *Journal of Gerontological Nursing, 33*(11), 47–56.

Cropley, S. (2012). The relationship-based care model: Evaluation of the impact on patient satisfaction, length of stay, and readmission rates. *Journal of Nursing Administration, 42*(6), 333–339. doi: 10.1097/NNA.0b013e31825738ed

de Witte, L., Schoot, T., & Proot, I. (2006). Development of the client-centered care questionnaire. *Journal of Advanced Nursing, 56*(1), 62–68. doi:10.1111/j.1365-2648.2006.03980.x

Disch, J. (2012). Are we really ready for patient-centered care? *Nursing Outlook, 60,* 237–239. doi: 10.1016/j.outlook.2012.07.001

Doak, C. C., Doak, L. G., & Root, J. H. (1996). *Teaching patients with low literacy skills* (2nd ed.). Philadelphia, PA: Lippincott. Available at http://www.hsph.harvard.edu/healthliteracy/resources/teaching-patients-with-low-literacy-skills/

Eldh, A. C., Ekman, I., & Ehnfors, M. (2006). Conditions for patient participation and non-participation in health care. *Nursing Ethics, 13*(5), 503–514. doi:10.1191/0969733006nej898oa

Enehaug, I. H. (2000). Patient participation requires a change of attitude in health care. *International Journal of Health Care Quality Assurance, 13,* 178–181.

Epstein, R. M., & Street, R. L. (2011). The values and value of patient-centered care. *Annals of Family Medicine, 9*(2), 100–103. doi: 10.1370/afm.1239

Eysenbach, G., & Jadad, A. R. (2001). Evidence-based patient choice and consumer health informatics in the Internet age. *Journal of Medical Internet Research, 3*(2), e19. Retrieved from http://www.jmir.org/2001/2/e19/HTML

Fiester, A. (2012). What "patient-centered care" requires in serious cultural conflict. *Academic Medicine, 87*(1), 20–24. doi: 10.1097/ACM.0b013e31823ac84b

Fights, S. D. (2012). Do we really provide patient-centered care? *Medsurg Nursing, 21*(1), 5–6.

Fredericks, S., Lapum, J., Schwind, J., Beanlands, H., Romaniuk, D., & McCay, E. (2012). Discussion of patient-centered care in health care organizations. *Quality Management in Health Care, 21*(3), 127–134. doi: 10.1097/QMH.0b013e31825e870d

Gagliardi, A., & Jadad, A. R. (2002). Examination of instruments used to rate quality of health information on the Internet: Chronicle of a voyage with an unclear destination. *British Medical Journal, 324,* 560–573.

Hansten, R. (2005). Relationship and results-oriented healthcare. *Journal of Nursing Administration, 35,* 522–524.

Hewitt-Taylor, J. (2003). Issues involved in promoting patient autonomy in health care. *British Journal of Nursing, 12,* 1323–1330.

Hickson, G. B., Federspiel, C. F., Pichert, J. W., Miller, C. S., Gauld-Jaeger, J., & Bost, P. (2002). Patient complaints and malpractice risk. *Journal of the American Medical Association, 287,* 2951–2957.

Institute of Medicine. (2001). *Crossing the quality chasm: A new health system for the 21st century.* Washington, DC: National Academies Press.

Institute of Medicine. (2003). *Health professions education: A bridge to quality.* Washington, DC: National Academies Press.

Jenkins, S. D., Kerber, C. S., & Woith, W. H. (2013). An intervention to promote civility among nursing students. *Nursing Education Perspectives, 34*(2), 95–100. doi: 10.5480/1536-5026-34.2.95

Kleiman, S. (2007). Revitalizing the humanistic imperative in nursing education. *Nursing Education Perspectives, 28,* 209–213.

Knoerl, A. M., Esper, K. W., & Hasenau, S. M. (2011). Cultural sensitivity in patient health education. *Nursing Clinics of North America, 46*(3), 321–333. doi: 10.1016/j.cnur.2011.05.008

Landers, M. G., & McCarthy, G. M. (2007). Person-centered nursing practice with older people in Ireland. *Nursing Science Quarterly, 20*(1), 78–84. doi:10.1177/0894318406296811

Lee, P. (2007). What does partnership in care mean for children's nurses? *Journal of Clinical Nursing, 16,* 518–526. doi:10.1111/j.1365-2702.2006.01591.x

McCance, T., McCormack, B., & Dewing, J. (2011). An exploration of person-centeredness in practice. *OJIN: The Online Journal of Issues in Nursing, 16*(2), Manuscript 1. doi: 10.3912/OJIN.Vol16No02Man01

McCauley, K., & Irwin, R. S. (2006). Changing the work environment in ICUs to achieve patient-focused care: The time has come. *Chest, 130,* 1571–1578. doi:10.1378/chest.130.5.1571

McCormack, B. (2004). Person-centeredness in gerontological nursing: An overview of the literature. *Journal of Clinical Nursing, 13*(3a), 31–38.

McCormack, B., & McCance, T. V. (2006). Development of a framework for person-centered nursing. *Journal of Advanced Nursing, 56*(5), 472–479. doi:10.1111/j.1365-2648.2006.04042.x

McGilton, K. S., Heath, H., Chu, C. H., Bostrom, A-M, Mueller, C., Boscart, V. M., . . . Bowers, B. (2012). Moving the agenda forward: A person-centered framework in long-term care. *International Journal of Older People Nursing, 7,* 303–309. doi: 10.1111/opn.12010

Medina, J. (2006). A natural synergy in creating a patient-focused care environment: The critical care family assistance program and critical care nursing. *Chest, 128,* 99–102. doi:10.1378/chest.128.3_suppl.99S

Nailon, R. E. (2007). The assessment and documentation of language and communication needs in healthcare systems: Current practices and future directions for coordinating safe, patient-centered care. *Nursing Outlook, 55*(6), 311–317. doi:10.1016/j.outlook.2007.04.005

NANDA International. (2012). *Nursing diagnoses definitions and classification 2012–2014.* Ames, IA: Wiley-Blackwell.

National Diabetes Education Program. (n.d.). *What we want to achieve through systems changes.* Retrieved from http://ndep.nih.gov/hcp-businesses-and-schools/practice-transformation/

Nielsen-Bohlman, L., Panzer, A. M., & Kindig, D. A. (Eds.). (2004). *Health literacy: A prescription to end confusion.* Washington, DC: National Academies Press. Available at http://www.nap.edu/catalog/10883.html

Nolan, M. R., Davies, S., Brown, J., Keady, J., & Nolan, J. (2004). Beyond "person-centered" care: A new vision for gerontological nursing. *Journal of Clinical Nursing, 13*(3a), 45–53.

O'Donovan, A. (2007). Patient-centered care in acute psychiatric admission units: Reality or rhetoric? *Journal of Psychiatric and Mental Health Nursing, 14*, 542–548.

Peplau, H. E. (1952). *Interpersonal relations in nursing: A conceptual frame of reference for psychodynamic nursing.* New York, NY: Putnam.

Plain Writing Act, H.R. 946 Pub. L. No. 111-274 (2010).

Pope, T. (2012). How person-centred care can improve nurses, attitudes to hospitalised older patients. *Nursing Older People, 24*(1), 32–36.

Redman, R. W. (2008). Whither patient-centered care? *Research and Theory for Nursing Practice: An International Journal, 22*(1), 5–6. doi:10.1891/0889-7182.22.1.5

Ridpath, J. R., Greene, S. M., & Wiese, C. J. (2007). *PRISM readability toolkit* (3rd ed.). Seattle, WA: Group Health Research Institute. Available at www.tinyurl.com/prismtoolkit

Rosemond, C. A., Hanson, L. C., Ennett, S. T., Schenck, A. P., & Weiner, B. J. (2012). Implementing person-centered care in nursing homes. *Health Care Management Review, 37*(3), 257–267. doi: 10.1097/HMR.0b013e318235ed17

Saha, S., Beach, M. C., & Cooper, L. A. (2008). Patient centeredness, cultural competence and healthcare quality. *Journal of the National Medical Association, 100*(11), 1275–1285.

Sand-Jecklin, K., Murray, B., Summers, B., & Watson, J. (2010). Educating nursing students about health literacy: From the classroom to the patient bedside. *OJIN: The Online Journal of Issues in Nursing, 15*(3). doi: 10.3912/OJIN.Vol15No03PPT02

Sidani, S. (2008). Effects of patient-centered care on patient outcomes: An evaluation. *Research and Theory for Nursing Practice: An International Journal, 22*(1), 24–37. doi:10.1891/0889-7182.22.1.24

Slater, L. (2006). Person-centeredness: A concept analysis. *Contemporary Nurse, 23*, 135–144.

Speros, C. I. (2011). Promoting health literacy: A nursing imperative. *Nursing Clinics of North America, 46*(3), 321–333. doi: 10.1016/j.cnur.2011.05.007

Stichler, J. F. (2011). Patient-centered healthcare design. *Journal of Nursing Administration, 41*(12), 503–506. doi: 10.1097/NNA.0b013e3182378a3b

Tellis-Nayak, V. (2007). A person-centered workplace: The foundation for person-centered caregiving in long-term care. *Journal of the American Medical Directors Association, 8*, 46–54. doi:10.1016/j.jamda.2006.09.009

Townsend, M. S. (2011). Patient-driven education materials: Low-literate adults increase understanding of health messages and improve compliance. *Nursing Clinics of North America, 46*, 367–378. doi:10.1016/j.cnur.2011.05.011

U.S. Department of Health and Human Services Office of Disease Prevention and Health Promotion. (2010a). *Healthy people 2020.* Retrieved from http://www.healthypeople.gov/2020/topicsobjectives2020/overview.aspx?topicid=18

U.S. Department of Health and Human Services Office of Disease Prevention and Health Promotion. (2010b). *National action plan to improve health literacy.* Washington, DC: Author.

Van Mossel, C., Alford, M., & Watson, H. (2011). Challenges of patient-centered care: Practice or rhetoric. *Nursing Inquiry, 18*(4), 278–289. doi: 10.1111/j.1440-1800.2011.00523.x

Vangeest, J. B., Welch, V. L., & Weiner, S. J. (2010). Patients' perceptions of screening for health literacy: Reactions to the newest vital sign. *Journal of Health Communication, 15*, 402–412. doi: 10.1080/10810731003753117

Weiss, B. D., Mays, M. Z., Martz, W., Castro, K. M., DeWalt, D. A., Pignone, M. P., . . . Hale, F. A. (2005). Quick assessment of literacy in primary care: The newest vital sign. *Annals of Family Medicine, 3*, 514–522. doi:10.1370/afm.405

Williams, M. D., Gish, K. W., Giuse, N. B., Sathe, N. A., & Carrell, D. L. (2001). The patient informatics consult service (PICS): An approach for a patient-centered service. *Bulletin of the Medical Library Association, 89*, 185–193.

Wolf, M. S., Williams, M. V., Parker, R. M., Parikh, N. S., Nowlan, A. W., & Baker, D. W. (2007). Patients' shame and attitudes toward discussing the results of literacy screening. *Journal of Health Communication, 12*, 721–732. doi: 10.1080/10810730701672173

Woolley, J., Perkins, R., Laird, P., Palmer, J., Schitter, M. B., Tarter, K.,... Woolsey, M. (2012). Relationship-based care: Implementing a caring, healing environment. *Medsurg Nursing, 21*(3), 179–184.

Ziebland, S., & Herxheimer, A. (2008). How patients' experiences contribute to decision making: Illustrations from DIPEx (personal experiences of health and illness). *Journal of Nursing Management, 16*, 433–439. doi:10.1111/j.1365-2834.2008.00863.x

CHAPTER 7

Critical Thinking and Interdisciplinary Teams

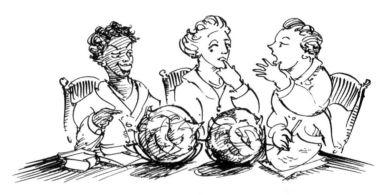

`I DON'T THINK THAT'S WHAT THEY MEANT`

"Two Heads Are Better Than One."

It's hard to imagine anyone who has not heard this saying. The basic idea is that the combined thinking of two individuals produces better outcomes than trying to solve a problem from only one perspective. Now, we know you are thinking, "Yeah, well, lots of times if I want to get it done properly, I just have to do it myself!" You are right; there are those times, but the key is to be able to use your critical thinking (CT) to discriminate between the best times for individual thinking and the best times to use interdisciplinary team (IDT) thinking to produce the best outcomes.

Participants in an Institute of Medicine (IOM) study (2003) strongly believed that combining "heads" was essential to improving health care and therefore included "work in interdisciplinary teams" as one of their five competency recommendations for practice and education. They envisioned IDTs as having the ability to "cooperate, collaborate, communicate, and integrate care in teams to ensure that care is continuous and reliable" (p. 45). These teams are composed of members from different professions who are able to "integrate their observations, bodies of expertise, and spheres of decision making" (p. 54). This team approach is particularly important today. "Interdisciplinary teams are critical in dealing with the increasing complexity of care, coordinating and responding to multiple patient needs, keeping pace with the demands of new technology, responding to the demands of payers, and delivering care across settings" (p. 54).

The IOM did not address CT directly. But let's use some *logical reasoning* here. How can individuals, let alone IDT members, address all the factors in the last IOM quote without solid CT skills? Look at the language used by the IOM: "dealing with," "coordinating," "responding," "integrate their observations," "expertise," "decision making." CT is the engine that drives those activities. All 17 dimensions are required, but consider just a few examples. *Open-mindedness* and *flexibility* are needed to consider alternative approaches and suggestions from other disciplines. *Logical reasoning* and *perseverance* are needed to consider solutions beyond those that first come to mind. *Confidence* helps members know that the IDT solutions are well reasoned based on the expertise of all team members.

We suspect that the IOM was simply assuming we could see the underlying CT. But such assumptions contribute to why details of thinking are frequently overlooked in complex processes such as IDT work. When we make these basic assumptions and do not emphasize the underlying CT, we make IDT work harder to learn and harder to teach others.

The theme of interdisciplinary collaboration is very strong in the IOM 2011 document on the future of nursing. "Care teams need to make the best use of each member's education, skill, and expertise and all health professionals need to practice to the full extent of their license and education" (IOM, 2011, pp. 72, 76). Shared decision making and collaboration need to be improved, with nurses being full partners in these processes.

Over the past decade, many authors have acknowledged the need for thinking in IDT activities (Apker, Propp, Ford, & Hofmeister, 2006; Erickson, Ditomassi, & Jones, 2008; Falise, 2007; Rossen, Bartlett, & Herrick, 2008). Some have even used the terms *inquiry* and *information seeking* as operational concepts important for IDT work (O'Daniel & Rosenstein, 2008). The growing awareness of the need for IDT activities has been demonstrated through the increase in national conferences sponsored by healthcare foundations. For example, the Josiah Macy Jr. Foundation, American Board of Internal Medicine, and the Robert Wood Johnson Foundation (2011) sponsored a national conference, Team-Based Competencies: Building a Shared Foundation for Education and Clinical Practice in February 2011. This conference addressed the paradigm shift needed to move from thinking in disciplinary silos to team thinking in both healthcare education and healthcare practice.

This chapter begins with an explanation of IDT work and a brief discussion of IDT in both practice and education. This background will help us understand the complexity of the thinking embedded in IDT work. We then explore the uniqueness of IDT thinking and the growing examples of IDT work and thinking in health care. In the last two sections, we focus your thinking on these questions: What interferes with IDT thinking, and what cultivates it?

What Is Interdisciplinary Teamwork?

Before examining the thinking necessary for teamwork, let's identify what IDT work is. Basically IDT work occurs when folks from different backgrounds or disciplines (two or more heads) work together to accomplish a task. Employing an interdisciplinary approach to work and recognizing the value of team thinking began long ago. Civilization as we know it would not have survived without the collaborative thinking of folks with different skills needed to save the clan from saber-toothed tiger attacks, to harvest crops, to build factories, and to fly into space. We have vivid examples of teamwork today in the Amish culture, for example, where large tasks such as barn raising are accomplished only by teams. Other recent examples are the IDTs of health professionals, first responders, contractors, volunteers, and others who come together to help in times of major disasters, such as recent hurricanes in the United States, the tsunami in Southeast Asia, and earthquakes in other countries around the world.

There are many levels of working together. Shortly we will discuss the different levels of working together in the healthcare arena. First, let's clarify some terminology issues.

Changing IDT Terminology

In 2000, the IOM convened a panel of 17 experts representing 11 disciplines involved in health care to review over 750 citations using the term *interdisciplinary health care*. The term *interprofessional* was recommended by the National Academies of Practice (Simpson et al., 2001) and is seen more commonly in the literature today, but the majority of the literature continues to use the term *interdisciplinary* (Erickson et al., 2008; Falise, 2007; Reeves & Freeth, 2006; Rossen et al., 2008).

The goal of the National Academies of Practice was "to promote the implementation of cost-effective interprofessional health practice that leads to better healthcare outcomes" (Simpson et al., 2001, p. 6). They focused on three recommendations for achieving the goal: (1) disseminating information on successful models of IDT practice, (2) increasing opportunities for healthcare professionals to make referrals to one another and practice collaboratively, and (3) advocating for changes in legal and reimbursement policies to support IDT practice. For this chapter we will use the abbreviation IDT, while recognizing that most of the current literature uses the term *interprofessional*.

IDT Work in Healthcare Practice

Although much of healthcare delivery in the past traditionally has been done within professional silos, the current emphasis is on how to transition into more collaborative practice models. The IOM (2011) clearly supported this movement for nursing with its recommendations for equal partnerships in providing care. The American Academy of Nursing's Care Coordination Task Force recommended the importance of "thinking about care coordination" (Cipriano, 2012, p. 330), with interprofessionalism being one of the team's guiding principles. In her editorial, Rycroft-Malone cited the need "for more creative approaches and thinking" (2013, p. 67) as we design programming for multidisciplinary teamwork.

There are growing numbers of articles addressing IDT in practice settings from ICUs (Rose, 2011) to geriatric care (Young et al., 2011). To explore the thinking and efforts in IDT practice, we encourage you to consider doing a literature review that captures articles from the *Journal of Interprofessional Care*.

IDT Work in Healthcare Educational Settings

Health professions education has essentially taken place in disciplinary silos similar to the silos of practice. In fact, education probably has been even more silo-focused than practice. At least in practice there are multiple opportunities throughout the workday to interact. In academic settings, however, multiple external constraints (curricular scheduling, clinical learning environments, credit hour restrictions, etc.) interfere with productive collaboration time. We might talk to healthcare educators from other disciplines at conferences or when we are supervising students in a clinical setting, but it is by no means the foundation for effective IDT work.

But we are in luck! Interprofessional education (IPE) is becoming a growing movement in the United States and internationally since the previous edition of this text. The IOM recommendations (2003) have lit a fire! For example, the Interprofessional Education Collaborative (IPEC), composed of six leading professional health education organizations, has developed core competency domains, one of which is Interprofessional Communication (Schmitt, Blue, Aschenbrener, & Viggiano, 2011). Their website (http://ipecollaborative.org/About_IPEC.html) includes news, resources, funding opportunities, conferences, and events to guide educators into thinking more collaboratively and moving toward IPE thinking.

Do student nurses really need help with interprofessional collaboration? Two studies indicate the answer is yes. Popkess and McDaniel (2011) found, in their secondary analysis of data from a national survey of college students, that nursing students and other health profession majors scored lower than education majors in the area of active and collaborative learning. In her literature review of 18 studies focused on interdisciplinary education, Dufrene found through anecdotal comments that nursing students "felt unprepared to communicate with other health care disciplines" (2012, p. 212). Because communication is key to interprofessional activities, this inadequate preparation is a concern. And, because thinking is the foundation for effective communication, such findings point to a need to actively engage nursing and other healthcare students in exploring their thinking skills and habits of the mind.

So how are today's health professions' curricula embracing interprofessional thinking and doing? IPE curricula and course work are actually growing exponentially across the United States. Research into IPE is also expanding. For example,

Hawala-Druy and Hill (2012) designed a mixed methods study to examine the impact of an interprofessional course for 106 pharmacy, nursing, and allied health sciences students on cultural competency. The results of the qualitative portion of the study reflected students' growing awareness of their thinking biases. A pilot study conducted by Lyons and colleagues (2012) at Thomas Jefferson University, Virginia, demonstrated the value of designing an Interprofessional Grand Rounds Seminar for senior nursing and fourth-year medical students. This research team found that thinking together during the debriefing at the end of the experience was critical to both groups of students and promoted further collaborative thinking that could be carried from the educational setting to the practice setting.

All these efforts in interprofessional practice and education require not only the 17 CT dimensions of the individuals, but also an expanded version of those dimensions to achieve team thinking and systems thinking.

Teamwork and Team Thinking in Healthcare Practice

We will elaborate on the thinking aspects of IDT thinking in practice and education later in the chapter, but before we tell you our ideas, we'd like you to reflect on IDT thinking. Perhaps you've seen the application of team thinking in practice similar to this. (See **TACTICS 7-1**.)

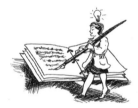

TACTICS 7-1: Practice-Setting Team Meeting and Thinking

1. Read **Scenario 7-1**.
2. Find the thinking that occurred.
3. Identify the thinking done by the individuals by comparing the scenario descriptions with CT vocabulary.
4. Make a list of what you would do to make the team more interprofessional and, by yourself or with a colleague, explain the CT needed to do it more effectively.
5. Think about the kind of thinking that may have occurred beyond individual thinking. This task is challenging at this point in the chapter because we have not yet begun a discussion of team thinking, but all good thinkers enjoy a challenge, so see how you do.

Scenario 7-1: Practice-Setting Team Meeting and Thinking

CD is a 75-year-old married male admitted to a subacute unit for rehabilitation following a mild right-sided ischemic stroke, attributed to atrial fibrillation, that has affected his left side. He agreed to a short stay to improve his strength and functional abilities. Medications were adjusted prior to discharge from the hospital. Now, a week later, he is participating in the care conference, which includes his physical therapist (PT), occupational therapist (OT), speech and language pathologist (SLP), registered nurse (RN), registered dietitian (RD), physician (MD), social worker (SW), and charge nurse. Fortunately, his regular doctor and nurse practitioner (NP) are on staff and round at this facility regularly. No other family members are present. He says, "I want to go home tomorrow. I am really feeling good and I don't see any sense in wasting everyone's time."

Going home has been a recurrent theme since he arrived. The SW has done his evaluation and learned that CD is the primary caregiver to his wife, who has dementia. She is being cared for by their son, who flew in when CD was hospitalized. The SW reports that CD is a retired engineer with good insurance benefits.

PT, OT, and SLP all report that CD has made great progress this past week. He is ambulating 50 feet with contact guard. He is a bit impulsive in his movements and decision making; he needs frequent cues to attend to tasks at hand. He makes his needs known. They believe he could benefit from at least 2 more weeks of therapy, twice daily, for safety and strength reasons. SLP says that his swallowing problems are also improving, and he has advanced to a Dysphagia II diet. He continues to take his meals in his room to avoid distractions, maintaining aspiration precautions. He eats impulsively, gulping and not chewing his food completely. The RD tells the group that CD's weight has been stable, and his nutritional needs are being met based on a completed calorie count.

The RN identified the following problems: impaired physical mobility, toileting self-care deficit (requires postvoid residual bladder scanning and clean intermittent catheterizations), unilateral neglect, impaired skin integrity (Stage 3 pressure ulcer on coccyx), and knowledge deficit regarding medical condition. High risk for falls was identified on admission; she notes that he fell last night while confused. The NP saw him; no injuries were found, but he is still quite confused this morning. Because he had an indwelling catheter while hospitalized and is still not emptying his bladder, she is checking for a urinary tract infection. The nurse is also worried because his Coumadin (warfarin) dose is still not stable, and his recent international normalized ratio (INR) was 4.0. The NP ordered this to be checked STAT today because of his fall. If he needs an antibiotic, it may further affect his INR. If his confusion worsens, he will have to go back to the hospital to be evaluated for a bleed.

Discussion

The scenario is abbreviated, but you get the idea. On a scale of a good–better–best ranking in terms of team CT and the two heads are better than one approach, how would you rate it?

This typical team meeting in the clinical arena gives everyone some input and provides opportunities for bringing up problems and concerns, but that is about the extent of its function. Most team meetings in practice best match the characteristics of a multidisciplinary team, or what Bensimon and Neumann would classify as a "utilitarian team," whose activities consist of delivering information, coordinating and planning, and making decisions (1993).

We are sure you came up with a long list to make the team interaction a better fit with interprofessional care. For starters, those changes might include (1) openly discussing with CD his desire to go home and the implications for his safety and that of his wife if he plans to continue caring for her, (2) discussing options with CD for community resources available for his wife's care, and (3) helping CD see the patterns of impulsive behavior and their implications for his safety. All issues discussed in the meeting are important to patient care, but the team did not transition from simply sharing information to true collaborative thinking.

Teamwork and Team Thinking in Healthcare Education

One might assume that academic nurse educators engage in teamwork and team thinking as a natural part of their scholarly endeavors. Unfortunately, nurses in academe appear to be even less skilled at IDT thinking than nurses in practice. In reality, educators have very little opportunity to collaborate across disciplines. The traditional reward systems in higher education favor independent, not interdependent, thinking. That tradition is changing as institutions of higher learning begin to recognize the value of interdisciplinary work. That change is being facilitated by external funding sources (national and private) that are prioritizing funding to interdisciplinary projects.

Here is an opportunity to examine an educator's team meeting and see how thinking occurs. (See **TACTICS 7-2**.) Again, this is just an example to help your thinking expand, knowing that we have lots more to discuss about thinking in teams later in the chapter.

TACTICS 7-2: Educator Team Meeting and Thinking

1. Read **Scenario 7-2** and reflect on the following:
   a. The thinking being demonstrated by the individuals
   b. The process of thinking as a team
   c. The outcome of the thinking for achieving one of their goals: increasing nursing student understanding of IDT work
2. Make a list of what you would do differently, and, by yourself or with a colleague, explain why. Again, use the thinking vocabulary of the 17 dimensions to reflect or share your thinking with a peer.

Scenario 7-2: Educator Team Meeting and Thinking

Janet is the lead nursing faculty member in the community health nursing courses. Bob and TaNisha are the other tenured nursing faculty. There are three part-time nursing faculty who teach in the clinical sections of the course. Janet, Bob, and TaNisha each teach a third of the classroom portion of the course. Janet calls a meeting with Bob and TaNisha to review the syllabus for the following year and asks for input.

Bob reminds the others that the paper assignment needs to be changed; it requires too much grading, and he isn't sure that students even read all of his extensive feedback on each paper.

TaNisha wants to change the textbook and has a recommendation. TaNisha also shares a need to change how they teach primary, secondary, and tertiary prevention, based on the feedback in student evaluations and the low scores on test items in that area.

Janet brings up the need to deal with the new program objective related to increasing students' abilities to work in IDTs. She reminds the others of the faculty decision to incorporate that aspect of the IOM recommendations.

Bob suggests a plan to have guest speakers from occupational therapy, physical therapy, and social work make presentations to the class and explain the role of each in patient care.

TaNisha says, "I don't know how we will ever fit that in; we have so much critical information to teach already. I can't give up any of my time. Maybe you or Janet can."

In the end they decide to do the following:
1. *Change the paper assignment to include a peer-reviewed first draft component.*
2. *Change to a newer textbook.*
3. *Add some additional readings on IDT work to each topic in the course.*

Discussion

What thinking occurred? With regard to individual thinking, we can make a case for *reflection* when Bob and TaNisha looked back at the past year and identified assignments and textbooks that needed modifications. TaNisha also used *logical reasoning* when she inferred that a different teaching approach was needed to present primary, secondary, and tertiary prevention concepts, based on low student evaluations of that assignment and low test scores in that content area.

But where is the evidence of team thinking? How did the three think differently as a team than as individuals sharing information? Was team thinking necessary, or was this group interaction enough?

This scenario does not even approach the multidisciplinary level of work, let alone IDT thinking, because there are no other disciplines represented. The team in Scenario 7-2 consists of only the three educators who teach the classroom content. It does not include the part-time nursing faculty who work with students in the clinical setting to apply classroom concepts. Their insights could have significantly affected the team thinking. Students, or even alumni, could have added valuable insights as well.

Even with these additional members, however, the thinking would still be limited to nurses. Including faculty from other disciplines, such as occupational or physical therapy or social work, would have increased the probability of an interdisciplinary thinking perspective for both ideas and solutions.

What Is Interdisciplinary Team Thinking?

The literature on IDT work in health care is growing but still offers little to describe the CT needed either individually or jointly by IDT members. To better understand team thinking, we must first examine the literature from other disciplines. Studies of organizations and leadership in business and industry, education, and adult learning provided useful guidance for arriving at descriptions of IDT thinking that we can apply to healthcare settings with some TACTICS. Then we need to look at the growing body of healthcare literature that (1) acknowledges the complexity of thinking in interdisciplinary healthcare teams and (2) begins to provide examples of how IDT work is making a difference.

IDT Thinking Outside Healthcare Settings

It is important at this juncture to make a distinction between team thinking and *groupthink*. According to Bensimon and Neumann (1993), groupthink was a negative term that described what happens when groups mistakenly assume that harmony is the way to achieve group goals. Originating in the early 1970s, groupthink described a phenomenon of assumed consensus that discouraged group members from voicing their concerns, doubts, or points of view, or sharing data that did not fit with the predominant conclusions. Groupthink does not describe thinking as a team; instead, it describes a quick method to reach a conclusion, frequently directed by an individual with power. Groupthink is a very different phenomenon from IDT thinking.

Are there ways for team members to pool their thinking without settling for groupthink? The answer is yes, and one solution is systems thinking. Senge (1990) explained how to use systems thinking to create team-oriented learning organizations in business. As shown in **Box 7-1**, systems thinking goes beyond the thinking of the individual and helps counter some of the linear thinking habits that adults have developed over the years. Systems thinking is ideally suited for IDT work.

Senge believed that the key to systems thinking was dialogue among members of the team as they "enter into a genuine 'thinking together'" (1990, p. 10). Genuine thinking together requires that thinkers suspend assumptions (*open-mindedness* and *flexibility* are helpful here) and allow for "free flowing of meaning through the

Box 7-1   Senge's View: Systems Thinking Is . . .

- A discipline of seeing wholes, seeing interrelationships rather than things, seeing patterns of change versus static snapshots.
- Recognizing that members are part of that pattern, not separate from the patterns.
- Seeing relationships versus linear cause and effect chains of actions.
- The ability to avoid merely shifting problems around and making today's solutions tomorrow's problems.
- Recognizing that our basic skills in systems thinking are underdeveloped or repressed by formal education in linear thinking. Reality is made up of circles, but we tend to see only straight lines that limit our systems thinking.
- A process that requires more dialogue than discussion, interactions of the mind as opposed to simply sharing information.

Source: Senge, 1990.

group, allowing the group to discover insights not attainable individually" (p. 10). Senge, Smith, Kruschwitz, Laur, and Schley (2010) expanded on Senge's earlier work by discussing not only how most problems are interconnected, but also the necessity to "think differently" to see those connections (p. 43). They described how thinking together avoids "reactive problem solving" (p. 44) and moves teams and thinkers toward more creative problem solving and improved "commitment, imagination, patience, and perseverance" (p. 44). They believed that moving to this level of thinking requires three learning capabilities or skill sets, "seeing systems, collaborating across boundaries, and creating desired futures" (p. 44). All three core skills are necessary for effective problem solving, but we are most concerned in this chapter about collaborating across boundaries. The IOM (2003) used the language of system mindedness to capture this same idea: cooperation and thinking together.

Ubbes, Black, and Ausherman (1999) wrote that systems thinking is a tool for thinkers to modify their "value dualisms" of linear thinking (yes–no, black–white, body–mind) to more real-world dimensions of yes–no–maybe, black–white–gray, mind–body–spirit. They described systems thinking as the means to see multiple perspectives and broaden understanding by recognizing relationships between and among pieces of data. (*Contextual perspective* and *transforming knowledge* dimensions should come into play.)

Bensimon and Neumann (1993) have used the term *team thinking* in their writings about collective thinking. **Figure 7-1**, based on their findings, is an illustration of the continuum of team types and the different thinking at the ends of that continuum. The ideal is on the far right and may not be realistic for all organizations in

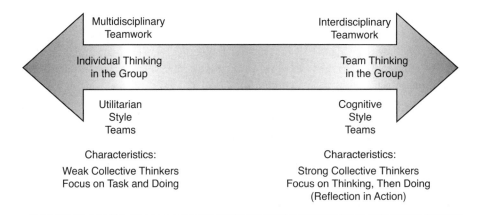

Figure 7-1 Continuum of thinking in teams.

health care or education, but it gives us something to strive for. Remember, in reality, clinicians and educators often need to adapt ideas and create hybrid teams to work in their worlds (*creativity* needs to emerge!). Use this illustration to visualize some of the gradations of IDT thinking before reading about them in more detail.

Bensimon and Neumann (1993) used the terminology of *team thinking* to represent "the art of thinking together" (p. 55), a condition necessary to move from "utilitarian"-style teams to "cognitive"-style teams. Utilitarian-style teams simply achieve tasks, and their members are generally weak at collective thinking. Cognitive-style thinking teams achieve more than task completion. These authors believed that accomplishing a task was only the tip of the iceberg of real teamwork. The inner workings of real teams, not visible in task outcomes, include "team members' thinking, talking, wondering, asking, speculating, arguing, correcting, trying, rethinking, creating, trying again" (p. 55). (It looks like they were recommending that all members use at least *inquisitiveness, information seeking, analyzing, logical reasoning*, and *transforming knowledge* as a group!)

According to Bensimon and Neumann (1993), real teams functioning at the cognitive level recognize their purpose as "sense making." In a real team,

> its members are collectively involved in perceiving, analyzing, learning, and thinking . . . [;] the team is a brain-like social structure that enlarges the intelligence span of individual team members . . . [and] allows the group to behave as a creative system . . . a) viewing problems from multiple perspectives, b) questioning, challenging, and arguing, and c) acting as a monitor and feedback system. (p. 41)

Brookfield and Preskill (1999) offered another perspective on team thinking. They referred to "'group talk' as a blending of conversation, discussion and dialogue

. . . to create new meanings, [incorporating] reciprocity . . . , exchange and inquiry, cooperation and collaboration" (p. 6). They described thinking habits of collaboration that include critical analysis and reflective speculation. Bensimon and Neumann (1993) and Brookfield and Preskill recommended group self-assessment and *reflection* to monitor thinking and its outcomes.

Some additional options for improving team thinking come from the education literature. Harvey and Daniels (2009) have written a book for school-age children. The book focuses on thinking in small groups. One chapter is titled, "Think and Wonder about Images." Another older, but very useful, educational text, *Learning Circles: Creating Conditions for Professional Development* (Collay, Dunlap, Enloe, & Gagnon, 1998) was written for college-age adults. This too guides readers in the strategies of not only working together, but also thinking together for more effective problem solving. We can learn a lot from our education colleagues.

Applying IDT Thinking to Nursing Situations

Let's see how this group thinking assessment might work. We have created a Team Thinking Inventory (**Box 7-2**) based on the works of Bensimon and Neumann (1993), Brookfield and Preskill (1999), and Senge (1990) to help clinicians and educators discriminate how team thinking is different from individual thinking. **TACTICS 7-3** helps us assess team thinking and use the CT dimension of *discriminating* to sort out the differences and similarities.

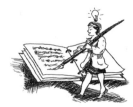

TACTICS 7-3: Team Thinking Assessment

This activity can be performed by both clinicians and educators.

1. Select a team of which you are a member.
2. Think about the function of that team, its purpose, the way it operates, and the ways in which its members participate. Compare the team functioning to Figure 7-1 and see where on the Utilitarian–Cognitive Continuum your team fits.
3. Using the Team Thinking Inventory (Box 7-2), assess that team.
4. Using your critical thinking skill of *discriminating*, identify differences and similarities between individual thinking and team thinking.

Discussion

What did you discover? Does your team function at the utilitarian or the cognitive end of the continuum, or somewhere in between? How did the team thinking manifest itself on the Team Thinking Inventory? What can you and the others on the team do to modify your team thinking? When you used *discriminating*, were you able to see some similarities and the differences between individual thinking and team thinking?

Box 7-2   Team Thinking Inventory

---

1. What strategies are used to help team members think about the big picture as well as the parts?
2. What strategies are used to help team members see the situation from different perspectives?
3. What strategies are used to help team members see their biases and assumptions?
4. What strategies help team members think about patterns and interrelationships of issues and parts of problems?
5. What strategies are used to help team members think beyond cause and effect consequences?
6. Does the thinking that occurs in the team resemble simple sharing of information or discussion and dialogue? Why? How can you move in the direction of discussion and dialogue?
7. What is done to encourage team members to share their thinking or feel comfortable enough to talk about it?
8. How is conflict managed in the team to promote thinking instead of discouraging it?
9. What other sources of gratification are available for team members to socialize, obtain recognition, and interact, besides interdisciplinary teamwork?
10. How were the interdisciplinary team members prepared for their thinking roles?
11. How does the team deal with ambiguity? How long can they tolerate not having a solution?
12. How does the team examine its own thinking processes (e.g., *how* it works, not *what* it is doing and *who* is doing it)?

Sources: Bensimon & Neumann, 1993; Brookfield & Preskill, 1999; Senge, 1990.

These are tough questions, and the answers probably require more than just your CT. It may be time to share this activity with the team and initiate some team thinking to answer these questions.

An Example of IDT Thinking in a Healthcare Setting

An example of interprofessional and cross-institutional thinking is exemplified in this story from Jane Duerr, a nurse practitioner.

Our interprofessional project is a hybrid Acute Care of Elders (ACE) unit. It is a collaborative unit between a large university hospital and a community teaching hospital designed to care for frail elders aged 65 years and older. It is staffed by physicians from both institutions who are board certified in geriatrics and palliative care, nurse practitioners (NPs), RNs who have completed Nurses Improving Care for Healthcare Elders (NICHE) certification, patient care technicians, a social worker (SW), a pharmacist who specializes in geriatrics, and a registered dietitian (RD). All members of the team were hand picked, united in their desire to work only with the elderly.

The full team gathers every morning to review each patient. The MD gives a brief overview of the patient, followed by the RNs who address nursing needs using a SPICES tool (Skin, PO intake, Incontinence, Confusion, Evidence of falls, and Sleep) and assess depression as measured by a geriatric depression scale. Nurses also address safety concerns and functional issues. Nurses also use screening data collected on admission—Mini Cog, Alzheimer's Clock, Katz Functional Status, Braden Scale skin assessment, Morse Falls Risk, and delirium. Medications are reviewed by the pharmacist, who identifies problems with dosing, drug interactions, and drug choices. She advises the practitioners on discharge medications, dosing, and length of treatments. The RD addresses nutritional issues, and the SW is informed of discharge needs and updates the team on related concerns. Referrals are routinely made to the Physical Therapy Department to evaluate safety issues, home care needs, and further recommendations for discharge. The morning group meeting is the time for every team member to have an equal say and to think together to arrive at goals and interventions for each patient.

As the NP, I am pivotal in keeping the team's collaborative goals at the forefront throughout the day and communicating with family, nursing, and medical staff. Many hours are spent talking to families about the realities of their elder's declining status and what they can expect while they are on the unit. I also interact closely with the RN staff, especially in terms of using nonpharmaceutical interventions as much as possible, such as reorientation, heat, and massage. Nurses are empowered to offer alternative suggestions for medications, especially in terms of sleep aids. Cross-cover physicians sometimes order diphenhydramine, Ambien, or Restoril for sleep, all of which contribute to delirium and psychosis in frail elders, so I need to help them think about alternative meds to better fit this population.

The uniqueness of this unit lies in the team thinking and communication. All members of the team have important contributions to the joint decision making. Because these patients are so complex, the usual approaches seen on general medicine units— care farmed out to several separate specialties, without much coordination—would not work. Many of the patients have numerous problems—generally 10 or more and up to 20. These include complications of infections, heart failure exacerbated by infection, Systemic Inflammatory Response Syndrome (SIRS), dementia, delirium, metabolic abnormalities, dehydration, falls, diabetes, heart disease, obesity, and sleep apnea (undiagnosed and diagnosed, treated and untreated). Most patients are taking multiple medications and few families have little understanding of the importance of bringing medications or even a list of medications with them. It's our job to keep this whole big picture in our minds and to engage patients and their families in the thinking to plan customized care.

My hope is this unit will show the power of nursing as equal participants in team-based care. The unit is new; right now, we are just beginning this journey in interprofessional practice.

It's time for another TACTIC. Let's explore how our individual thinking dimensions also work with IDT thinking. (See **TACTICS 7-4**.)

TACTICS 7-4: Matching Some CT Dimensions with IDT Thinking

1. Reflect on the definitions of the dimensions addressed in **Table 7-1**.
2. Read **Scenario 7-3**.
3. Study Table 17-1, and compare and contrast the differences between the thinking examples as they relate to the scenario.
4. Fill in the areas next to *Applying Standards* and *Transforming Knowledge*.
5. Share your ideas with colleagues at work or in class and discuss your different approaches to thinking.
6. What are your conclusions about the similarities and differences in individual thinking and IDT thinking?

TABLE 7-1 Comparing Individual and IDT Thinking

CT Dimension	Individual Thinking	IDT Thinking
Flexibility	Physical therapist thinks about ways to customize PT activities for JW to minimize complications with his asthma.	The team thinks about ways to customize all of JW's care to fit his needs regarding recidivism, housing, finances, nutrition, activity, pain management, respiratory health, medication, and health teaching.
Open-mindedness	Nutritionist acknowledges that JW's food preferences are not always the healthiest but that he has the right to choose.	The IDT acknowledges their temptation to judge JW for frequent visits to the ED and for not getting his prescriptions filled for his asthma medication.
Applying Standards		
Transforming Knowledge		

Scenario 7-3: JW

JW is a 48-year-old Hispanic male with a diagnosis of asthma and chronic low-back pain. He is currently homeless. He has just been admitted to the inpatient unit from the ED to get his asthma under control. This is his third hospitalization within the past 6 months. During his stay, he receives care from an IDT consisting of an SW, a nurse, a pulmonologist, a nutritionist, and a PT.

Discussion

What did you discover? The use of the thinking dimensions by groups is not so different from their use by individuals, is it? What is different is using the thinking dimension on a larger scale and with more input. It is also helpful to use the dimensions very overtly. Comments such as, "Let's use our *flexibility* thinking for a minute here and see if we can't" or "If we all put on our thinking caps and use some *inquisitiveness*, what are some of the things we need to know but don't know?" or "If we try a recommendation, what can we *predict* as possible outcomes?" or "What part of the big picture (*contextual perspective*) are we missing?" or "We really need to break this down and look at the parts (*analyzing*) before we try to draw any conclusions (*logical reasoning*) about how to fix things."

For more practice, try adding other dimensions and different scenarios to discriminate the subtle and overt differences between thinking from an IDT perspective and an individual perspective.

The next sections address some of the barriers to, as well as what helps, IDT thinking. The better we understand the factors that influence IDT thinking, the better we are able to use our individual thinking to modify and enhance it.

What Interferes with IDT Thinking?

The literature cites numerous factors that interfere with IDT thinking. We have classified these barriers to IDT thinking into the following categories: (1) time, resources, and support; (2) professional preparation; and (3) personality, including communication skills and behavioral patterns. Communication and behavior are paramount because IDT work and thinking are totally dependent on our ability (or inability) to interact with one another.

Time, Resources, and Support

The lack of time constantly plagues healthcare providers. With all the work that needs to be done, it is difficult to convince people that more time needs to be found for meetings within the discipline, let alone interdisciplinary ones. It is even harder to convince folks if their only experience with meetings is wasting time. What's that old saying? A meeting is where you keep minutes but lose hours. Creative solutions for IDT thinking without meetings are proposed later in the chapter. We bet that piqued your interest!

Lack of resources and support can also restrict movement toward IDT work and thinking (O'Daniel & Rosenstein, 2008). A few examples of resources and support include the following:

1. Physical space for IDTs to meet, where staff can talk and think together with limited distractions
2. Designated time for team activities and thinking
3. Functioning computers and Internet access so that physicians, nurses, SWs, PTs, and so on, can continually update their knowledge about their discipline and how others are using IDT work to improve patient outcomes
4. Leadership, policies, and procedures that acknowledge the value of IDT work and thinking, and empower IDT members to work together

Professional Preparation

Most professional disciplines pride themselves on their discipline autonomy. Nurses have been working very hard since the 1950s to establish their profession as unique and separate from medicine. They have achieved that goal through the development of a solid knowledge base, discipline-specific research, a code of ethics, and standards of care. However, in the process, they may have also promoted clinicians who avoid collaborative thinking for fear of being traitors to the nursing profession. Nursing, like other disciplines, is a bit ethnocentric—or should we say, discipline-centric? We have been educated in our own domains with our own paradigms for thinking and problem solving separately instead of together. The literature refers to this as working in disciplinary silos (Herbert et al., 2007; Kuehn, 1998; Verma, Paterson, & Medves, 2006). It is time to apply new professional standards—interdisciplinary work standards—that include strategies for IDT thinking. There are new standards, but we still do not see specific standards for thinking. For example, the core competencies for interprofessional care that were developed by the American Academy of Nursing's Care Coordination Task Force (Cipriano, 2012) demonstrate a positive movement toward standards, but the thinking is only implied.

Thinking and working together is not easy; it requires preparation for teamwork both in the educational arena and in the practice arena. Lack of preparation for teamwork significantly hinders team members from thinking together, let alone working together. Although teamwork has been given lip service over the past few decades, unidisciplinary teams are still the most common. For the most part, nurses talk with nurses, doctors talk with doctors, nurse educators talk with nurse educators, and so on. This isolation limits thinking to the paradigms of the discipline.

Because of the nature of their work, SWs, case managers, discharge planners, and community health nurses are probably the groups most skilled at engaging more than one discipline in team thinking and activities. Their jobs require extensive collaboration to connect clients with necessary resources. Doing that job effectively demands communication and thinking collaboration with other disciplines.

Personality

President Harry S. Truman once commented, "It is amazing what you can accomplish if you do not care who gets the credit" (Quotations Page, n.d.). If team members need to feel important, believe they have the best ideas, or have difficulty accepting good ideas from other members, team thinking suffers. If team members use the team's thinking time to meet their personal needs for socialization, team thinking suffers. IDT thinking requires the *intellectual integrity* to go beyond one's beliefs and assumptions and seek a better truth.

Low tolerance for ambiguity hinders folks from taking extra time to go beyond acceptable to better or best solutions. A lack of *open-mindedness*, *flexibility*, and *contextual perspective* contributes to low tolerance for ambiguity. If team members are uncomfortable because there are no obvious answers to problems, they are more likely to rush to quick solutions. Quick solutions may ease the anxiety of the team, but they are not always the best choices.

Comfort level in working together is another personal factor to consider. How comfortable are you with team membership? For example, what about when patients are present? Will the presence of patients prevent you from saying what you really think for fear of hurting their feelings, creating unnecessary worries, or challenging data? How much you value *contextual perspective* may influence your comfort with the patient being part of the context.

And perhaps one of the most essential personality factors is emotional intelligence (EI). Goleman (1995) asserted that EI is critical to success in any area of life. EI is particularly critical in developing the collaboration needed for effective IDT thinking (McCallin & Bamford, 2007; McQueen, 2004). In a nutshell, EI is a constellation of personality characteristics that requires several thinking dimensions. Individuals with high levels of EI are better team thinkers because team thinking is complex. The more complex a situation is, the more knowledge and thinking need to converge, moving from one point of view to a synthesis (Kuehn, 1998). That sure sounds like *transforming knowledge* to us!

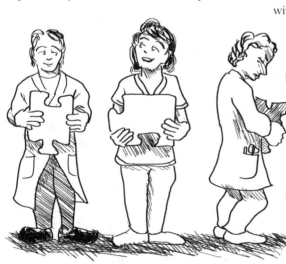

© Jesse Rubenfeld

McCallin and Bamford (2007) referred to the thinking skill needed for the complexity of IDT work as pluralistic dialogue. Pluralistic dialogue allows IDT members to use *reflection*, *open-mindedness, contextual perspective, transforming knowledge,* and *confidence* to break through stereotypes, come to grips with different ways of approaching problems, synthesizing, and exploring alternative solutions, and be assured that their reasoning is sound. Without EI, effective team thinking is difficult, if not impossible.

Communication Skills

The medium for IDT collaborative thinking is language. Discipline-specific language and jargon are cited repeatedly as limiting factors for working in IDTs (Case, 1998; O'Daniel & Rosenstein, 2008; Schofield & Amodeo, 1999). Converting to the language of thinking may become the unifying factor for IDT communication and collaboration.

When individuals in the same or different disciplines communicate, conflict is inevitable. One's inability to handle conflict can hinder CT and IDT work. Conflict creates anxiety, which prevents higher-order thinking (Hart, 1983). The secret is not to try to eliminate conflict (which, by the way, is impossible), but to use conflict to improve the effectiveness of teams (Northouse & Northouse, 1985; O'Daniel & Rosenstein, 2008; Sessa, 1998). Strategies for improving your ability to use conflict constructively depend on *confidence* in your reasoning, *flexibility,* and *intellectual integrity.*

An analysis of the current interaction style in healthcare practice and education indicates a developmental delay. Many providers' interaction styles might best be described as parallel play or, at best, multidisciplinary. Parallel play refers to the interaction style used by 2- and 3-year-old toddlers as they begin their socialization process beyond self. Toddlers using parallel play are aware of others; they enjoy being in the vicinity of others, but basically they do their own thing, not having figured out how to play together. Does this sound like the way we operate sometimes in health care? Moving beyond parallel play to collaborative interactions will likely require *perseverance* to learn better ways to work and think as teams instead of in silos.

The current literature on IDT work and IDT thinking repeatedly emphasizes that communication skill has the most important impact on whether outcomes of IDT work are positive or negative (Charlton, Dearing, Berry, & Johnson, 2008; O'Daniel & Rosenstein, 2008; Reader, Flin, Mearns, & Cuthbertson, 2007; Risser, Simon, Rice, Salisbury, & Morey, 2011; Schmitt et al., 2011; Seago, 2008; Williams, Vares, & Brumbaugh, 2006).

Behavioral Patterns

Our behavioral patterns can reflect our thinking. For example, some of us behave by removing ourselves to a quiet place to think. Others behave by pausing to think before offering ideas. And many behave as active listeners, respectfully absorbing the information that others are sharing before responding.

Our behavioral toward others is a primary measure of how well we have been socialized as thinking human beings in a civilized society. Disruptive, counterproductive behavioral patterns that have been around for years in health care and elsewhere are finally being identified as totally unacceptable. These patterns are particularly problematic because they literally make IDT thinking and IDT work impossible.

These patterns have been referred to as disruptive or bad behavior (O'Daniel & Rosenstein, 2008), lateral violence (Martin, Stanley, Dulaney, & Pehrson, 2008; Sincox & Fitzpatrick, 2008), and incivility (Clark, 2008a, 2008b; Jenkins, Kerber, & Woith, 2013). Whether it is covert (passive aggressiveness, ignoring, rudeness) or overt (yelling, belittling, bullying, physical violence), this behavior represents flagrant disrespect for colleagues. Disruptive behavior, lateral violence, or incivility in health care can occur between any individuals—nurses and nurses, physicians and nurses, administrators and healthcare workers, nursing faculty and nursing students, and so on. The Center for American Nurses (2008) prepared a position paper calling for zero-tolerance policies related to disruptive behavior and lateral violence. IDT thinking can work only with a foundation of respect and trust for one another. Confronting negative behaviors and modeling positive behaviors are essential for quality patient outcomes.

What Cultivates IDT Thinking?

Brookfield and Preskill (1999) made a strong case for how discussion enhances learning through the cultivation of critical *reflection* and thinking. They offered strategies promoting CT through discussion with exercises called Critical Incident Questionnaires (p. 49), Telling Tales from the Trenches (p. 77), and Circle of Voices (p. 80), to name just a few.

Thinking in an effective team environment does not happen automatically; it takes time, effort, and a commitment to think beyond your discipline's knowledge bases, aspirations, and values (McCormack, 2001; Salmon & Jones, 2001). It also takes a shift in organizational culture to mutually respect working partnerships (Coombs, 2001). The bottom line is that cultivating IDT thinking is hard work. We do not have any magic bullets, but we have some helpful suggestions.

For starters, not all IDT thinking requires meetings. The IOM talks about IDT work, not IDT meetings. This is an important distinction and helps us think outside that old box! This awareness can lead to all kinds of *creativity* and *flexibility* to change the IDT work environment mindset for clinicians and educators.

Clinicians

The IOM (2003) summarized eight conditions necessary for effective IDT work in the practice setting. Although they do not specifically mention thinking, we believe that if you examine **Box 7-3**, you will decide that it is impossible to achieve anything on the list without thinking. These too can all occur in providers' daily interactions in addition to meetings.

Case (1998) identified several similar factors that need to be in place for teamwork to occur in the practice setting: (1) a common language, (2) a common knowledge base, (3) shared core values, (4) understanding the roles of the team members,

---

Box 7-3   IOM Conditions for Effective IDT Work

- Learn about other team members' expertise, background, knowledge, and values.
- Learn individual roles and processes required to work collaboratively.
- Demonstrate basic group skills, including communication, negotiation, delegation, time management, and assessment of group dynamics.
- Ensure that accurate and timely information reaches those who need it at the appropriate times.
- Customize care and manage smooth transitions across settings and over time, even when the team members are in entirely different physical locations.
- Coordinate and integrate care processes to ensure excellence, continuity, and reliability of the care provided.
- Resolve conflicts with other members of the team.
- Communicate with other members of the team in a shared language, even when the members are in entirely different physical locations.

Source: Reproduced with permission from *Health Professions Education: A Bridge to Quality*, 2003 by the National Academy of Sciences, Courtesy of the National Academies Press, Washington, D.C.

(5) respect for team members, and (6) mutual sharing among the members. Case encouraged staff development specialists to pay attention to these factors when they promote IDT work. Note that Case did not say "meetings." All of her recommendations can occur in corridor discussions as long as privacy is not violated, of course.

An excellent example of nonmeeting IDT thinking is offered by Halm, Goering, and Smith (2003), with the use of interdisciplinary rounds (IDR). These are enhanced discharge planning rounds in which each discipline reviews the patient record, identifies problems from the discipline's perspective, shares information with the team, collaborates on approaches, identifies barriers to the approaches, and identifies individual and team learning needs. The goals for IDR were timely and safe discharges, improved documentation of collaborative care, and increased awareness of each discipline's skills and resources.

They implemented IDR in a large midwestern hospital on medicine, orthopedics, neurology, rehabilitation, surgery, cardiology, oncology, behavioral health, and birthing center units. The plan was to use IDR as a means of engaging all disciplines in discharge planning. Participating clinical nurse specialists used the Internet to collaborate with other institutions using similar processes. Sharing of ideas and constant modifications took place as new information became available. At the end of 6 months, outcomes of the IDR included "greater participation by all the disciplines in achieving patient and family outcomes, increased early recognition of patients at risk, and improved communication among members of the healthcare team" (Halm et al., 2003, p. 133).

Seago (2008) reviewed 36 studies focused on professional communication. She found empirical evidence of the strong relationship between effective communication and positive patient outcomes. O'Daniel and Rosenstein (2008) synthesized findings focused on teamwork and team thinking. They identified 13 components of successful teamwork and focused very clearly on issues of open communication, a respectful atmosphere, and processes for acknowledging and dealing with conflict, among others. One effective strategy they cited was SBAR (situation–background–assessment–recommendations) as a guide for nurse–physician reporting. Developed at Kaiser Permanente and becoming increasingly popular, this simple approach not only facilitates communication but also "helps develop desired critical-thinking skills" (p. 2-277). You can see how thinking would be enhanced by the reminders. Consider how some of the CT dimensions come through:

Situation: What is going on with the patient? What *information seeking* have I done? How has my *discriminating* helped me clarify signs and symptoms?

Background: What is the clinical background or *contextual perspective*?

Assessment: What do I think the problem is? What are the results of my *analysis* and *logical reasoning*?

Recommendation: What would I do to correct it? What would I *predict*?

Educators

The IOM conditions for effective IDT in Box 7-3 and the issues identified by O'Daniel and Rosenstein (2008) are also valuable for thinking about implementing IDT work in the educational setting. Implementation in the academic arena, however, has some additional challenges because IDT activities are not generally rewarded in that arena. Value in education has traditionally been given to independent work. These traditions must be changed to prepare educators and students of all the professions for IDT practice in the real world.

Rice (2000) recommended a dual socialization process in academic education. For example, nursing students would not only learn their profession, but also have courses and clinical experiences together with students from other disciplines; as a result of thinking and working together as groups, they would learn to share and respect each other from the start. Rice based her recommendation on her experience as an SW and her extensive literature review of 302 articles.

We have firsthand knowledge of one IDT course that has been very successful. Faculty from the School of Nursing, the School of Social Work, and the School of Associated Health Professions at Eastern Michigan University worked collaboratively to develop and teach a course called Aging to Infancy: A Retrospective Approach to Life. The disciplines involved were nursing, social work, occupational therapy, and dietetics. All four faculty participated before, during, and after the class periods to coordinate their teaching, discuss issues arising in class, and assess students' learning. A major goal of this course was to demonstrate to students how the disciplines collaborate in both thinking and doing to address healthcare issues across age groups. The course enrollment increased from 25 students the first year to over 100 students 2 years later.

Since this text was first published, numerous articles and texts have emerged that address the need for educational models to promote interdisciplinary thinking. Verma et al. (2006) identified core competencies for curricula and ideas for assessing interdisciplinary learning outcomes, elaborating on the stages of learning and how to work and think collaboratively. Reeves and Freeth (2006) discussed the development of a model of IPE in community mental health in England. Golanowski, Beaudry, Kurz, Laffey, and Hook (2007) offered a model for interdisciplinary decision making. Dellasega, Milone-Nuzzo, Curci, Ballard, and Kirch (2007) described a discipline-neutral model, in which all professionals are on equal ground. This model was used in a humanities course to explore interdisciplinary thinking and problem solving. Weaver (2008) proposed a model for examining the antecedents, processes, and outcomes that need to be addressed for successful IDT. All aspects of this model require what Weaver described as "integration of thought" and "synergy" (p. 112). As we mentioned earlier, readers should look at the *Journal of Interprofessional Care* for the most current literature.

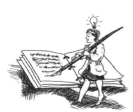

TACTICS 7-5: How Do My Interprofessional Teammates Think?

Clinicians

Identify a health professional outside of nursing you have worked with, but not regularly. Set up a plan to have coffee, or better yet, lunch, to learn more about each other. Explain that the purpose of this interaction is to better understand each other's role and thinking as a means of becoming more collaborative in designing patient care. After some small talk, focus the interaction on each of you answering the following six questions:

1. At what point do you have to put your thinking cap on when you start patient care?
2. How do you assess and collect information on your patients, and how would you label the thinking you use to assess and collect information?
3. How do you label the health concerns you identify for patients, and how would you label the thinking you use to identify health concerns?
4. How do you decide on priorities for care, and how would you label the thinking you use to prioritize?
5. What are some words you would use to describe all the different kinds of thinking you use with patient care?
6. What could we do to do a better job of thinking together for patient care?

At the end of the interaction, share briefly what you have learned that you didn't realize before and thank your colleague for participating in this activity. Consider sharing this experience with your other nursing colleagues.

Educators

Pair up your students with other students or healthcare professionals from a different discipline. Have them meet as previously described and ask the same six questions of each other.

After completing that portion of this TACTICS, meet with all your students to address these questions:

1. What do you know now about the other discipline's approach to care that you didn't know before?
2. What did you learn about the differences and similarities in your thinking skills and habits of the mind?
3. How can you use what you learned to improve future interprofessional collaboration and thinking?

Discussion for Both Clinicians and Educators

Continue to unpack the learning that occurred. Clinicians might do this with colleagues on the unit. Educators would do this during the postconference discussions. These additional questions might stimulate more interprofessional thinking:

- How can you deal with different approaches that conflict with your perspectives?
- What are some of the nonverbal behaviors in the individuals that promote or inhibit thinking?
- What are some of the strategies for helping both disciplines recognize each other's thinking skills and habits of the mind?
- What would you like to do next to expand your understanding of interprofessional collaboration with your peers or colleagues?

Perseverance Is Needed

Whether in practice or education, initial efforts to enhance IDT work will take time, energy, and CT. It may seem overwhelming; you will want to fall back on, it's easier to do it myself. At first we will likely continue using hybrid versions of IDT. But once IDT thinking is integrated into daily activities that go beyond having more meetings, the time factor will become less of an issue.

Before finishing this chapter, let's return to the two heads are better than one idea and expand on it. Consider this: compare the positive outcomes of IDT thinking to a molecule of sugar!

Think back to your organic chemistry course. For some, this may be a bit painful, but bear with us a minute. Remember how the elements of carbon, hydrogen, and

$$
\begin{array}{c}
H\diagdown C\diagup\!\!\!\!=O \\
| \\
H-C-OH \\
| \\
HO-C-H \\
| \\
H-C-OH \\
| \\
H-C-OH \\
| \\
H-C-OH \\
| \\
H
\end{array}
$$

Figure 7-2   Dry glucose molecule.

oxygen combine to make sugar? Each of the elements has unique properties and is distinct. But when certain conditions exist, those elements work together to create sugar, a whole new entity (**Figure 7-2**).

Sugar is a totally different substance from any of its three elements: carbon, hydrogen, and oxygen. Sugar is something new (and much tastier than any of the three elements by themselves) that results from the combined efforts of energy, the right amounts of elements, and the right conditions. But even as sugar, the elements of carbon, hydrogen, and oxygen maintain their basic molecular integrity.

IDT work and IDT thinking work in similar (sweet?) ways. Healthcare providers (the elements) collaborate using energy to combine their thinking and disciplinary knowledge (the necessary conditions) to create quality patient outcomes (sugar). And, as with the sugar molecule, all the healthcare providers (elements) maintain their unique identity, disciplinary knowledge, and thinking skills.

Now, if you are really into organic chemistry, you know there are lots of different types of sugar and starches that result from combining these elements in different amounts. IDT work and thinking have the same kinds of results, if not more. Imagine the quality patient outcome possibilities that IDT thinking could create.

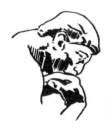

© Jesse Rubenfeld

PAUSE and Ponder

Future Implications of IDT Thinking

According to growing evidence, moving toward IDT thinking is no longer a choice; it is a necessity. IDT thinking is the catalyst for moving us from disciplinary silos to collaborative outcomes. Our job is to better understand IDT work and IDT thinking. We must value IDT thinking, overcome the barriers to it, nurture the factors that cultivate it, respect each other's thinking, teach it, and model it as we strive for quality patient outcomes. You and your peers will be the new generation of leaders in practice and education to achieve that goal. Today's clinicians may have to learn IDT thinking on the job, but it is hoped that tomorrow's clinicians will have learned IDT thinking in school.

REFLECTION CUES

- IDTs are essential for dealing with the increasing complexity of health care.
- Most team meetings in practice best match the characteristics of a multidisciplinary team or a utilitarian team whose activities consist of delivering information, coordinating and planning, and making decisions.
- IDTs focus on collaborative problem identification and problem solving.
- IDTs occur less frequently in academic settings than in practice settings.
- Multiple factors—time, resources, support, professional preparation, personality, communication skills, and behavioral patterns—can interfere with team thinking.
- Discipline autonomy tends to promote working and thinking in silos.
- Lack of preparation and training to work in IDTs is a major impediment to IDT work.
- Thinking in IDTs is more than simply adding ideas together; IDT thinking blends ideas and creates new ones that individuals would not have considered independently.
- Not all IDT thinking requires meetings; IDR is one alternative.
- New educational models and research are demonstrating effective IDT strategies and outcomes.
- IDT work takes time and energy, effective leadership, and critical thinking to be successful.

REFERENCES

Apker, J., Propp, K. M., Ford, W. S. Z., & Hofmeister, N. (2006). Collaboration, credibility, compassion, and coordination: Professional nurse communication skill sets in health care team interactions. *Journal of Professional Nursing, 22*(3), 180–189. doi:10.1016/j.profnurs.2006.03.002

Bensimon, E. M., & Neumann, A. (1993). *Redesigning collegiate leadership: Teams and teamwork in higher education.* Baltimore, MD: Johns Hopkins University Press.

Brookfield, S. D., & Preskill, S. (1999). *Discussion as a way of teaching: Tools and techniques for democratic classrooms.* San Francisco, CA: Jossey-Bass.

Case, B. (1998). Competency development: Critical thinking, clinical judgment, and technical ability. In K. J. Kelly-Thomas (Ed.), *Clinical and nursing staff development: Current competency, future focus* (2nd ed., pp. 240–281). Philadelphia, PA: Lippincott.

Center for American Nurses. (2008). *The Center for American Nurses calls for an end to lateral violence and bullying in nursing work environments.* Retrieved from http://www.mc.vanderbilt.edu/root/pdfs/nursing/center_lateral_violence_and_bullying_position_statement_from_center_for_american_nurses.pdf

Charlton, C. R., Dearing, K. S., Berry, J. A., & Johnson, M. J. (2008). Nurse practitioners' communication styles and their impact on patient outcomes: An integrated literature review. *Journal of the American Academy of Nurse Practitioners, 20*, 382–388. doi:10.1111/j.1745-7599.2008.00336

Cipriano, P. (2012). The imperative for patient-, family-, and population centered interprofessional approaches to care coordination and transitional care: A policy brief by the American Academy of Nursing's Care Coordination Task Force. *Nursing Outlook, 60*, 330–333. doi: 10.1016/j.outlook.2012.06.021

Clark, C. M. (2008a). Faculty and student assessment of and experience with incivility in nursing education. *Journal of Nursing Education, 47*, 458–465.

Clark, C. M. (2008b). Student voices on faculty incivility in nursing education: A conceptual model. *Nursing Education Perspectives, 29*, 284–289.

Collay, M., Dunlap, D., Enloe, W., & Gagnon, G. W., Jr. (1998). *Learning circles: Creating conditions for professional development.* Thousand Oaks, CA: Corwin Press.

Coombs, M. (2001). Towards collaborative and collegial caring: A comparative study. *Nursing in Critical Care, 6*, 23–27.

Dellasega, C., Milone-Nuzzo, P., Curci, K. M., Ballard, J. O., & Kirch, D. G. (2007). The humanities interface of nursing and medicine. *Journal of Professional Nursing, 23*, 174–179.

Dufrene, C. (2012). Health care partnerships: A literature review of interdisciplinary education. *Journal of Nursing Education, 51*(4), 212–216. doi:10.3928/1484834-20120224.01

Erickson, J. I., Ditomassi, M. O., & Jones, D. A. (2008). Interdisciplinary Institute for Patient Care: Advancing clinical excellence. *Journal of Nursing Administration, 38*, 308–314.

Falise, J. P. (2007). True collaboration: Interdisciplinary rounds in nonteaching hospitals—it can be done! *AACN Advanced Critical Care, 18*, 346–351.

Golanowski, M., Beaudry, D., Kurz, L., Laffey, W. J., & Hook, M. L. (2007). Interdisciplinary shared decision-making: Taking shared governance to the next level. *Nursing Administration Quarterly, 31*, 341–353.

Goleman, D. (1995). *Emotional intelligence: Why it can matter more than IQ.* New York, NY: Bantam Books.

Halm, M. A., Goering, M., & Smith, M. (2003). Interdisciplinary rounds: Impact on patients, families, and staff. *Clinical Nurse Specialist, 17*, 133–142.

Hart, L. A. (1983). *Human brain and human learning.* New York, NY: Longman.

Harvey, S., & Daniels, H. (2009). *Comprehensive collaboration: Inquiry circles in action.* Portmouth, NH: Heinemann.

Hawala-Druy, S., & Hill, M. H. (2012). Interdisciplinary: Cultural competency and cultural congruent education for millennials in health professions. *Nurse Education Today, 32*, 772–778. doi:10.1016/j.nedt.2012.05.002

Herbert, C. P., Bainbridge, L., Bickford, J., Baptiste, S., Brajtman, S., Dryden, T., . . . Solomon, P. (2007). Factors that influence engagement in collaborative practice: How 8 health professionals became advocates. *Canadian Family Physician, 53*, 1318–1325.

Institute of Medicine. (2003). *Health professions education: A bridge to quality.* Washington, DC: National Academies Press.

Institute of Medicine. (2011). *The future of nursing: Leading change, advancing health.* Washington, DC: National Academies Press.

Jenkins, S. D., Kerber, C. S., & Woith, W. H. (2013). An intervention to promote civility among nursing students. *Nursing Education Perspectives, 34*(2), 95–100. doi: 10.5480/1536-5026-34.2.95

Josiah Macy Jr. Foundation, American Board of Internal Medicine, & Robert Wood Johnson Foundation. (2011). Team-based competencies: Building a shared foundation for education and clinical practice. *Conference proceedings.* Retrieved from http://ipecollaborative.org/uploads/IPEC-Team-Based-Competencies.pdf

Kuehn, A. F. (1998). Collaborative health professional education: An interdisciplinary mandate for the third millennium. In T. J. Sullivan (Ed.), *Collaboration: A health care imperative* (pp. 419–465). New York, NY: McGraw-Hill.

Lyons, K. J., Giordano, C., Isenberg, G., Arenson, C., Speakman, E., Ward, J., . . . Anthony, R. (2012, October). *An assessment of an interprofessional clinical rounding experience.* Paper presented at Association of Schools of Allied Health Professions Annual Conference, Lake Buena Vista, Florida.

Martin, M. M., Stanley, K. M., Dulaney, P., & Pehrson, K. M. (2008). The role of the psychiatric consultation liaison nurse in evidence-based approaches to lateral violence in nursing. *Perspectives in Psychiatric Care, 44*(1), 58–60.

McCallin, A., & Bamford, A. (2007). Interdisciplinary teamwork: Is the influence of emotional intelligence fully appreciated? *Journal of Nursing Management, 15*, 386–391.

McCormack, B. (2001). Clinical effectiveness and clinical teams: Effective practice with older people. *Nursing Older People, 13*(5), 14–17.

McQueen, A. C. H. (2004). Emotional intelligence in nursing work. *Journal of Advanced Nursing, 47*, 101–108.

Northouse, P. G., & Northouse, L. L. (1985). *Health communication: A handbook for health professionals.* Englewood Cliffs, NJ: Prentice Hall.

O'Daniel, M., & Rosenstein, A. (2008). Professional communication and team collaboration. In R. G. Hughes (Ed.), *Patient safety and quality: An evidence-based handbook for nurses* (Vol. 2, pp. 2-271–2-284). Rockville, MD: Agency for Healthcare Research and Quality. (AHRQ Publication No. 08-0043)

Popkess, A. M., & McDaniel, A. (2011). Are nursing students engaged in learning? A secondary analysis of data from the national survey of student engagement. *Nursing Education Perspectives, 32*(2), 89–94.

Quotations Page. (n.d.). *Quotations by author.* Retrieved from http://www.quotationspage.com/quotes .php3?author+Harry+S+Truman

Reader, T. W., Flin, R., Mearns, K., & Cuthbertson, B. H. (2007). Interdisciplinary communication in the intensive care unit. *British Journal of Anaesthesia, 98*(3), 347–353. doi:10.1093/bja/ael372

Reeves, S., & Freeth, D. (2006). Re-examining the evaluation of interprofessional education for community mental health teams with a different lens: Understanding presage, process and product factors. *Journal of Psychiatric and Mental Health Nursing, 13*, 765–770.

Rice, A. H. (2000). Interdisciplinary collaboration in healthcare: Education, practice and research. *National Academies of Practice Forum, 2*(1), 59–73.

Risser, D. T., Simon, R., Rice, M. M., Salisbury, M. L., & Morey, J. C. (2011). A structured teamwork system to reduce clinical errors. In P. L. Spath (Ed.), *Error reduction in health care: A systems approach to improving patient safety* (pp. 297–334). San Francisco, CA: Jossey-Bass.

Rose, L. (2011). Interprofessional collaboration in the ICU: How to define? *Nursing in Critical Care, 16*(1), 5–10. doi: 10.1111/j.1478-5153.2010.00398.x

Rossen, E. K., Bartlett, R. B., & Herrick, C. A. (2008). Interdisciplinary collaboration: The need to revisit. *Issues in Mental Health Nursing, 29*, 387–396.

Rycroft-Malone, J. (2013). Reflecting back, looking forward: 10 years of *Worldviews on Evidence-Based Nursing. Worldviews on Evidence-Based Nursing, 10*(2), 67–68. doi: 10.1111/wvn.12006

Salmon, D., & Jones, M. (2001). Shaping the interprofessional agenda: A study examining qualified nurses' perceptions of learning with others. *Nurse Education Today, 21*, 18–25.

Schmitt, M., Blue, A., Aschenbrener, C. A., & Viggiano, T. R. (2011). Core competencies for interprofessional collaborative practice: Reforming health care by transforming health professionals' education. *Academic Medicine, 86*(11), 1351. doi: 10.1097/ACM.0b013e3182308e39

Schofield, R. F., & Amodeo, M. (1999). Interdisciplinary teams in healthcare and human service settings: Are they effective? *Health and Social Work, 24*, 210–219.

Seago, J. A. (2008). Professional communication. In R. G. Hughes (Ed.), *Patient safety and quality: An evidence-based handbook for nurses* (Vol. 2, pp. 2-247–2-269). Rockville, MD: Agency for Healthcare Research and Quality. (AHRQ Publication No. 08-0043)

Senge, P., Smith, B., Kruschwitz, N., Laur, J., & Schley, S. (2010). *The necessary revolution: Working together to create a sustainable world.* New York, NY: Broadway Books.

Senge, P. M. (1990). *The fifth discipline: The art and practice of the learning organization.* New York, NY: Doubleday.

Sessa, V. (1998). Professional development initiative: Using conflict to improve effectiveness of nurse teams. *Orthopaedic Nursing, 17*(3), 41–46.

Simpson, G., Rabin, D., Schmitt, M., Taylor, P., Urban, S., & Ball, J. (2001). Interprofessional healthcare practice: Recommendations of the National Academies of Practice expert panel on healthcare in the 21st century. *Issues in Interdisciplinary Care, 3*(1), 5–19.

Sincox, A. K., & Fitzpatrick, M. (2008). Lateral violence: Calling out the elephant in the room. *Michigan Nurse, 81*(3), 8–9.

Ubbes, V. A., Black, J. M., & Ausherman, J. A. (1999). Teaching for understanding in health education: The role of critical and creative thinking skills within constructivism theory. *Journal of Health Education, 30*(2), 67–72.

Verma, S., Paterson, M., & Medves, J. (2006). Core competencies for health care professionals. *Journal of Allied Health, 35,* 109–115.

Weaver, J. E. (2008). Enhancing multiple disciplinary teamwork. *Nursing Outlook, 56,* 108–114. doi:10.1016/j.outlook.2008.03.013

Williams, J., Vares, L., & Brumbaugh, M. (2006). Education to improve interdisciplinary practice of health care professionals: A pilot project. *Medicine & Health Rhode Island, 89,* 312–313.

Young, H. M., Siegel, E. O., McCormick, W. C., Fulmer, T., Harootyan, L. K., & Dorr, D. A. (2011). Interdisciplinary collaboration in geriatrics: Advancing health for older adults. *Nursing Outlook, 59,* 243–251. doi:10.1016/j.outlook.2011.05.006

CHAPTER 8

Critical Thinking and Evidence-Based Practice

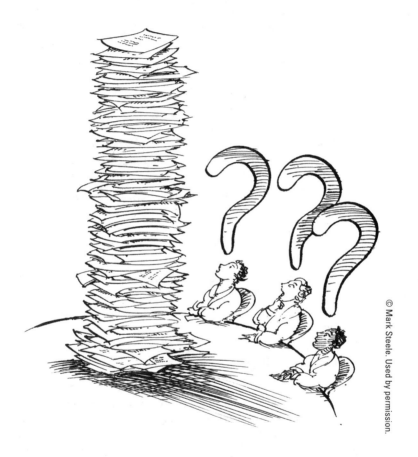

© Mark Steele. Used by permission.

"All this research and we still have questions."

Evidence-based practice (EBP) is a very important paradigm shift in how health care is practiced and taught. Publications on EBP have exploded in the past few years. Various definitions of EBP and its cousins (e.g., evidence-based medicine and evidence-based nursing) have emerged. Common among the many definitions of EBP is the idea of moving away from practice based merely on tradition—doing things the way they've always been done without questioning whether that is the best approach—toward practice decisions based on the best available knowledge (evidence). This chapter is designed to introduce nurses, nurse educators, and nursing students to the thinking required to base practice on evidence.

The Institute of Medicine (IOM) described EBP as "the integration of best research evidence, clinical expertise, and patient values in making decisions about the care of individual patients" (2003, p. 56). The IOM clarified "best research evidence" as quantitative evidence such as that obtained through clinical trials and laboratory experiments, evidence from qualitative research, and evidence from experts in practice. Clinical expertise comes from knowledge and experience over time. Patient values are those unique circumstances of each patient. The IOM enumerated several tasks necessary to EBP: (1) knowing where and how to find the best evidence, (2) formulating clinical questions, (3) searching for answers to those questions with the best evidence and determining the validity and appropriateness of that evidence for patient populations, and (4) determining how and when to integrate those new findings in practice. Each task is primarily a thinking process. Specifically implied is the use of the critical thinking (CT) skills of *analyzing, applying standards, discriminating, information seeking, logical reasoning, predicting,* and *transforming knowledge,* and habits of the mind, such as *contextual perspective, inquisitiveness, intellectual integrity,* and *open-mindedness.*

Call it what you want, but EBP is a way of thinking. Increasingly, we are seeing links between thinking and EBP in the literature; even when the links aren't explicit, there is an implication that the very nature of EBP necessitates CT. A collection of some of those statements is in **Box 8-1**. The history of this movement is very helpful for understanding its importance and how closely it has been aligned with CT since its inception.

Historical Overview of EBP

Nurses have a quintessential picture of EBP in their founder, Florence Nightingale, who collected and analyzed evidence to show how deaths of Crimean War soldiers could be drastically reduced. Using that evidence, she enabled a change in health care that persists even today (Hayes, 2005). It is too bad that more references don't put Nightingale at the top of the list of those credited with the EBP movement. We nurses must remember to brag about her more.

More often, the historical roots of EBP are credited to the forward thinking of Archie Cochrane, a British physician who, in the 1970s, saw a need to examine the economics of health care and determine the cost–benefit of treatments. In 1993, Cochrane and others founded the Cochrane Collaboration, which has become the core of EBP (Cochrane Collaboration, 2013). The Cochrane Collaboration focuses on interventions and precise and thorough searches for and evaluation of evidence, and it considers the randomized controlled trial (RCT) as the gold standard of research evidence (Jennings & Loan, 2001).

Box 8-1   Links between EBP and Thinking in the Literature

Avis & Freshwater, 2006:
"Critical analysis of the concept suggests that EBP overemphasizes the value of scientific evidence while underplaying the role of clinical judgement and individual nursing expertise." (p. 216)

Bucknall & Hutchinson, 2006:
"The use of evidence in practice is dependent upon cognitive competence." (p. 137)

Finn, 2011:
"Rational—or critical—thinking is an essential clinical skill and important complement to EBP in our profession." (p. 69)

Fonteyn, 2005:
"Nurses' ability to think well and understand research is essential to evidence-based practice and, correspondingly, involvement in evidence-based practice and scholarly activities is important for honing nurses' thinking skills and enhancing their ability to comprehend research." (p. 439)

Hancock & Easen, 2006:
"As both the extension of nursing practice and the demand for evidence-based practice increase, the quality of the decision making of nurses becomes imperative." (p. 694)

Harbison, 2006:
"What turns 'information' into 'evidence'? A process of reasoning is undergone, whereby information is selected and assessed in relation to its relevance and weight in the individual case." (p. 1490)

Holmes, Murray, Perron, & McCabe, 2008:
"The BPG [Best Practice Guideline] movement is ideologically driven, giving us 'ready-made tools,' 'rules' and 'guidelines' that ultimately impede nurses' critical thinking and serve as disciplinary technologies to govern nursing work." (p. 395)

Hudson, Duke, Haas, & Varnell, 2008:
"Multiple ways of knowing, or evidence, for informed clinical decision making must be considered based on situational context." (p. 409)

Mantzoukas, 2008:
"EBP is a decision-making process that enables the practitioner to consciously and explicitly choose the best treatment option for individual patients." (p. 221)

(continues)

Box 8-1 Links between EBP and Thinking in the Literature (continued)

McWilliam, 2007:
"As evidence-based practice gains momentum, continuing education practitioners increasingly confront the need to develop and conduct events promoting the uptake of research findings. Recently this challenge has changed . . . [;] the current expectation is one of knowledge translation." (p. 72)

Nickerson & Thurkettle, 2013:
"Nursing students and practicing nurses require a high level of cognitive maturity to be adequately disposed to clinical inquiry, research utilization, and EBP." (p. 21)

Pierce, 2007:
"A prerequisite to becoming an evidence-based rehabilitation nurse is to become a reflective professional." (p. 203)

Profetto-McGrath, Hesketh, Lang, & Estabrooks, 2003:
"Nurses who have the attributes consistent with the ideal critical thinker, and especially those who are open-minded, inquisitive, and systematic, are more likely to use research findings in their work as nurses." (p. 334)

Rycroft-Malone, 2008:
"Evidence-informed practice is a problem-solving process in which practitioners are active stakeholders." (p. 407)

Sams & Gannon, 2000:
"Evidence-based practice is well suited to the information age because it demands critical thinking, integration of work efforts, ongoing knowledge-based queries, continual outcome improvement, and interdisciplinary work." (p. 126)

Sandelowski, 2004:
"Qualitative health research offers the best chance of producing truly transformative knowledge and fully activating the knowledge transformation cycle foundational to the evidence-based practice paradigm." (p. 1382)

Scott-Findlay & Pollock, 2004:
"We hope to improve clinical decision making by increasing practitioners' reliance on research findings while acknowledging the important part played by other forms of knowledge in the decision-making process." (p. 96)

Stetler et al., 1998:
"Inherent to EBP are critical thinking and research utilization competencies." (p. 49)

On this side of the ocean, coining the term *evidence-based medicine* in the 1980s were Canadians at McMaster Medical School in Hamilton, Ontario, who made this new critical approach to medical education and practice a reality (Straus, Richardson, Glasziou, & Haynes, 2005). The McMaster approach heralded a move away from valuing authority to valuing research as a basis of learning.

Meanwhile, in the United States, the federal government committed money in the early 1990s to set up the Agency for Health Care Policy and Reform (AHCPR), which established interdisciplinary teams to gather and assess available literature and develop evidence-based clinical guidelines for several important areas of health care. Examples of early guidelines were *Pressure Ulcer Treatment, Depression in Primary Care*, and *Management of Cancer Pain*. Those of us who grabbed these guidelines as if they were gold soon realized that we had reached a new era of practice. It wasn't just up to us to keep up with the latest research; someone else valued our desire to provide the best care using the best evidence. Nurses were prominent members of the interdisciplinary teams who did this early work. AHCPR became the Agency for Healthcare Research and Quality (AHRQ) in the mid-1990s (http://www.ahrq.gov); it now has a clearinghouse for clinical guidelines (http://www.guideline.gov) and has established numerous centers and offices having to do with EBP and research (AHRQ, 2013).

Other aspects of nursing history are also very important to the EBP movement. In the late 1970s and early 1980s, nursing groups started focusing on research utilization. Of particular note is the Conduct and Utilization of Research in Nursing project in Michigan. Seventeen hospitals in Michigan participated in developing research-based protocols in pre- and postoperative teaching, in reducing diarrhea in tube-fed patients, and in several other areas (Haller, Reynolds, & Horsley, 1979). Unfortunately, although this group and its many followers pushed for increased use of research in nursing, a gap between research and practice in the field persisted. However, the research utilization movement provided fertile ground for nursing to wholeheartedly embrace the EBP movement.

In 1994, Sigma Theta Tau International started publishing *Worldviews on Evidence-Based Nursing*. In 1998, the *Evidence-Based Nursing Journal* was published by a Canadian and British group. In Australia, the Joanna Briggs Institute (JBI) became a model of nursing-focused EBP, conducting systematic reviews, developing evidence-based best practice guidelines, and maintaining an excellent website used by nurses all over the world (http://www.joannabriggs.edu.au). The Registered Nurses' Association of Ontario has developed a similar online nursing resource, creating and posting evidence-based best practice guidelines (http://www.rnao.org).

Today, one can find vast amounts of material on the Internet relative to EBP. We have compiled in **Box 8-2** a few of our favorite sites. If you look at these sites, you can find links to hundreds more. Because the EBP and informatics movements are growing so rapidly, by the time you read this text, there likely will be many other sites to be found, and some may no longer exist. A general Internet search for the

---

Box 8-2 Some Favorite Internet Sites for EBP

Agency for Healthcare Research and Quality:
http://www.ahrq.gov

American Diabetes Association:
http://www.diabetes.org

Appraisal of Guidelines for Research and Evaluation (AGREE):
http://www.agreetrust.org/

Centers for Disease Control and Prevention:
http://www.cdc.gov/CDCForYou/healthcare_providers.html

Centre for Health Evidence (McMaster University):
http://www.cche.net

Cochrane Collaboration:
http://www.cochrane.org

Cochrane Consumer Network (CCNet):
http://www.cochrane.org/consumers/homepage.htm

Cochrane Qualitative and Implementation Methods Group:
http://cqim.cochrane.org/

DISCERN (instrument for critique):
http://www.discern.org.uk

Evaluation of Information Sources:
http://www.vuw.ac.nz/staff/alastair_smith/evaln/evaln.htm

Evidence-Based Nursing:
http://www.ebn.bmj.com

Healthfinder: National Health Information Center, U.S. Department of Health and Human Services:
http://www.healthfinder.gov

Institute for Quality and Efficiency in Health Care:
http://www.informedhealthonline.org

Joanna Briggs Institute:
http://www.joannabriggs.edu.au

Leapfrog Group:
http://leapfroggroup.org/

Medical Library Association:
http://www.mlanet.org/resources/consumr_index.html

MedlinePlus (good links to other sites and good consumer information):
http://www.medlineplus.gov/

National Guideline Clearinghouse:
http://www.guideline.gov

National Institute for Health and Care Excellence:
http://www.nice.org.uk

New Zealand Guidelines Group:
http://www.nzgg.org.nz

RAND Health:
http://www.rand.org/health/

Registered Nurses' Association of Ontario:
www.rnao.org

Turning Research into Practice (Trip):
http://www.tripdatabase.com/index.html

World Health Organization:
http://www.who.int/en/

words *evidence-based practice* will give you lots of strong hits. You need very little *information-seeking* ability to find EBP resources. However, you will need all your other thinking dimensions to sift through them intelligently.

A recent trend in nursing literature is an EBP debate focused on the interpretation of evidence. On one side, you have the advocates of EBP, who define evidence in terms of hierarchies, with randomized controlled studies on top. On the other side, you have the deconstructionists, who question the assumptions that controlled trials are the epitome of evidence (Rolfe, 2005). These debates have great value because they force readers to think about their interpretation of EBP. With our view through CT-colored lenses, we believe many of the debates would be mollified by keeping this thought topmost: EBP is a thinking process! Once you remove or deemphasize the thinking part, the polarization over evidence becomes greater.

Why Is EBP So Important?

It really doesn't require much *logical reasoning* to see why EBP is so important. It just makes sense to base health practices on the best evidence because most of the time it costs less, and almost all the time there are better patient outcomes. You'll note that we don't say it's always less expensive; sometimes the best approaches are costlier because they are newer. However, when we factor in costs of not using the best evidence in practice, the few times it costs more will be far outnumbered by the overall cost savings. What constitutes better patient outcomes must be clarified with caution—we must always take into account the patient's wishes, values, and so forth. Once in a while, for all kinds of reasons, patients will refuse what providers see as the best evidence-supported approaches. Ultimately, we must respect patient wishes as long as we know their decisions are based on the best available information.

Clinicians: On What Evidence Do You Base Your Practice?

Before we launch into details of the thinking that accompanies EBP, stop for a minute and think about your practice arena. Is your practice and that of clinicians around you based on knowledge you learned in school? How long ago was that? Is your practice based on your unit's protocols? What are those protocols based on? How many nursing journals do you read? What drives you to read them? What determines when you consider a change in your practice? Does it come from you or from some outside source? How often do you search the Internet for medical and nursing information? What are your sources of information?

Many clinicians will admit that they often do things because of past practice. Something stuck in their minds that worked. We are all very influenced by extreme events that stand out vividly in our memories—those in which something very positive or very negative occurred. Nursing practice is often directed by such events. Although learning from past peak experiences is important, there is danger in allowing those critical events to direct our practice too much, as you will see in **TACTICS 8-1.**

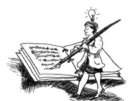

TACTICS 8-1: Clinicians: On What Evidence Do You Base Your Practice?

Reflect on these issues:

1. What in your past has been a critical event in your nursing practice? (Examples: A patient fell after you gave him a vaccination. A patient started to yell loudly when you touched her arm. A patient told you he could always breathe better after drinking a glass of cold water. A clogged percutaneous endoscopic gastrostomy (PEG) tube opened up miraculously when you flushed it with Coca-Cola.)
2. Was it a positive or negative event?
3. When and under what circumstances did it occur?
4. How much has this event influenced how you practice in similar situations?

After answering these questions, think about the CT dimensions you used and why. Then, for even more detailed thinking, consider how to search for evidence to support or negate what you are doing in that area of practice. You may want to read the rest of this chapter before you start your search because we'll discuss the thinking that will help you with that search.

Discussion

Without *reflection* such as this, we can go merrily along without realizing what a tenuous basis there is for our actions. We have a saying that you've probably used yourself: "She's basing that practice on an 'N of one.'" The danger, of course, in basing actions on an N of one is that the event may have been a fluke. Flukes are definitely not part of EBP (except perhaps to fishermen?) . . . Groan. What worked well for one patient does not provide evidence for generalizing to other patients.

Educators: On What Evidence Do You Base the Information You Teach AND How You Teach?

Just as we've asked clinicians to reflect on their practice, we ask educators to consider the knowledge base they use for teaching. (See **TACTICS 8-2.**) How old is it? Are you teaching the most current evidence, and are you encouraging your students to seek out the best evidence? Are your teaching methods based on evidence that those methods facilitate student learning outcomes?

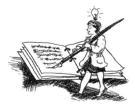

TACTICS 8-2: Educators: On What Evidence Do You Base the Information You Teach AND How You Teach?

How are you doing with promoting EBP? Look at your last teaching plan and answer these questions:

1. Am I handing down information, or helping students seek knowledge?
2. How old is the information I'm using?
3. How many times do I use the words *evidence* or *EBP*?
4. Have I searched for the latest evidence on this topic?
5. If I searched, how did I evaluate the evidence I found?
6. Do any of my course objectives address EBP and thinking?
7. What pedagogical evidence base supports my teaching methods?

Discussion

Most educators would like to think they teach the most up-to-date information, but it is easy to get in a rut and use the same notes year after year. That can no longer be an option. If we expect clinicians to access and use the best evidence for practice, we need to teach them how to do just that. We need to demonstrate how we are finding and evaluating new information. In the next section, which links CT with EBP, you will see how teaching can promote that thinking.

If you really want to embrace teaching based on the best evidence, ask yourself not just about the content you teach, but also these questions about your teaching methods: How is my teaching? Am I simply teaching with strategies I've used for years? Where is the research on teaching and learning that could enhance my process of teaching? *Reflection* on evidence-based teaching as an equal partner with teaching evidence-based content is essential for developing the nurses of today and tomorrow.

Links Between Critical Thinking and EBP

Not only are there specific thinking strategies involved in EBP, but the whole notion of practice based on evidence is a shift of thinking. Consider this comparison of old and new thinking in **Box 8-3**. Once you have the new thinking mindset, you can think about the tasks and link them with CT dimensions.

A clear connection between all dimensions of CT and EBP can be made. In **Figure 8-1**, eight steps as thinking landings on the path of EBP are identified, and superimposed on the path are all the CT skills and habits of the mind. Because CT skills and habits of the mind are used in harmony, there is no absolute step or stop in the EBP process in which only one or two CT dimensions are used alone. However,

---

Box 8-3   Comparing Old and New Thinking

Old Thinking	**New Thinking**
Follow the usual practice until an authority hands down a new policy.	Question practice constantly. Is this the best, most efficient, most cost-effective, safest way to do _____?
Knowledge is static.	Knowledge is dynamic. There's always something new being discovered.
Practice is discipline specific.	Practice is interdisciplinary.
Practice guidelines and policies are developed by management.	Practice guidelines and policies are developed by all nurses and other disciplines too.
Searching for evidence to support practice is someone else's job.	Searching for evidence to support *my* practice is *my* job.
Knowledge is factual information.	Evidence-based practice means *transforming knowledge*—judging and adapting it.

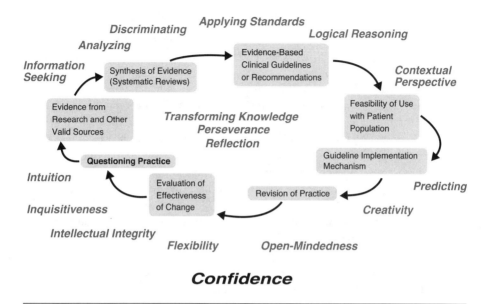

Figure 8-1 Inter-relationships of CT skills and habits of the mind and components of EBP.

certain parts of the EBP process demand more of some skills and habits of the mind than others. Look back to the beginning of this chapter to the four tasks set forth by the IOM (2003) as necessary to EBP. There are many such lists of tasks or steps to this process; most have a sequence of asking questions, looking for evidence, appraising evidence, using the evidence to improve practice, and evaluating the effectiveness of the practice revision. Although such lists appear linear, EBP is not simple; it's a set of complex tasks, all of which require CT. We have simplified the task list in Figure 8-1 to superimpose the thinking dimensions onto the components of EBP. Let's walk through that process. Before continuing, look again at Figure 8-1 to appreciate the whole, then start at the bold **Questioning Practice** point on the left.

Questioning Practice

This questioning is the absolute essential starting point on the path of EBP; one must approach health care, specifically nursing practice, as a dynamic process that changes as our knowledge base grows and patients' situations change. Anyone can question practice, but "hospital-based nurses are well positioned to identify clinical practice problems encountered daily at the bedside for needed research and should be supported to help generate the evidence for their practice" (Kelly, Turner, Speroni, McLaughlin, & Guzzetta, 2013, p. 22). The initial question might have to do with almost anything: an intervention (e.g., what's the best way to flush PEG tubes?), a specific patient population characteristic (e.g., what's the ideal blood pressure for this diabetic patient?), a potential complication (e.g., if I turn this patient more often than every 2 hours, can I prevent a pressure ulcer?), an expected outcome (e.g., what is the likelihood of this patient getting a urinary tract infection?), or a specific task (e.g., do I need to do this dressing as a sterile procedure?).

Once a question arises, it is important to ask it in a way that will help you search for answers. Straus and colleagues (2005) have helpful lessons for this task. First, use your *discriminating* skill to distinguish between *background questions* and *foreground questions*. A background question is the kind that one asks in a new situation—for example, how does acetaminophen work? An answer to that question could be found in a drug reference book. Foreground questions are more specific and are those posed for EBP—for example, which works best to reduce fever, acetaminophen or ibuprofen?

To help one's thinking while formulating foreground questions, many authors (e.g., Melnyk & Fineout-Overholt, 2011) advocate arranging thoughts in the PICO format: P—Patient population of interest, I—Intervention of interest, which could be a treatment, patient perception, test, prognosis, and so on; C—Comparison of interest, such as the usual practice or another intervention; and O—Outcome of interest.

Are you ready to try your hand at these kinds of questions? Down with passivity! Use these CT habits of the mind: *inquisitiveness* (be curious), *intellectual integrity* (look for answers even if they might go against what you're presently comfortable with), and *intuition* (listen to your gut). For a simple start, think about your area of practice and consider this question: Is there a better, more efficient, safer, less expensive way to do _____? Here are some examples to help you get in the groove:

- For elderly patients (P), does exercise (I) work as well as laxatives (C) to decrease constipation (O)?
- How do women (P) with fibromyalgia (I) perceive changes (C) in their quality of life (O)?
- For elderly patients with pressure ulcers (P), are wet-to-dry dressings (I) as effective as mechanical debridement (C) in time of healing (O)?

Inquisitiveness makes that questioning process come alive when clinicians wonder if they are practicing in the best possible way. Nurses who are eager to know and seek knowledge and understanding because they are naturally curious will more than likely seek the best knowledge and evidence all the time. They are the seekers of knowledge, not the takers. Seeking is an active process; taking is a passive process.

Intellectual integrity augments that *inquisitiveness*; nurses who value EBP will seek the truth of best practice evidence even when that questioning makes more work and increases discomfort as the status quo is shaken up. Nurses with strong *intellectual integrity* will give up traditional care approaches when there is clear evidence for considering changes in practice. An N of one will not be considered a legitimate source of evidence.

Another part of questioning practice is *intuition*. Think about nurses who have gut feelings that there must be a better way to do something. It's a fairly common phenomenon that is often not acknowledged because on the surface it seems not to be part of EBP. However, those vague feelings that there should or might be better approaches often drive nurses to go further, searching for those improved possibilities.

Only after clinicians' questions become focused can they look for the best evidence to find answers. Although we have the CT dimension of *discriminating* a little further along the path, clinicians definitely use it to help them hone the question. Focusing on a problem or question makes way for the exploration and learning that follows in this EBP process.

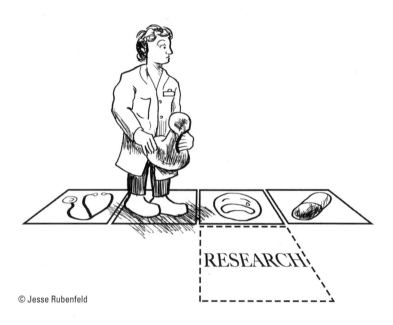

© Jesse Rubenfeld

Thinking While Searching for and Evaluating Evidence

Move to the next EBP landing in Figure 8-1. Evidence comes from many sources, starting with evidence from the patient situation right in front of you. Does your institution and unit collect evidence on patient outcomes, such as satisfaction, readmissions, and so forth? How do you use that evidence to change practice? Because these evidence sources are very specific, we have focused our chapter on outside sources of evidence. We have listed three sources of evidence that require thinking. The search for evidence can be approached in many different ways. Some start with information in its most synthesized, usable form, which for nurses is usually an evidence-based clinical practice guideline. Others build up from specific reports of research studies. The search process and its accompanying thinking can be a convoluted path.

The best evidence doesn't magically appear in front of each clinician; there must be some effort at *information seeking*. In the old way of thinking, nurses practiced one way until a manager came along and handed out a new policy. Today, with EBP, there will be management-level mandates for change, but each individual nurse cannot wait for that information to be distributed. There is too much evidence appearing constantly. Nurses must individually and collectively exercise professional role accountability and promote *information seeking* to find the best practice standards. They must move beyond expecting to find answers in their immediate environments—a book or a colleague—and learn how to find for themselves the best information from multiple sources. Did you catch that? Don't be tempted to stop after finding one source!

At first this *information-seeking* process seems very complex and may be overwhelming to nurses with limited backgrounds in research language and methods. However, increasingly there are excellent resources that offer assistance in how to find, analyze, and critique the quality of evidence (for example, DiCenso, Guyatt, & Ciliska, 2005; Melnyk & Fineout Overholt, 2011). We also have lots of help from technology today as we do online searches for new evidence. Think about your abilities relative to search technologies. Have you searched a CINAHL or Medline database on a computer? Can you define a topic narrowly or broadly enough to be successful in finding evidence-based articles?

Beyond the availability of computer searches and new technology, nurses must approach gathering evidence with their *analyzing* skills in top form. The process of searching for evidence is easier when the question has specific parameters. The best search techniques must be sought and used, and when difficulties in finding evidence arise, the searcher must again turn to *analysis* to figure out how to further break down the search problems. Librarians, especially those with health sciences or medical specialties, are a wonderful resource to help with searches.

Evidence from Research and Other Valid Sources

We're sure all our readers have done some searching for articles. Nevertheless, to illustrate this process, let's look at an example: Say you're a nurse on a surgical floor, and you're interested in decreasing postoperative infections and finding the best way to do wound dressings. You might frame the question in PICO language like this: In adult patients, which postoperative wound care results in low infection rates? You could take a traditional approach to searching that you probably learned in school. Go to a health-related database (PubMed is our current favorite) and do a literature search. What words would you use in your search? We logged in to our university library, pulled up the PubMed database, and typed in these subjects: "wound care" and "nursing." A total of 9,500 results came up, with article titles as diverse as "skin bacteria" and "nipple trauma in breastfeeding." Using *analyzing* to break things down more, we added a time frame of the past 2 years and added criteria for clinical trials and review. A total of 139 articles were then listed. Subjects were still pretty diverse, such as "perioperative shaving and surgical site infections" and "tranexamic acid (TXA) use in trauma." Nevertheless, we were able to scan through 139 titles, marking those that seemed to relate to wounds and nursing. After downloading and reading a few articles, we did not feel we had a good grasp on the body of evidence out there, but we certainly were using our thinking dimensions of *information seeking* and *analyzing*. Using more analysis, one decides if articles are research based and, using *discriminating* and *applying standards*, one decides on the quality of that research. **Box 8-4** contains a simple set of criteria for judging a research article.

As an aside, we need to note that we are assuming most readers have a working knowledge of the scientific research process and are able to recognize a research study and read it critically. It is obviously beyond the scope of this text to go into all of that. If you need to refresh that part of your knowledge, we recommend you review a research textbook or find a colleague with more experience or education, such as a clinical nurse specialist, and ask for help *analyzing* the article.

Continuing with our searching example, we decided that our quest to find the best evidence on wound care should focus on infections. Our next step was to visit the Cochrane Library to look for systematic reviews of evidence related to postoperative infections.

Box 8-4   Judging the Quality of Research Articles

Is the study valid?
> What type of study is it?
>> Did the researchers clearly state their purpose?
>
> What do I know about this method of study?
>> Did the researchers follow the rules of the method?
>>
>> Were there factors that may have interfered with the integrity of the research?
>
> What resources do I need to help me determine if this is a valid study?

What does the study tell me?
> What are the results?
>
> Are there clear links between the data collected and the conclusions reached?
>
> What resources do I need to interpret the results?
>
> How do these results compare with results found in similar studies?

Can I use the results of the study?
> Can the results be generalized?
>
> Is the study population similar to my patient population?
>
> What do the researchers say about applicability of results?

Source: This article was published in *Evidence-based nursing: A guide to clinical practice*, Copyright Elsevier 2005. Reprinted by permission of Elsevier.

We'll discuss the thinking surrounding systematic reviews and then come back to this example as we move through our CT skills and habits of the mind.

Evidence from Synthesized Sources (Systematic Reviews)

Fortunately, today there are many professional groups that collect research findings, do analyses, and compile syntheses of evidence bases, often called systematic reviews. We mentioned some of these sources earlier—AHRQ and the Cochrane Collaboration are popular examples. These groups are doing the time-consuming job of collecting evidence (articles and so forth), making judgments about the quality of that evidence, and compiling it into reports.

The Cochrane Collaboration is currently the largest organization that produces and maintains systematic reviews in health care, and its library can be accessed by any organization with a subscription. We found, for example, one systematic review on pressure-relieving interventions for diabetic foot ulcers (Lewis & Lipp, 2013) and another on perioperative hair removal to reduce surgical site infection (Tanner, Norrie, & Melen, 2011).

So where does that take us relative to EBP? Can we shut down our thinking a bit because we have found reviews by the prestigious Cochrane group? The answer must be no, of course. Whether nurses are finding specific research reports or finding compilations of research (systematic reviews), those sources must be read with *discrimination*. Nurses must *analyze* reports and *discriminate* the quality of the evidence. There are standards to help clinicians do just that, and nurses are *applying standards* as they judge the quality of the evidence and the conclusions reached by those conducting reviews.

A very important part of understanding and *discriminating* systematic reviews is determining how the evidence was gathered and judged for strength. There are standards that should have been applied, and you need to look for them. The various standards for systematic reviews were addressed by the IOM when they set up a committee to standardize the procedures for "producing scientifically valid, transparent, and reproducible SRs" (Eden, Levit, Berg & Morton, 2011, p. 3). Systematic reviews, if they are indeed systematic, must report how the evidence was collected so that you, the reader, can judge whether it was thorough and systematic. Theoretically, you should be able to reproduce what they found by following the report of their search process. You must be able to see the strength of the evidence and how that strength was judged. The Cochrane Library has a reputation that is equaled by no other group for excellence in doing reviews, so you might be able to trust their reviews a bit more than those of other organizations. Nevertheless, keep that keen *analytical* and *discriminating* ability in high gear at all times.

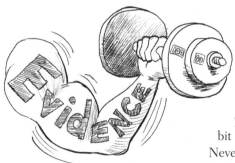

© Jesse Rubenfeld

Now, how about the issue of strength of evidence? There are heated debates over what constitutes legitimate or best evidence. All systematic reviews should report the evidence hierarchy used. There are no universal evidence hierarchies, but one similar to this example from Stetler and colleagues (1998) is commonly seen:

  I. Meta-analysis of multiple controlled studies
 II. Individual experimental study
III. Quasi-experimental study
 IV. Nonexperimental study (for example, descriptive, qualitative, and case studies)
  V. Systematically obtained, verifiable quality improvement program evaluation of case report data
 VI. Opinions of nationally known authorities based on their experience or the opinions of an expert committee, including the interpretation of non-research-based information; regulatory or legal opinions

You will note that this hierarchy has meta-analysis of multiple controlled studies at the top. Many groups, such as the Cochrane Collaboration (Higgins & Green, 2011), have specified RCTs as the gold standard for the best evidence. Recently, methods of judging evidence have been questioned because in some areas of practice we have only expert opinions and no research; also, there is a vast amount of research that is noncontrolled, descriptive, qualitative, and so forth. Groups such as the Cochrane Collaboration, with stringent standards for evidence, therefore include fewer nursing studies in their reviews. The danger of evidence hierarchies that place controlled, quantitative research findings at the top is that other forms of evidence may be eliminated (Holmes, Perron, & O'Byrne, 2006). Caution in being too rigid is being advocated (Romyn et al., 2003). Some nurses advocate revised hierarchies because there are few RCTs in nursing (Cesario, Morin, & Santa-Donato, 2002). Hudson and colleagues went so far as to say, "Nursing is too contextual to have a fixed hierarchy" (2008, p. 414).

The Cochrane group does acknowledge the importance of qualitative evidence. The 2011 Cochrane reviewers' handbook has this to say, while acknowledging that they focus primarily on systematic reviews of RCTs: "evidence derived from qualitative studies complements systematic reviews of quantitative studies" (Higgins & Green, 2011, Part 3: Special Topics, 20.1 Introduction). Recently, the Cochrane Qualitative and Implementation Methods Group (http://cqim.cochrane.org/) has been established. Further assistance in addressing qualitative evidence is emerging. Bearman and Dawson (2013) provided three qualitative synthesis methodologies—thematic analysis, meta-ethnography, and realist review—that may help with thinking in judging the quality of such reviews.

We are still debating the issue of evidence and its relative strength. We are not at the point at which we have widely accepted standards. Perhaps we will have more standardization by the time you read this, but more than likely, because nursing is always *contextual* and evidence comes from many sources, several approaches will remain for determining strength of evidence.

Box 8-5 Judging the Quality of Systematic Reviews

■ Did a reliable, qualified person or group conduct the review?
■ Did reviewers address potential conflicts of interest?
■ Is the method used for collecting and including studies clearly stated?
■ Did reviewers state specific strategies used to evaluate studies?
■ Is a hierarchy of strength of evidence clearly described?
■ Was the method of synthesizing evidence clearly articulated?
■ What is the likelihood that valid studies were missed?
■ When was the review done? What studies may have occurred since then?
■ What conclusions were made?
■ Can the conclusions be tracked back to specific studies?
■ Will the results help with patient care?

Sources: Eden et al., 2011; Melnyk & Fineout-Overholt, 2011.

Readers of systematic reviews must always look for criteria used to determine the strength of evidence. Because there are no hard-and-fast rules about what constitutes the best evidence, the reader's thinking is crucial. Readers must have *discriminating* abilities to see similarities and differences in the various studies and the conclusions about the body of evidence. They must look for and *apply standards* while thinking. We have provided a set of standards in **Box 8-5** to start this thinking process.

Evidence from Clinical Guidelines or Recommendations

Ultimately, because EBP is all about improving practice, clinicians need evidence translated into practice recommendations or clinical guidelines. Many groups that do systematic reviews go the next step and develop those guidelines. If you visit some of the websites in Box 8-2, you will find lists of evidence-based clinical guidelines or links to sites with guidelines. However, you can't turn off your brain after you find a guideline. You must use those thinking dimensions we discussed in the preceding section and add *logical reasoning*. All conclusions reached about what should be done in practice must be supported by the evidence and your *logical reasoning*. When using prepared guidelines, one must look to see if the trail from evidence to recommendations can easily be tracked. Only after that are you ready to consider if the guidelines fit with your patients' situations.

Many groups offer standards for evaluating clinical guidelines. We've compiled a list of them in **Box 8-6** using the references we included in that box. We recommend that you access the AGREE Enterprise for a more comprehensive instrument that has been tested for validity and reliability (AGREE Enterprise, 2009).

Box 8-6 Judging Clinical Practice Guidelines

- Is the process of guideline development transparent?
- Is the guideline too vague to be usable?
- Is the guideline too specific to be practical with your patient group?
- Who developed the guideline?
- Are the developers qualified to develop this guideline?
- How broad is the representation of the group?
- Were healthcare consumers part of the group?
- Are there any potential conflicts of interest because of developers or sponsors of the guideline?
- Is there a clear explanation of the evidence used to develop the guideline?
- Was a systematic review of the evidence done?
- Is the systematic review available for retrieval?
- How strong is the evidence supporting the guideline's recommendations?
- What is the date of this guideline? Is it current?
- When was it last updated? Is there a reasonable pattern of updates?
- Has it been tested? By whom?
- Are there other guidelines available in the same area? If so, how consistent are they?

Sources: The AGREE Collaboration, 2009; Centre for Health Evidence, 2001; Graham, et al., 2011; Grol, Dalhuijsen, Veld, Rutten, & Mokkink, 1998; National Guideline Clearinghouse, n.d.; Ransohoff, Pignone, & Sox, 2013; Shekelle, Woolf, Eccles, & Grimshaw, 1999; Thomson, Lavendere, & Madhok, 1995.

Recently, responding to the growth of guidelines without a concurrent lack of consistent quality among those guidelines, the IOM formed a committee to promote the standardization of guideline quality (Graham et al., 2011). They specified a new definition of clinical practice guidelines as "statements that include recommendations intended to optimize patient care that are informed by a systematic review of evidence and an assessment of the benefits and harms of alternative care options" (p. 4). One must never assume that guidelines are based on the best evidence, even if a seemingly trustworthy group developed them. We have to use *analyzing* and *logical reasoning* and *apply standards* to make our own judgments about how evidence-based those guidelines are. There is much potential for harm if guidelines are used without careful evaluation (Woolf, Grol, Hutchinson, Eccles, & Grimshaw, 1999).

Feasibility of Use with Patient Population

Once evidence-based clinical guidelines are found or established, one must determine the feasibility and desirability of using those guidelines in a specific practice setting. This activity certainly requires a *contextual perspective*. One must consider the patient population, their preferences, and their values. One must consider the institution in which the guidelines are to be used. How feasible is it to implement those guidelines? What resources are available for implementing them?

Considering the feasibility of using evidence-based guidelines with specific patient groups is best done by those providers working directly with patients and by patients themselves. Academics cannot stand afar and say that certain guidelines must be used with all patients. People who know patients best should make these decisions. However, those folks—providers and patients—must be educated about EBP and what constitutes good, better, and best evidence. Making decisions about the feasibility of evidence-based guidelines is a CT process.

Some might say that EBP is the antithesis of CT, viewing EBP as following the recommendations or guidelines that are formulated (often by groups outside one's personal arena) in cookbook fashion. Sackett, Rosenberg, Gray, Haynes, and Richardson responded to this best. "Evidence-based medicine is not 'cook-book' medicine. Because it requires a bottom-up approach that integrates the best external evidence with individual clinical expertise and patient-choice, it cannot result in slavish, cookbook approaches to individual patient care" (1996, para 6). We need to be cognizant of the temptations, however. More and more, we can find quick references that tell us they have the best evidence (e.g., Slawson, Shaughnessy, Ebell, & Barry, 2007). Taking such a reference and changing practice based on its recommendations without CT will result in cookbook approaches. Such behaviors cannot be called EBP.

If, in an ideal world, we had evidence-based guidelines that appeared in front of us in a timely manner, there still would be a need for the *contextual perspective* of CT. As with any standardized approach, such as assessment guidelines or clinical pathways, there will always be those who have an image of patient assembly lines and who just do the job and go home. However, as most nurses realize, thankfully, the individuality of patients supersedes all such imagery and forces even the most slothful nurse to think. Evidence-based guidelines actually provide clinicians with tools that augment rather than impede CT. Consider this example: You go to the Registered Nurses' Association of Ontario website and find a best practice guideline, Prevention of Constipation in the Older Adult Population (Registered Nurses' Association of Ontario, 2005), and you see that increasing fiber in the diet is recommended. Now, if you don't look at the context of your patient, you may do more harm than good. Have you considered the patient's other health issues? Can the patient drink enough fluid to keep the fiber from hardening? If you haven't considered the whole *context*, you may be worsening the problem and causing an impaction.

Guideline Implementation Mechanism

Predicting as a CT skill is imperative as nurses move toward a specific plan or mechanism to implement evidence-based guidelines. As anyone who has promoted change will quickly tell you, this process also requires *creativity*. How do you get clinicians, educators, and patients to value evidence-based guidelines enough to commit to implementing those guidelines? How do you devise a system easy enough to follow that the system of implementation doesn't bog down? Sometimes it's as simple as thinking about the people who will be implementing the guideline and talking to them about what they think is the best mechanism.

Recently at a conference on EBP, one of the speakers was discussing such mechanisms. Being gung-ho informatics advocates, we expected this educator to say that he was developing some elaborate plan for his medical students to download guidelines onto their personal digital assistants. When asked, he replied, "Oh no, I'm thinking along the lines of a laminated card for students and residents to carry in their pockets." It's hard to predict, but maybe the old-fashioned approaches still work the best; because we are asking people to change what they do, maybe we will have more luck if we keep the mechanism of implementing that change simple.

Revision of Practice

Ultimately, if practice is to be revised to be consistent with best evidence, all those involved in the process must be *open-minded* and *flexible* in their thinking. The persons advocating the change in practice must not demoralize those who prefer to hang on to tradition, but use *creativity* to help them increase their *flexibility*. This is, of course, no easy task. It is beyond the scope of this chapter and this text to describe all the dynamics of the change process, but certainly anyone contemplating a true commitment to EBP will want to think about all the nuances and strategies for successful change. Before we leave this subject, we'd like you to reflect on your reaction to the last change proposed at your institution. (See **TACTICS 8-3**.)

TACTICS 8-3: How Have You Reacted to Past Practice Changes?

Clinicians and Educators

Take a few minutes and think about a practice or teaching–curriculum change that you either supported or resisted— a ban on acrylic nails, moving IV flushes from heparin to saline, changing skills check-off lists to a less rigid format, moving from sterile to clean techniques for dressings, and so on. Use these questions to guide your *reflection*:

1. Did I support this or not?
2. If I did, how did I show my support?
3. If I didn't, how did I react?
4. Were my comments and actions proactive or reactive?
5. Was my response emotional or based on my thinking, or a combination of both?

6. How much knowledge did I have in making my decision to support or not support this?

7. How confident was I in my reasoning?

Discussion

Although we haven't talked much about the change process in this chapter, it is clear that approaching practice and education with an evidence-based perspective requires some change on our part. Neither practice nor education is static; both are dynamic. It behooves us all to think about how we deal with change generally, and how we deal with practice changes specifically. Change not only requires effort in thinking, but it also takes time. Change can be uncomfortable; discomfort will interfere with thinking and decision making. Recognizing this fact helps us plan changes.

Evaluation of Effectiveness of Change

Evaluating the effectiveness of a specific change of practice based on evidence is very important. Besides showing us if this was a good move, the evaluation process reminds us to continue questioning practice. We should no more think that a new approach to practice allows us to rest on our laurels than we should continue blindly doing what we've always done. We must critically evaluate what's been done and how it can be done even better.

Judging the effectiveness of a change requires planning ahead (*predicting*) to determine important data to collect, when to collect them, and for how long. It requires *logical reasoning* as one makes conclusions about this change. The skeptics will sit up and take notice when we can show, with objective data, why this change saved money, increased patient satisfaction, decreased complications or length of stay, and so forth.

Back to the Whole Picture of Critical Thinking and EBP

EBP is not for the fainthearted. That's why CT *confidence* is written across the bottom of Figure 8-1 as the sine qua non of this process. We hope you have developed *confidence* in your thinking skills as you have learned to embrace EBP. Three other CT dimensions cross over and are used through the entire EBP process: *transforming knowledge*, *reflection*, and *perseverance*.

EBP is *transforming knowledge*. The whole EBP process is the quintessential example of that CT skill. We are taking evidence and adapting it to our uses. McWilliam (2007) described the role of continuing education in EBP as one of "transformative knowledge translation."

EBP is also a process of *reflection* at each stop along the way. One must constantly *reflect* on practice, the need for change, the change process, the results of the change, and so forth. And, as anyone who has tried to practice nursing with an EBP approach realizes, *perseverance* in one's thinking processes is also essential. There will certainly be obstacles, some big and some small, depending on how large a change is required based on the evidence available. Ultimately, although the picture of the interrelationships of the CT components and the components of EBP might look like a neat oval process, it is, of course, not that clean, nor are the steps mutually exclusive. Just as happens when nurses use the nursing process, there is a lot of back and forth, modifying, adjusting, thinking, and rethinking along the way.

Big, Small, Individual, and Group Moves Toward EBP

As we have been discussing EBP so far, aside from our little foray into searching for information on wound care, we have not specified examples of EBP in action. Individual nurses can move to EBP thinking as a daily process, and they can focus on moving their teams in that direction. It is certainly ideal to work with a team that values EBP. That group will share evidence they find; they will plan changes together and support each other in the process. We often think that CT is an individual phenomenon, but look at the thinking points in Figure 8-1 from the perspective of your group. Then, if you're really brave, keep your EBP hat on and look at it from the perspective of interdisciplinary teams.

Now, consider EBP in terms of magnitude. Sometimes a major change in policies and procedures is called for as we get new evidence. Take, for example, the recent strong evidence of the benefits of glycemic control for diabetics that has transformed that area of practice (American Diabetes Association [ADA], 2013).

Let's bring that big example of widespread EBP down to a narrower scale—one nurse with an EBP mindset. Imagine this scenario: A nursing assistant on an adult medical–surgical unit takes vital signs on all patients. Nurse A glances at the results, sees nothing very far above 140/90 (the traditional normal), tells the aide to record them, and goes on with the day. Now, using *analysis* and a *contextual perspective*, Nurse B might think about the data as they relate to the specific patient, evaluating the normalcy of each reading.

If Nurse B is thinking about EBP, the diabetic patient with a blood pressure of 140/90 will stand out as needing attention because that nurse will be aware of the best evidence to direct practice and will apply that knowledge to the patients she is taking care of. The ADA, in its recommendations for hypertension management in diabetics, used strong research evidence as a basis for recommending that blood pressures of less than 130/80 be maintained for diabetics (2013).

Any nurse working with diabetics—and these days, that includes virtually all nurses—must vow to keep abreast of the enormous body of diabetes research evidence that has exploded over the past few years and that continues to change. Fortunately, groups such as the ADA continually review that research systematically and translate the evidence into clinical guidelines that are reviewed and updated yearly. All guidelines are freely available on the ADA website (http://www.diabetes.org). Nevertheless, many clinicians who work with diabetic patients continue to practice with information they learned in school or with 5-year-old protocols. We should question why that is so.

In this example, we used the CT skill of *analyzing* and the *contextual perspective* habit of the mind to illustrate a first step toward EBP. However, nurses in similar situations would need to use far more CT skills and habits to fully accomplish a goal of EBP. As we discussed earlier, two of the most important habits of the mind to promote those early steps toward EBP are *inquisitiveness* and *intellectual integrity*.

TACTICS 8-4: Clinical Practice Question of the Month

Clinicians

Try this on your unit: Each month, create a contest for the best clinical practice question. You might want to make cards with an explanation of the PICO components to help people word their questions succinctly. Encourage nurses to search for guidelines or evidence to support or negate usual practice, and post them in a specific place such as the gathering room. Rewards can be whatever is most coveted by that group—time off, money for conferences, a new uniform, or chits that can be saved and turned in for things such as being taken off the float list for 6 months. Such behavior could be built into performance evaluation criteria.

Take that a step further and post criteria for evaluating the strength of evidence of a summary report or a clinical guideline. (Consider using the AGREE instrument described earlier.) Have a contest for who can most accurately judge the strength of evidence for changing practice. If you want to really take it further, have nurses identify the thinking skills and habits of the mind used in this activity.

Educators

Use the same strategy with students. Whatever course you're teaching, build into your syllabus credit for students formulating questions about practice, finding the latest evidence, evaluating it, and discussing if and how that evidence should be used.

Discussion

As educators, we have used this tactic to teach EBP principles. In our nursing research classes, we have students write their major paper on a clinical issue they explore for the latest evidence. They show their knowledge of the research process in discussing the evidence they found. **Box 8-7** has several other general suggestions for activities to promote EBP, both in clinical and classroom situations. We hope they will help you think of specific TACTICS that will work for you.

Box 8-7 Suggestions for Promoting EBP in Clinical and Classroom Settings

---

- Incorporate *reflection* activities into assignments that require thinking about EBP.
- Have students or nurses work in groups to do an EBP activity of their choice and identify how the 17 dimensions of CT were used in that activity.
- Create an EBP tracking thinking diagram modeled after Figure 8-1, or let students create one.
- Build EBP expectations into evaluation criteria for promotions or grades.
- Make a list of how you can socialize a group to emphasize not only EBP but also the underlying thinking skills needed to operationalize EBP.
- Take a guideline that is familiar to most students and nurses, such as the *Guideline for Hand Hygiene in Health-Care Settings* (Centers for Disease Control and Prevention, 2002), have them find several of the studies used as evidence for the recommendations, and discuss how the Centers for Disease Control and Prevention decided on strength of evidence.
- Develop a rubric for assessing evidence-based guidelines in your setting.

One Nurse's Story of Successful EBP

Before we end this chapter, we'd like to share an EBP thinking story. (See **TACTICS 8-5**.) Sherry Bumpus, RN, PhD, FNP-BC, is a nurse practitioner and assistant professor.

Note that she makes reference (without prompting, we might add) not only to EBP but also to other IOM competencies, such as interdisciplinary practice and quality improvement.

TACTICS 8-5: Find the Thinking and EBP Components in Sherry's Story

Clinicians and Educators

As you read the story, circle the parts that illustrate thinking dimensions and those that exemplify EBP.

When I was invited to share an experience of evidence-based practice, I knew exactly what would fill the bill. At the time I wasn't aware of all the thinking dimensions that were being used, so I inserted them in brackets to highlight how critical the thinking was to this project that developed an evidence base for medical cardiac discharge care.

It was in a meeting with central scheduling that the director of Cardiovascular Medicine Clinical Operations/nurse manager first learned of the problem. It was shocking,
really. It seemed that the very patients at highest risk for adverse events after hospital
discharge were the same patients being lost to close follow-up care. According to the
schedulers, these high-risk patients, who were told to follow up with their healthcare
provider within 2 weeks of discharge, were in fact being scheduled for an appointment
50–60 days after discharge. Many of these patients thus ended up in the ER and were
frequently readmitted to the hospital before they even made it to their first follow-up visit.
[Those schedulers, using their logical reasoning, applying standards and confidence,
saw the incongruence of the current standard and expectation with the reality and the
resulting ineffective care model.]

Something had to be done. The director of Cardiovascular Medicine Clinical Opera-
tions/nurse manager, with the support of the senior cardiology faculty in this teaching
institution, called together an interprofessional team to examine this unacceptable
situation. [She was using some information seeking along with collaboration to start
analyzing the situation.] The team required the thinking of inpatient nurse managers,
inpatient clinical assistants in charge of assisting the residents with discharge scheduling,
nurse practitioners (NPs), residents, and the call center staff. The purpose of this combined thinking was to consider a new discharge model for patient care, based on evidence
and perhaps create an evidence-based standard for transitional care for cardiac patients.
[The thinking of this group required all 10 of the CT habits of the mind: confidence;
contextual perspective; creativity; flexibility; inquisitiveness; intellectual integrity;
intuition; open-mindedness; perseverance; and reflection; and most likely some, if not
all, of the seven CT skills.]

As with any major change in a this-is-the-way-we-have-always-done-this approach
to care, the key stakeholders had to buy into first exploring something different and then
agreeing to try something different. To make a long story short, the interprofessional team
looked at the existing evidence, which included actual days to cardiology follow-up postdischarge, hospital readmission rates for cardiac patients and the then-current guidelines
for care. Then they identified what their ideal outcome would be and set out to develop
these discharge standards. At the time, evidence-based guidelines only broadly suggested
that seeing patients earlier postdischarge would be beneficial in reducing adverse events.
It was not until 2010 that Hernandez and colleagues (2010) demonstrated that 7-day
follow-up for heart failure patients reduced readmissions in the first 30 days. Today, evidence-based guidelines for postdischarge follow-up of acute coronary syndrome (acute
myocardial infarctions and unstable angina) and atrial fibrillation are still lacking.

Many additional meetings were needed to sort out procedural issues (who did what,
when, and how), power issues (physicians agreeing to allow NPs in the newly designed
BRIDGE program to manage the discharge care of their patients), and how to collect
data to determine if this new pilot program had positive patient outcomes. Ultimately,

our BRIDGE model consists of a single postdischarge visit within 14 days of hospital discharge, where the NPs act as an extension of the hospital discharge team. It's been an exciting thinking and doing adventure for me and the other NPs involved. Creating an evidence-based standard for care requires lots of critical thinking, lots of time, and lots of collaboration, but the outcome was worth the effort.

*BRIDGE, by the way, stands for **BRI**dging the **D**ischarge **G**ap **E**ffectively and has now been in operation for over 5 years. The program is managed by five expert cardiology NPs and has received high praise from former opponents of the program, physicians, administrators, and patients. In our preliminary study we showed nearly a 20% reduction in 30-day readmissions for patients discharged after an acute coronary event. Several other research projects have been generated using this model of care, and results are being showcased at conferences nationally. Outcome data from this 5-year project clearly provide an evidence base for this model and, with replication elsewhere, could be developed into an evidence-based guideline for practice.*

Discussion

We bet many of you would like to work with Sherry. Are you fortunate enough to work with nurses like her? Are you a nurse like her? She exemplifies EBP, doesn't she?

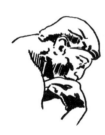

© Jesse Rubenfeld

PAUSE and Ponder

Where Should Our EBP Thinking Go?

OK, so you're totally convinced that EBP is the bandwagon you should be on, right? We hope you can approach this not as a bandwagon, but as a thinking journey for excellence in practice. It is a more enlightened and exciting approach that gets us away from tradition as a driving force. However, it is changing very fast, and we must be clear on what we are promoting when we say *EBP*. As Estabrooks cautioned, there is a lot of jargon: "research utilization, knowledge utilization, innovation diffusion, technology transfer, evidence-based practice, knowledge translation, knowledge transfer and knowledge mobilization" (2003, p. 62). It is all about using the best thinking and knowledge we have for practice and that knowledge will not just be handed down. Knowledge must be sought actively. Recognizing when we need it, accessing it, evaluating it, using it, and evaluating its usefulness is a constant cycle requiring CT. CT also helps us recognize that not all current knowledge is bad. We need to be careful that we don't throw the baby out with the bath water. But we have to apply the standards of EBP to support what we keep, what we pitch, and what we update.

REFLECTION CUES

- EBP is an important paradigm shift away from practice based on tradition to one based on the use of the best knowledge available.
- The IOM envisioned EBP as several tasks: knowing where and how to find the best evidence, formulating clinical questions, searching for and evaluating the evidence to answer those questions, and determining how and when to integrate that evidence into practice.
- Links between CT and EBP can be easily tracked.
- The history of EBP shows an international movement that primarily started in the 1980s and continues today.
- There is increasing focus on health consumers' part in the EBP movement.
- EBP is important because most of the time it saves money and other resources and promotes better patient outcomes.
- Clinicians and educators need to reflect on how they use evidence in their daily practice.
- EBP requires the use of all 17 dimensions of CT.
- Questioning practice is augmented by *inquisitiveness, intellectual integrity*, and *intuition*.
- Searching for evidence necessitates the use of informatics and the thinking dimensions of *discriminating, information seeking*, and *analysis*.
- Synthesis of evidence in systematic reviews is done by several groups today, notably the Cochrane Collaboration.
- Users of systematic reviews must evaluate them with *discrimination*, use *analyzing* skills, and *apply standards* for judging quality.
- Mechanisms to judge strength of evidence are currently being studied extensively.
- Using evidence-based clinical guidelines requires *logical reasoning* so that recommendations for practice can be traced back to the evidence.
- A *contextual perspective* is imperative when considering the feasibility of using evidence-based guidelines with patient populations.
- EBP is not cookbook health care.
- Implementing EBP requires *predicting* and *creativity*.
- Revising practice is best done with *open-minded, flexible* thinking.
- Evaluating effectiveness of practice changes requires *logical reasoning* and *predicting*.
- The whole process of EBP requires *confidence* in one's thinking, *reflection*, and *perseverance*.
- EBP is a process of *transforming knowledge*.
- EBP can be done with large innovations or in small, day-to-day increments.
- One nurse's story about how she is using EBP helps us appreciate how this is possible and how important CT is to this process.

■ Clinicians and educators must take care not to approach EBP with a bandwagon mentality, but with CT fully engaged.

REFERENCES

Agency for Healthcare Research and Quality. (2013, July). Centers and offices. Retrieved from http://www.ahrq.gov/cpi/centers/index.html

AGREE Enterprise. (2009). The AGREE II Instrument [Electronic version]. Retrieved from http://www.agreetrust.org

American Diabetes Association. (2013). Standards of medical care in diabetes—2013. *Diabetes Care, 36*(Suppl. I), S11–S66. doi: 10.2337/dc13-S011

Avis, M., & Freshwater, D. (2006). Evidence for practice, epistemology, and critical reflection. *Nursing Philosophy, 7*, 216–224.

Bearman, M., & Dawson, P. (2013). Qualitative synthesis and systematic review in health professions education. *Medical Education, 47*(3), 252–260. doi: 10.1111/medu.12092

Bucknall, T., & Hutchinson, A. M. (2006). Editorial. *Worldviews on Evidence-Based Nursing, 3*, 137–138.

Centers for Disease Control and Prevention. (2002). Guideline for hand hygiene in health-care settings: Recommendations of the healthcare infection control practices advisory committee and the HICPC/SHEA/APIC/IDSA hand hygiene task force. *Morbidity and Mortality Weekly Report, 51*(RR-16), 1–47.

Cesario, S., Morin, K., & Santa-Donato, A. (2002). Evaluating the level of evidence of qualitative research. *Journal of Obstetric, Gynecologic, & Neonatal Nursing, 31*, 531–538.

Cochrane Collaboration. (2013, July). Archie Cochrane: The name behind the Cochrane Collaboration. Retrieved from http://www.cochrane.org/about-us/history/archie-cochrane

Cullum, N., & Guyatt, G. (2005). Health care interventions and harm: An introduction. In A. DiCenso, G. Guyatt, & D. Ciliska (Eds.), *Evidence-based nursing: A guide to clinical practice* (pp. 44–70). St. Louis, MO: Elsevier Mosby.

DiCenso, A., Guyatt, G., & Ciliska, D. (2005). *Evidence-based nursing: A guide to clinical practice*. St. Louis, MO: Elsevier Mosby.

Eden, J., Levit, L., Berg, A., & Morton, S. (Eds.). (2011). *Finding what works in health care: Standards for systematic reviews*. Washington, DC: National Academies Press.

Estabrooks, C. A. (2003). Translating research into practice: Implications for organizations and administrators. *Canadian Journal of Nursing Research, 35*(3), 53–68.

Finn, P. (2011). Critical thinking: Knowledge and skills for evidence-based practice. *Language, Speech, and Hearing Services in Schools, 42*, 69–72. doi: 10.1044/0161-1461(2010/09-0037)

Fonteyn, M. (2005). The interrelationships among thinking skills, research knowledge, and evidence-based practice. [Editorial]. *Journal of Nursing Education, 44*, 439.

Graham, R., Mancher, M., Wolman, D. M., Greenfield, S., & Steinberg, E. (Eds.). (2011). *Clinical practice guidelines we can trust*. Washington, DC: National Academies Press.

Grol, R., Dalhuijsen, J., Veld, C., Rutten, G., & Mokkink, H. (1998). Attributes of clinical guidelines that influence use of guidelines in general practice: Observational study. *British Medical Journal, 317*, 858–861.

Haller, K. B., Reynolds, M. A., & Horsley, J. A. (1979). Developing research-based innovation protocols: Process, criteria and issues. *Research in Nursing and Health, 2*, 45–51.

Hancock, H. C., & Easen, P. R. (2006). The decision-making processes of nurses when extubating patients following cardiac surgery: An ethnographic study. *International Journal of Nursing Studies, 43*, 693–705.

Harbison, J. (2006). Clinical judgement in the interpretation of evidence: A Bayesian approach. *Journal of Clinical Nursing, 15*, 1489–1497. doi:10.1111/j.1365-2702.2005.01487.x

Hayes, R. A. (2005). Introduction to evidence-based practices. In C. E. Stout & R. A. Hayes (Eds.), *The evidence-based practice methods, models, and tools for mental health professionals* (pp. 1–9). Hoboken, NJ: Wiley.

Hernandez, A. F., Greiner, M. A., Fonarow, G. C., Hammill, B. G., Heidenreich, P. A., Yancy, C.W., . . . Curtis, L. H. (2010). Relationship between early physician follow-up and 30-day readmission among Medicare beneficiaries hospitalized for heart failure. *JAMA, 303*(117), 1716–1722. doi: 10.1001/jama.2010.533

Higgins, J. P. T., & Green, S. (Eds.). (2011). *Cochrane handbook for systematic reviews of interventions version 5.1.0.* Retrieved from http://handbook.cochrane.org

Holmes, D., Murray, S. J., Perron, A., & McCabe, J. (2008). Nursing best practice guidelines: Reflecting on the obscene rise of the void. *Journal of Nursing Management, 16,* 394–403. doi:10.1111/j.1365-2834.2008.00858.x

Holmes, D., Perron, A., & O'Byrne, P. (2006). Evidence, virulence, and the disappearance of nursing knowledge: A critique of the evidence-based dogma. *Worldviews on Evidence-Based Nursing, 3*(3), 95–102.

Hudson, K., Duke, G., Haas, B., & Varnell, G. (2008). Navigating the evidence-based practice maze. *Journal of Nursing Management, 16,* 409–416. doi:10.1111/j.1365-2834.2008.00860.x

Institute of Medicine. (2003). *Health professions education: A bridge to quality.* Washington, DC: National Academies Press.

Jennings, B. M., & Loan, L. A. (2001). Misconceptions among nurses about evidence-based practice. *Journal of Nursing Scholarship, 33,* 121–126.

Kelly, K. P., Turner, A., Speroni, K. G., McLaughlin, M. K., & Guzzetta, C. E. (2013). National survey of hospital nursing research, part 2: Facilitators and hinderances. *The Journal of Nursing Administration, 43*(1), 18–23. doi: 10.1097/NNA.0b013e3182786029

Lewis, J., & Lipp, A. (2013). Pressure-relieving interventions for treating diabetic foot ulcers. *Cochrane Database of Systematic Reviews, 1* (Article No. CD002302). doi: 10.1002/14651858.CD002302.pub2

Mantzoukas, S. (2008). A review of evidence-based practice, nursing research and reflection: Leveling the hierarchy. *Journal of Clinical Nursing, 17,* 214–223. doi:10.1111/j.1365-2702.2006.01912.x

McWilliam, C. L. (2007). Continuing education at the cutting edge: Promoting transformative knowledge translation. *Journal of Continuing Education in the Health Professions, 27*(2), 72–79. doi:10.1002/chp

Melnyk, B. M., & Fineout-Overholt, E. (2011). *Evidence-based practice in nursing and healthcare: A guide to best practice* (2nd ed.). Philadelphia, PA: Lippincott Williams & Wilkins.

National Guideline Clearinghouse. (n.d.). Guideline comparison template. Retrieved from http://guideline.gov/compare/comparison-template.aspx

Nickerson, C. J., & Thurkettle, M. A. (2013). Cognitive maturity and readiness for evidence-based nursing practice. *Journal of Nursing Education, 52*(1), 17–23. doi:10.3928/01484834-20121121-04

Pierce, L. L. (2007). Evidence-based practice in rehabilitation nursing. *Rehabilitation Nursing, 32,* 203–209.

Profetto-McGrath, J., Hesketh, K. L., Lang, S., & Estabrooks, C. A. (2003). A study of critical thinking and research utilization among nurses. *Western Journal of Nursing Research, 25,* 322–337.

Ransohoff, D. F., Pignone, M., & Sox, H. C. (2013). How to decide whether a clinical practice guideline is trustworthy. *JAMA, 309*(2), 139–140. doi: 10.1001/jama.2012.156703

Registered Nurses' Association of Ontario. (2005). Prevention of constipation in the older adult population. Retrieved from http://rnao.ca/bpg/guidelines/prevention-constipation-older-adult-population

Rolfe, G. (2005). The deconstructing angel: Nursing, reflection and evidence-based practice. *Nursing Inquiry, 12*(2), 78–86.

Romyn, D. M., Allen, M. N., Boschma, G., Duncan, S. M., Edgecombe, N., Jensen, L. A., . . . Warnock, F. (2003). The notion of evidence in evidence-based practice by the nursing philosophy working group. *Journal of Professional Nursing, 19,* 184–188.

Rycroft-Malone, J. (2008). Evidence-informed practice: From individual to context. *Journal of Nursing Management, 16,* 404–408. doi:10.1111/j.1365-2834.2008.00859.x

Sackett, D. L., Rosenberg, W. M. C., Gray, J. A. M., Haynes, R. B., & Richardson, W. S. (1996). *Evidence-based medicine: What it is and what it isn't.* Retrieved from http://www.ncbi.nlm.nih.gov/pmc/articles/pmc2349778/

Sams, L., & Gannon, M. E. (2000). Evidence-based practice and clinical work assessment. *Seminars in Perioperative Nursing, 9*(3), 125–132.

Sandelowski, M. (2004). Using qualitative research. *Qualitative Health Research, 14,* 1366–1386. doi:10.1177/1049732304269672

Scott-Findlay, S., & Pollock, C. (2004). Evidence, research, knowledge: A call for conceptual clarity. *Worldviews on Evidence-Based Nursing, 1,* 92–97.

Shekelle, P. G., Woolf, S. H., Eccles, M., & Grimshaw, J. (1999). Developing guidelines. *British Medical Journal, 318,* 593–596.

Slawson, D., Shaughnessy, A., Ebell, M., & Barry, H. (2007). *Essential evidence: Medicine that matters.* Hoboken, NJ: Wiley.

Stetler, C. B., Brunell, M., Giuliano, K. K., Morsi, D., Prince, L., & Newell-Stokes, V. (1998). Evidence-based practice and the role of nursing leadership. *Journal of Nursing Administration, 28*(7/8), 45–53.

Straus, S. E., Richardson, W. S., Glasziou, P., & Haynes, R. B. (2005). *Evidence-based medicine: How to practice & teach EBM* (3rd ed.). New York, NY: Elsevier Churchill Livingstone.

Tanner, J., Norrie, P., & Melen, K. (2011). Perioperative hair removal to reduce surgical skin infection. *Cochrane Database of Systematic Reviews, 11* (Article No. CD004122). doi: 10.1002/14651858. CD004122.pub4

Thomson, R., Lavendere, M., & Madhok, R. (1995). Fortnightly review: How to ensure that guidelines are effective. *British Medical Journal, 311,* 237–242.

Woolf, S., Grol, R., Hutchinson, A., Eccles, M., & Grimshaw, J. (1999). Potential benefits, limitations, and harms of clinical guidelines. *British Medical Journal, 318,* 527–530.

CHAPTER 9

Critical Thinking and Informatics

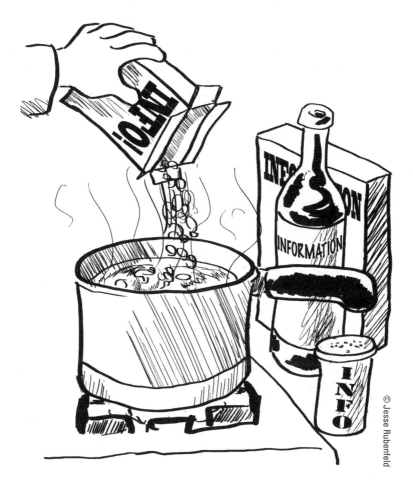

© Jesse Rubenfeld

The computer, the telephone, the Web, video—these, and all that is still to come, are unquestionably powerful tools. Used badly, they waste time and money, and dehumanize our interactions with each other. Used well, guided by a clear understanding of basic informatics principles, they are neither to be feared, loved, nor loathed. They are simply to be used. In the next century, the study of informatics will become as fundamental to the practice of medicine as anatomy has been to the last.

That poignant statement is from Enrico Coiera's paper, based on an article he wrote for the *Medical Journal of Australia* in 1998 and posted on the Internet as *10 Essential Clinical Informatics Skills* (1999). He is referring to *informatics*—a term that is now as much a part of nursing and healthcare delivery as the bedpan. Although it is commonplace, informatics is not a natural subject for most nurses; however, it is being thrust upon us as a necessity because computer technology and the information it processes are here to stay.

Health informatics is about how we process, use, and share information relative to healthcare delivery. The Institute of Medicine (IOM), with its conjoint emphasis on patient-centered care, evidence-based practice (EBP), quality improvement, and interdisciplinary practice, described the competency of utilizing informatics as "communicate, manage knowledge, mitigate error, and support decision making using information technology" (2003, p. 46). Informatics has remained an important focus for the IOM since that 2003 statement, with health information technology a recurrent theme in its 2011 document on the future of nursing. There is no part of health care and nursing that is untouched and not rapidly changing in terms of informatics. Nurses "are expected to use a variety of technological tools and complex information management systems that require skills in analysis and synthesis to improve the quality and effectiveness of care" (IOM, 2011, p. 7)

Informatics is a broad concept covering a wide range of technology—from simple email to complex clinical information systems, from the familiar electrocardiogram machine to electronic medical ordering systems, from PowerPoint presentations to complete computer-assisted instruction, to high-fidelity simulation learning in the laboratory setting. You get the idea. One can become narrow in view depending on what aspect of informatics one is most involved with. For example, if you are a nurse working in an institution that is going paperless, you are focused on the electronic health record; if you are a nurse working in a rural clinic, you might be focused on telehealth; if you are a nursing student, you might be focused on doing a thorough electronic search for evidence.

At any level of involvement, and clearly in the IOM and Coiera's statements, it is evident that critical thinking (CT) needs to be an integral part of using informatics. Most of Coiera's 10 skills start with words that imply thinking—"understand," "search for and assess," "interpret," "analyze and structure clinical decisions," "adapt and apply knowledge," "access," "assess," "select and apply," "structure and record data," and so forth. The IOM statement included "manage knowledge" and "support decision-making."

The relationship between informatics and thinking is a complex and uncharted one. One chapter cannot begin to explore the intricacies and unknown waters of the brain as it deals with the information explosion. However, there is one thing that is obvious: nowhere is CT more important than in relation to informatics. Informatics can enhance thinking, but thinking is also requisite to the effective use of informatics.

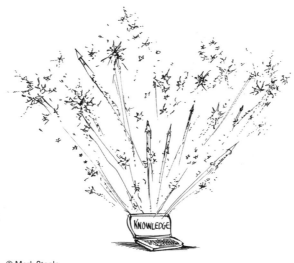

© Mark Steele

Context of Old Nurses and Young Informatics

Some younger readers may be tempted to skip this chapter because they think that anyone old enough to write a book cannot possibly teach you anything about informatics, which is as natural to you as breathing. We ask that you stick with us because you need to see the full spectrum of how nurses deal with informatics, be they young or old.

Some older readers may be tempted to skip this chapter because they think they won't understand informatics. Maybe it's something that just doesn't interest you. You probably get really angry at all the cell phone conversations in restaurants and stores and the exorbitant prices you pay for cable TV and computer games for your teenagers. Stick with us and you'll see that you are not alone in your frustration over informatics. We sympathize with you on a personal and professional level because we're also old nurses dealing with young informatics.

If you remember when we didn't use computers every day, you are possibly our age. When we started out in nursing in the late 1960s and early 1970s, computers were props in science fiction movies—big, cumbersome things that filled whole buildings, whirring and whizzing to help the spies. Thirty-some years later, we're unable to imagine life without these machines—now as small as peas—that we love and hate. (Yes, Dr. Coiera, in spite of what you say, we do love and hate them.) We love them because they make it so easy to access information. We hate them because when they go down, freeze up, flash blue-screen messages, lose our last 3 hours of writing, get viruses, and cause other situations too numerous to list, we are left with the realization that we are way too dependent on them. For most of us, that dependency is not only frustrating, but also scary, because so much of today's technology is mysterious. However, information technology is here to stay, and it's evolving more rapidly than we can fathom. As McBride said, "There is no aspect of nursing that will be untouched by the informatics revolution in progress" (2005, p. 188).

Those of us in the baby boom generation have lived through the birth and rapid growth of computers. We learned this foreign language later in life. For several years, we wrote with a pen and then typed things into the computer—the old typewriter mentality. (Don't worry, we've grown up; we're now typing original ideas here sans yellow pad.) We oldsters have had to change our ways to keep up with computers. For younger generations, computers are as common as electricity was for most of us back then. However, many nurses are our age and older. According to the U.S. Department of Health and Human Services Health Resources and Services Administration (2010), in 2008 the median age of nurses was 46; that age was rising steadily until recently, when it stabilized. The IOM, citing Buerhaus and colleagues, said, "From 1983 to 2009, the number of nurses over age 50 more than quadrupled, and the number of middle-aged nurses (aged 35-49) doubled to approximately 39 percent . . . These older and middle-aged nurses now represent almost three-quarters of the nursing workforce, while nurses younger than 34 now make up only 26 percent" (2011, p. 125). The majority of nurses did not grow up with computers in their homes; many used a computer for the first time in their places of employment. Many still anxiously stumble along using computers every day.

In an editorial in the *Online Journal of Nursing Informatics*, McGonigle hit the scary nail on the head when she wrote the following paragraph to illustrate the "abbreviation frenzy" that makes the language of informatics so foreign to many of us:

> When we speak of BI and look for VAP from the VAN it is not so surprising that we crunch IEs on our HPCs. Sometimes we use a DSS. At other times, we look for help from as many people as we can by using VNC, our VM or enlisting VOIP to contact the people "in the know" at the NHIN or RHIOs. Now doesn't that make it as clear as MUD with MOO? (2006, para 4)

She gave an abbreviation translation taken from a biomedical abbreviation server: BI is business intelligence; VAP is value-added process; VAN is value-added network; IE is information element; HPC is handheld personal computer; DSS is decision support system; VNC is virtual network computing; VM is virtual machine; VOIP is voice over Internet protocol; NHIN is national health information network; RHIO is regional health information organization; MUD is multiuser dimension/domain; and MOO is MUD, object oriented (McGonigle, 2006). We've given you this example not to scare you off, but to help you realize that you're not alone in thinking this new language is beyond you.

Almost everyone around us uses computers in some way—if not directly, at least indirectly. We have a U.S. government mandate that all Americans have electronic medical records by 2014, making computer competency an immediate reality (Ornes & Gassert, 2007). Electronic medical records are becoming common and are evolving. It may be that the whole face of medical records will be reworked in the next few years. These changes "range from simple, portable jump drive approaches that an individual person may carry and use to record health data such as immunizations, to highly sophisticated, integrated records that can amass many types of health data from various sources and can provide health education and health data exchange opportunities between the patient and caregiver" (Androwich, 2013, p. 38).

Consumers of health care have more access to information than they have ever had before. People who think they can survive in this world without integrating informatics into their lives are dinosaurs trying to survive in the 21st century. We're getting ahead of ourselves here, but we want to show you that reading this chapter is worth the effort even though it may be scary to some of us with middle-aged eyes. We apologize to our youthful readers, but, according to the statistics, you are a minority. Let's go back and set up more groundwork.

Healthcare Informatics Evolution

Lest we lead you down a confusing path, and before we join CT with informatics, we'll detour here to discuss the evolution of health informatics. It used to be that informatics meant computer technology, and so far we have focused many of our comments in that direction. Because computers were the instigators of this field, we often equate them with informatics. Today, however, the focus of this burgeoning field is more on information and the meanings of information in communicating, sharing knowledge, and decision making.

As you may deduce from that statement, not everyone defines informatics the same way. The term *informatics*, coined in the 1970s, initially referred to computers and their immediate context (Saba, 2001). Since that time, people have broadened the descriptions, some doing it according to discipline. For example, *nursing informatics*, according to Saba and McCormick, is

the use of technology and/or a computer system to . . . process . . . and communicate timely data and information in and across healthcare facilities that administer nursing services and resources, manage the delivery of patient and nursing care, link research resources and findings to nursing practice, and apply educational resources to nursing education. (2001, p. 226)

The American Nurses Association (ANA) supports the movement toward informatics in the practice arena and has developed a document called *Nursing Informatics: Scope and Standards of Practice* (2008). The ANA defined the specialty of nursing informatics in this way:

Nursing informatics (NI) is a specialty that integrates nursing science, computer science, and information science to manage and communicate data, information, knowledge, and wisdom in nursing practice. NI supports consumers, patients, nurses, and other providers in their decision-making in all roles and settings. This support is accomplished through the use of information structures, information processes, and information technology. (p. 1)

You may notice that the newer definition from the ANA has a broader focus than the earlier Saba definition. This change reflects the move from computers as the central idea to that of information.

The National League for Nursing (NLN) focused its support on the education arena as demonstrated by its 2008 position statement titled *Preparing the Next Generation of Nurses to Practice in a Technology-Rich Environment: An Informatics Agenda.* The position statement was triggered by an NLN survey indicating the following:

1. Only 50–60% of respondents identified informatics as being integrated into their curricula, and most of that was primarily in the clinical setting.
2. Only 60% of the programs surveyed had computer literacy as a program requirement.
3. Only 40% of the programs surveyed had an information literacy requirement.
4. Content on informatics was more commonly found in baccalaureate degree programs and higher.

The NLN concluded that

there was considerable confusion as to what nursing informatics entails and what constitutes the necessary knowledge to practice in an informatics-rich environment . . . [and] faculty, deans, administrators, and the NLN itself [must] advocate that all students graduate with up-to-date knowledge and skills in each of three critical areas: computer literacy, information literacy, and informatics. (2008, para 3, 4)

Perhaps because of the published results of that survey, or perhaps in spite of them, it seems that nurses in academic settings are embracing informatics in a big way. Nursing courses are being taught; national conferences are being held; articles, whole journals, and books are emerging; and nursing curricula across the country are integrating informatics with gusto.

Over the past decade a variety of terms have been used to label informatics in the healthcare arena, such as medical informatics, nursing informatics, patient informatics, and consumer health informatics. Most people have landed on *health informatics* as a common label. Clearly evident from these various descriptions is that informatics has to do with managing information and knowledge, communicating, and making decisions—all direct links to thinking. The IOM (2003, 2011) specifically noted the value of informatics in preventing errors, which fits with its emphasis on increased safety in health care.

The Changing Nature of Informatics

In considering how to approach the subject of CT and informatics, we were struck by the real probability that anything we said about informatics would be out of date by the time this text was published. Indeed, as one reads about informatics, one can readily see that unless informatics information has been posted on a website in the past 6 months, it is out of date. This rapid rate of change, of course, is due to the increasing sophistication of the technology we utilize to share and use information.

We're trying to get a feel for where informatics will be going in the near future, but by the time we sit down to write that, the future has become the present. Nevertheless, we'll try to keep as much of a futuristic view as possible in our comments about CT and informatics. The IOM, in its Quality Chasm series, *Patient Safety* (2004), called for three important foci for informatics that can contribute to increased quality in health care. It proposed increased support from government agencies and health-care systems to accelerate improvement of (1) data exchange formats, (2) structured terminologies, and (3) knowledge representation. These three areas will facilitate recording and accessibility of information, increase the intersystem and interdisciplinary communication, and facilitate decision making.

By 2011, the IOM focused more on nursing's role in informatics. As part of its second recommendation to expand opportunities for nurses, the IOM had this to say: "Health care organizations should engage nurses and other front-line staff to work with developers and manufacturers in the design, development, purchase, implementation and evaluation of medical and health devices and health information technology products" (2011, p. 11). Numerous examples of nurses' roles in informatics were presented, such as remote patient monitoring, which was seen to be "expanding exponentially" (p. 137).

Plenty of other examples of nursing's use of informatics can be found in the literature. For example, teleintensive care unit nursing, where nurses can remotely access information and assist bedside nurses, "is a developing subspecialty of critical care nursing and requires high-level critical thinking and analytical skills" (Williams, Hubbard, Daye, & Barden, 2012, p. 62). The use of tablet technology (Duffy, 2012), smartphones (Mitchell, 2012), and YouTube (Logan, 2012) are other such examples of nurses using informatics in everyday practice.

Another interesting view of the present and near future of informatics was articulated by Ball and Lillis (2000). Even though they published this article in 2000, which by informatics standards is very old, their observations about trends remain relevant. Using information from the Gartner Group Research Review, Ball and Lillis (2000) discussed eight trends in healthcare information technology that we can see occurring today. They began by listing how technology helps, not with just data, but with decision-making processes such as decision trees and algorithms. They note a second trend in which the concept of communication has moved to the broader concept of collaboration, as informatics allows for working together via phone conferencing, Skype, webcasts, etc., regardless of geographic locations. Some software even allows for language translations, but we need to beware of words and phrases that do not translate meaning effectively or accurately. Third, they noted how technology allows for the integration of information into usable knowledge as more synthesized sources become available at our fingertips with an Internet connection.

Ball and Lillis's fourth trend, "from network computing to ubiquitous computing" (p. 387) addressed the physical space where information is stored and its relative unimportance in today's world of portable devices. Even our grandchildren have handheld devices that they seem to manipulate better than we do. The fifth trend addressed the transition to more sophisticated interfaces, moving to areas such as speech recognition. An excellent example of this is how some smart phones recognize your voice and either call the person you want to call or give you verbal directions for where you want to go. Will automated diagnosticians and caregivers be next?

The sixth trend, the move to a more mobile approach to technology, allows for access in remote locations. For example, it is becoming common for rural centers to link to larger facilities for specific services. This is currently occurring across continents with some healthcare facilities. The seventh trend, from "physical to virtual" should simplify many procedures. We can't wait for our virtual colonoscopies! The eighth trend is toward a focus on consumers, rather than business. We hope this is occurring as part of the patient-centered care trend.

As you contemplate these trends, you can probably see yourself in the middle of those trends right now, and maybe even past them. The constant rapid rate of change of informatics and our panting as we run alongside to keep up are ultimately the reasons why addressing the thinking involved in informatics is so critical. All healthcare providers need to have a CT frame to go along with the rapid changes. That thinking frame will have built into it ways of dealing with the changes in those mechanisms that can enhance our thinking. Linear or dualistic thinking must be minimized; thinking must be primarily *contextual* and relativistic. Thinkers who are uncomfortable with uncertainty will either give up or they will suffer extreme stress. Stop for a minute and assess (*reflect*) on your style of thinking. Where are you on a continuum, with dualistic thinking (seeing the world dichotomously, such as only black or white, right or wrong) at one end, and relativistic thinking (able to recognize many shades of gray depending on the circumstances and the situation) at the other end? Many of us may be closer to the dualistic end, which helps explain the next paragraph.

It seems that nursing is lagging in its informatics competency (Fetter, 2008; National League for Nursing, 2008). Several initiatives have begun to focus on how we can catch up. The Technology Informatics Guiding Educational Reform (TIGER) Initiative (2013) hopes to close the gap by providing recommendations for, among other stakeholders, academic institutions and professional organizations. The Canadian Nurses Association has an "e-nursing strategy" (2006). Nursing is not alone in its perceived need to get going to increase its informatics competency. The U.S. government has set up the Office of Health Information Technology within the Department of Health and Human Services (Health Information Technology, 2013) to provide assistance to professionals and consumers regarding health information technology.

Critical Thinking and Health Informatics

We may be biased, but it doesn't seem like a leap to see that CT must be part of the informatics picture. Mastrian (2008), echoing Wang (2003), proposed "cognitive informatics" as a branch of informatics bridging artificial and natural intelligences. Turley's (1996) model showed nursing informatics as the overlap of three science circles: cognitive, information, and computer sciences. Our merging of thinking and informatics may be a bit simplistic when compared with the models by Wang or Turley, but we envision the merger coming from two directions. As seen in **Figure 9-1**, one can augment one's CT with informatics, but one must use CT to best choose and use informatics. Informatics is only slightly akin to a new piece of equipment (for example, needleless needles) that, once mastered, can be used to augment work.

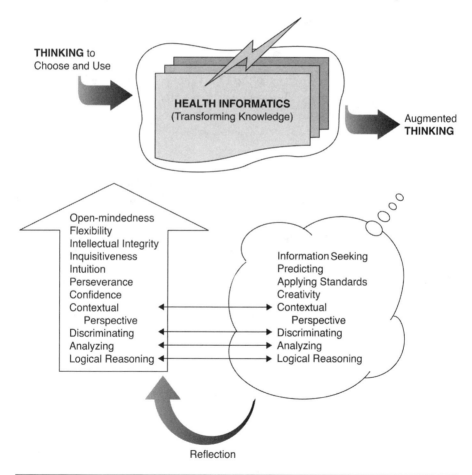

Figure 9-1 Relationship between critical thinking and health informatics.
© Jesse Rubenfeld

Informatics includes many processes, changing daily, that are there for our use if we know enough about them and are open-minded enough to choose them.

In Figure 9-1, we have listed several CT dimensions on the left side that help us choose and use informatics. The list on the right side indicates the dimensions augmented by informatics. There is some overlap of those dimensions, and we will address the reasons for that overlap shortly. You will also note that we have the dimension of *transforming knowledge* at the top with health informatics and *reflection* as the connecting dimension with the arrow at the bottom. Why have we done that?

TACTICS 9-1: Use Your Creativity and Logical Reasoning

Clinicians and Educators

Before reading further, stop a minute and look at Figure 9-1 and reflect on the 17 CT dimensions that we have revisited frequently throughout this text. Test your *creativity* and *logical reasoning* to consider why we might have placed the dimensions where we did.

Discussion

The next section will give you our explanation, but this TACTICs encourages you to construct your own meanings first. Then compare your meanings with our explanation to see if you thought of things that we forgot. It's quite possible that you put all 17 dimensions on both sides. As you realize by now, artificially separating CT dimensions is just that: artificial. In reality, we use all dimensions in most thinking situations. What we've done here is try to tease out those that are especially important to each side of the picture. Rest assured that there are other ways to interpret this; you may have come up with a much different configuration.

Informatics *as* Transforming Knowledge

Earlier we talked about the difference between information and knowledge. Informatics allows us to transform information into knowledge and allows us to *transform knowledge*, "changing or converting the condition, nature, form, or function of concepts among contexts" (Scheffer & Rubenfeld, 2000, p. 358). That's why we highlighted *transforming knowledge* in Figure 9-1. As an aside, have you noticed that *transforming knowledge* comes up frequently as a core thinking skill? We asked you to think of EBP as *transforming knowledge*, for example. EBP and informatics have a very symbiotic relationship. It is through the use of informatics that we can transform the evidence into practice.

Consider a computer application used by a nurse practitioner for prescribing medications. In the old days, the practitioner would have to consider other medications that the patient was taking and try to think of any potential interactions. She would spend time looking up such things, and there was a good chance that something could be missed because there were several places that could, and should, be checked. Today, when using electronic programs like Epocrates (http://www.epocrates.com) or Tarascon (http://www.tarascon.com/), for example, information on each drug is available so that, in one fell swoop, all potential interactions are noted, dosing for certain conditions is listed, and so on. The drug information has been transformed into usable knowledge in a very timely manner.

The very act of communicating within an informatics framework allows knowledge to be transformed much more easily. Let's take a simple example: writing on a computer as opposed to writing on a typewriter or on a pad of paper. Anyone who writes as we do—stream of consciousness first, then moving things around and editing—will definitely say that transforming information and knowledge is so much easier on a computer. You get the idea, right? Using informatics is *transforming knowledge*—sorting it, *analyzing* it, communicating it, and converting it into a practical, usable form.

Critical Thinking for Choosing and Using Informatics

On the left side of Figure 9-1 is a list of 11 CT dimensions that are particularly used to choose and use informatics. The last four on the list (*contextual perspective, discriminating, analyzing,* and *logical reasoning*) are repeated on the right side of the figure because, in addition to helping thinkers choose and use informatics, those dimensions are augmented by informatics. Those dimensions will be discussed here and in the "How Informatics Augments Critical Thinking" section later in this chapter.

Open-Mindedness *and* Flexibility

First and foremost are the *open-mindedness* and *flexibility* CT dimensions. Using informatics means changing from how one has been doing things, either using applications for the first time or keeping up with newer applications. We'll bet that many of you can remember, as we do, the first year we moved our teaching materials over to PowerPoint presentations. It seemed like such a big deal, and it would have been so much easier to stick with our handwritten notes and overhead transparencies. Today, we expect PowerPoint presentations and are shocked when someone doesn't use them.

Another area for *open-mindedness* and *flexibility* in the education arena is the movement toward high-fidelity simulations in the nursing clinical skills laboratory. There are growing numbers of adult, child, and infant simulators that are considered state-of-the-art necessities for nursing skills laboratories these days. These highly sophisticated devices can talk, breathe, react to medications, and even die (Leigh & Hurst, 2008). Simulation is an augmentation, not a substitute, for thinking in practice. It is most effective when it is couched in terms of situated cognition or learning in context (Onda, 2012). Focusing on the need to link thinking and simulation experiences, Lasater (2007) used the simulation environment to develop an instrument to measure clinical judgment. However, there remains a need to examine simulation in relationship to thinking, an area of study still in its infancy and, at best, equivocal (Maneval et al., 2012).

Learning how to use these devices has not been easy for nurse educators. Leigh and Hurst (2008) discussed the challenges of helping faculty to be *open-minded* and *flexible* in order to embrace these new teaching tools and maximize their benefits. Maintaining a flexible and open-minded approach to new methods of gathering, storing, sorting, *analyzing*, and using information and technology is a challenge because it seems that we are always at the start of a learning curve. In case you haven't caught on yet, that will never change; nursing and health care are too dynamic. Change is the name of the game!

Intellectual Integrity

Related to *open-mindedness* and *flexibility* is *intellectual integrity*—"seeking the truth through sincere, honest processes, even if the results are contrary to one's assumptions and beliefs" (Scheffer & Rubenfeld, 2000, p. 358). This is a tough one because it is so much easier to maintain the status quo: The way I do things now works just fine; I don't want to learn a new way; I don't have time or energy. We've all said those things, especially on a Friday after a long week. But *intellectual integrity* nudges us to think beyond our own needs and consider what is best for our patients and our students in the long run.

Just how does one maintain an *open mind*, the *flexibility*, and the *intellectual integrity* to embrace informatics? For starters, it helps to receive positive reinforcement for those thinking habits of the mind. Second, it's important to tell yourself that you can't survive in this field without informatics. (You can't, you know; it's definitely a force to be reckoned with.) Third, start talking about informatics to the people you work with and those who work at institutions like yours. Ask them what they know—their visions, fears, and reality—when it comes to information technology. Fourth, make yourself sit down at a computer and do something you haven't done before. To get you started with those four suggestions, try **TACTICS 9-2**.

TACTICS 9-2: Think How Informatics Could Ease Your Life

Clinicians and Educators

Take some time and reflect on informatics; then think about your daily activities. Even if you know nothing about computers or information technology, where do you think you could improve your job efficiency and accuracy with technology? Don't allow yourself to think about the specifics of changing over to such technology; that will shut down the open-minded side of your brain. Be a divergent thinker; let your thoughts expand!

Discussion

What did you come up with? Did you let your creative juices flow? As clinicians, we'd want voice-activated recording devices and handheld computer terminals that we could put in our pockets to access and record information. We'd want all patients to have a smart card with their health data on it—one that we could insert into our handheld device and retrieve and record information. Perhaps by the time you're reading this text, you'll laugh because you have such devices with you. Maybe you'll laugh even more because what you have goes far beyond our old-fashioned vision.

As educators, we would want teaching aids that talk to each other more easily. We'd want instant, surefire Internet access in every classroom. We also would want those handheld devices that we can carry around and use easily. We'd want functioning virtual classrooms where people can talk to each other around the world, all at the same time. We'd want students to have these handheld resources so that, if they have to do tracheostomy care, for example, they can pull up a virtual demonstration anytime and anywhere. We want to explore the use of simulation technology in the clinical laboratory, where students can learn from critical mistakes but bring patients back to life after an oops. You get the idea, right? Let your mind soar; almost anything our limited minds can envision will most likely be a reality very soon.

Inquisitiveness

Getting back to our dimensions for choosing and using informatics, it will help your *intellectual integrity* if you engage your *inquisitiveness* habit of the mind. Are you naturally inquisitive? If so, you've probably already explored the various information technologies available to you. If you are less inquisitive, try to tweak it more—but do it with fun activities. For example, get some movies that deal with informatics—not necessarily science fiction stuff, but stories about people who are touched by technology. If you need suggestions, here are some examples (in no particular order) listed by Tyler, one of our sons who is a movie buff: *Jumping Jack Flash*, *Being There*, *The Conversation*, *Blow Out*, *Apollo 13*, *Enemy of the State*, *The Net*, *Eternal Sunshine of the Spotless Mind*, *The Social Network*, *Me and You and Everyone We Know*, *Something the Lord Made*, and *Wag the Dog*.

Do you need more suggestions to get your *inquisitiveness* going? Get a computer program that's fun—a game or drawing program that you can really get into. Talk to kids about technology. Consider where you are first, though—that could scare you off because kids are really knowledgeable; they grew up with this stuff. Find the person in your environment you secretly call the "techno-geek" and strike up a conversation about why he or she is so into technology. Go on the Internet and look up people you know; you may be surprised what you find. Try to find friends from your past whom you've lost track of. Write emails to those persons. One of us, because of a simple email request, has had a wonderful renewed friendship with a childhood friend after being out of touch for 30 years. The point of these activities is to immerse yourself in technology and information exchange. It's hard for some of us to be *inquisitive* about something that we've never played around with. Start by putting your toes in the technology waters, and it won't be long before you'll love diving in so much, you'll lose track of time, even days!

Intuition

Intuition can help enhance one's choice and use of informatics. That may seem a bit strange at first glance because *intuition* seems so subjective and informatics seems so objective, but it really isn't that dichotomous. Computers can't be intuitive, but we can be. Without *intuition*, we wouldn't be able to use technology, including computers, as well as we can. Just because the computer program dictates that we do something a certain way doesn't necessarily mean it's the best or only thing to do in that situation. If it doesn't feel right, chances are it isn't.

To illustrate more subtle connections between *intuition* and informatics, let's get away from computers and use a simple, more familiar technology example: a computer order-entry program used by a physician to order enoxaparin. The enoxaparin comes from the pharmacy already loaded in its syringe—technical aids to your work. You double-check the dose (*applying standards*), and you go to administer it. How do you know how much pressure to use when you inject the short needle? Can you remember the first time you gave a subcutaneous injection? You may have not punctured the skin, or you may have done it so hard that you were almost past the hub. What guides you to know how much pressure to exert? That doesn't come from the instrument. Effken (2001) would call that "prospective control"—intuitive visual information. That information is so taken for granted by experts that many would not call it thinking. However, without that *intuitive* part of the process, the technology part cannot be fully used. Because *intuition* usually comes with experience, and because most of us are new to informatics, it's easy to forget about *intuition*. With repeated use of informatics and openness to gut responses, we allow *intuition* to help our CT.

Intuition can certainly help us identify areas in which we need technological interventions. A hospital that we have frequented as faculty used a carbon-copy medication order system; checking an order became a guessing game as one worked with partially visible orders, messy handwriting, and so forth. Every time we used it, we knew intuitively that this was a mistake waiting to happen. Fortunately, that system has now moved to a computer-based ordering system.

Perseverance

Perseverance is an absolute necessity for using informatics, especially if this field is new to you. Recently, in one of our early classes on EBP, students complained about the amount of time they spent searching the Internet to find the evidence reports they needed. They had horror stories of spending hours in one area, only to discover they could have saved that time if they had gone to another website first. Some students gave up, thinking that 8 hours on the computer was excessive. Many

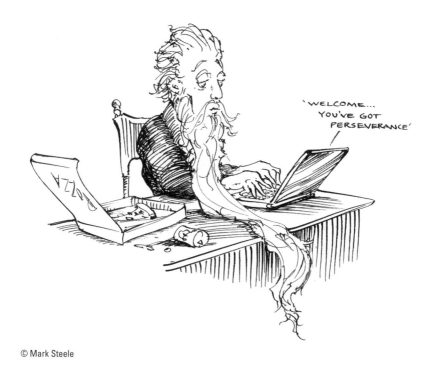

'WELCOME...
YOU'VE GOT
PERSEVERANCE'

© Mark Steele

were surprised when we didn't bat an eyelash and they heard similar stories from their classmates. We discussed the realities of time when using new technologies and how important *perseverance* is, especially in doing something new like evidence searches.

In our old ways of getting information—asking someone, finding a book, searching library index cards—there were fewer options for search paths. Less *perseverance* was needed to think from question to answer. Today, we noodle around on the Internet for hours before we find what we're looking for. (That's our favorite description— "noodle"—implying that it is not a straight, linear process.) Because we are new to computers and their mechanisms to address information, we are slower than we think we should be.

It's an interesting position to be in—most nursing leaders, as noted at the start of this chapter, were not raised in homes where computers were commonplace. We are constantly learning a new language and a new set of skills. Because we are experts in our fields already, we have trouble accepting that when it comes to today's technology, we are novices. Look at teenagers and young adults today—they can maneuver around a computer program so fast that we're left in the dust. Part of the reason youngsters can maneuver so well is their experience with computers and computer programs. They have developed an *intuitive* sense of where to move that cursor to get to the screens they want. We take much longer to do everything because it's still so new to us. We often say we don't have enough RAM to do things fast. (You can tell how in the know about computers your listeners are when they either laugh or don't laugh at that remark.) We must maintain *perseverance* and accept our novice status relative to informatics.

Confidence

Related to our novice technophile status is *confidence*. It is hard to have *confidence* in one's thinking in unfamiliar territory. This is an area in which it is helpful to separate *confidence* in doing something from *confidence* in one's thinking ability. We can accept our novice states and the reality of our clumsiness and anxiety when using new information technology, but we still have *confidence* in our ability to think. Actually, the latter will help the former. A confident thinker can often figure out unknown computer commands just by relying on his or her own logic, and sometimes *intuition*. Computer programs are, in spite of what we think sometimes, very logical (or at least as logical as the people who programmed them). However, they don't think, as such; they only follow our commands or the commands of the programmer. In that area, we are superior. Having a little sign over your desk that says "Computers can't think, but I can" is helpful to *confidence* building. Advances in computers with sophisticated artificial intelligence are growing, but for right now, your brains and CT are still what we want to count on for quality, safe nursing care.

So what interferes with your thinking *confidence* besides lack of experience? We cannot underestimate the negative effects of anxiety on our thinking *confidence*. If you are choosing and directing the implementation of a new technology for your work unit, for example, consider how you might decrease the anxiety of the staff as they begin this difficult process. First and foremost, we must acknowledge the negative effects of anxiety on thinking and that working with a new technology produces anxiety. There is nothing more anxiety producing than to anticipate looking stupid. We tend to respond in anger and use pretty low-level thinking skills. Let's get that on the table and acknowledge that we're all in that boat when we try something new.

Second, we must set up support services. Nurses take pride in their self-sufficiency; we have strong thinking skills and manage on our own quite well. Well, it's time to swallow that pride and accept the fact that we all need help with informatics. A technology or informatics expert should be available at all times to staff using something new. That person should be in place before the initiation of a new system. If you work in a system without this, demand one. You could also come up with rules to avoid technology-driven frustration. For example, Koeniger-Donohue (2008), while starting a project for students and faculty to use personal digital assistants (PDAs), had a 15-minute rule: they wouldn't struggle for longer than 15 minutes on a technical problem before calling in help.

We need to broaden our view of our teams when we increase our use of informatics. One thing we say to our students frequently is, "The librarian is your friend." As we set out to do things, such as finding evidence-based clinical guidelines or discovering what computer programs are available for our consideration, we forget that librarians are experts in such searches. Older people (we) often have this old-fashioned view of librarians as bespectacled, quiet people who stamp and sort books. For as much as nurses have had to fight the old stereotypes, so too have librarians. Our cartoon illustrates this change in vision that we'd like to see for nurses and librarians. Acknowledging that healthcare providers are not always good information seekers, Newland (2012) reminded readers to use the services of librarians who are part of the healthcare team. Have you talked to librarians recently, especially those with a specialty in healthcare informatics? They are phenomenal resources, and we need an updated vision of who they are and how they can be critical to our use of informatics.

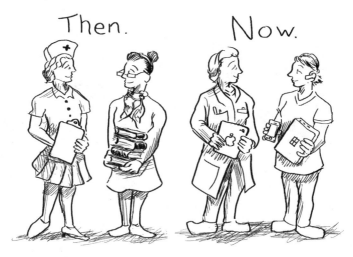

© Jesse Rubenfeld

Crumley and Koufogiannakis (2002) listed six domains of librarianship. Three of those six are providing service and access to information; helping users with library resources; and creating better methods to retrieve and access information. "The librarian's role has expanded to include the role of teacher or consultant as well as that of expert mediated searches" (Calabretta, 2002, p. 34).

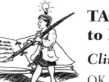

TACTICS 9-3: Take Your Librarian to Lunch

Clinicians and Educators

OK, this may seem a bit hokey, but bear with us here. If you know your librarian well and he or she often helps you, then you probably can skip this TACTICs. But if you've never thought of your institution's librarian in Calabretta's terms (just mentioned), go to the library, send an email, or call the librarian and ask that person to have lunch with you. Tell him or her that you would like to pick his or her brain about health informatics.

Discussion

If you did this, we'll bet you were pleasantly surprised in terms of what you learned about that person's knowledge and willingness to help. You will feel more *confident* in your thinking relative to informatics when you know you have this resource. You may also find someone who would be delighted to come to your unit or classroom to help with informatics. That's what we found when we started working more closely with our wonderful health sciences librarian, Elizabeth Bucciarelli, at our university. We talked to her about her relationship with nursing students and faculty in this time of informatics explosion. We have summarized some of her words of wisdom in **Box 9-1**.

Box 9-1 Words of Wisdom from Academic Health Sciences Librarian Elizabeth Bucciarelli

---

- Librarians are seekers of knowledge; they enjoy the whole research process, not just finding information. Roy Tennant, a keynote speaker at the Michigan Library Association's Academic Libraries Day, said it this way: "Librarians like to seek, most people like to find" (Tennant, 2008).
- The best approach for teaching library research skills is a tiered one, in which the librarian has multiple sessions with students. Each session builds on the previous ones, with some overlap to reinforce learning.
- Information literacy is a shared responsibility of faculty and librarians.
- Librarians need to meet with and be part of the teaching team to accomplish the following:
  - Better understand the subject
  - Better identify how to weave new technology and resources into courses
  - Make volumes of information streamlined and usable
  - Appreciate the necessity of leveling research skills for all students, from beginners to graduate students
  - Acknowledge the librarian's role as a guide for both students and faculty in the seeking process, not just finding things for them
  - Clarify that helping students synthesize knowledge is usually a teaching faculty, not a librarian, responsibility
- Handing information to students is not the best way for them to learn how to navigate research tools, but we have to realize that everyone learns differently. Sometimes we have to get to the end of their sidewalk and meet them.

Box 9-1   Words of Wisdom from Academic Health Sciences Librarian
Elizabeth Bucciarelli (continued)

- The librarian's job is to weave in new technology and streamline the extreme number of resources.
- Key areas for nursing faculty and librarians to address when they meet include the following:
  - Expectations for the course, including topics and, in particular, assignments that will require searches
  - Syllabi with due dates for projects
  - How this course fits into the overall sequence of classes within the program
  - Learning objectives for the library research session
- Key areas that librarians should address during a library research session include the following:
  - Role of librarians today and how it differs from yesterday
  - Student fears and concerns about using technology and searching
  - Rationale as to why students are learning these research skills, which addresses students who are thinking that they already know how to search because they use Google
  - Glossary of terms related to searching
  - Search process, including research databases
  - Time-saving tricks of the trade
  - Help students understand that searching is not a quick-and-dirty process; it takes a significant amount of the total time needed to complete a project or paper
  - Advise students to select the *best* resources, not simply the ones that are the easiest to retrieve
  - Encourage students to use databases beyond the ones with which they are familiar; using a variety of resources will produce a richer end product
  - Pass along the theoretical concept regarding the stream of information created and disseminated in nursing (e.g., a conference paper may become a journal article, which may become a review article, which may become a book)
- The thinking dimensions that are most needed with informatics and library searches are as follows:
  - *Information seeking*
  - *Analyzing* to evaluate the content of an article
  - *Discriminating*, which goes hand-in-hand with *analyzing* and determining quality

(continues)

Box 9-1 Words of Wisdom from Academic Health Sciences Librarian
Elizabeth Bucciarelli (continued)

- *Flexibility,* because you can't be linear; searching is very relational, going from one idea to another, such as with following up on bibliography references to gain more information
- *Inquisitiveness,* which means going beyond the basics
- *Intellectual integrity* in both academic and professional pursuits
- *Perseverance*
- *Open-mindedness;* you have to let go of an idea, broaden your thinking, and move on

Contextual Perspective

We have now arrived at the four dimensions that are on both sides of Figure 9-1. *Contextual perspective* is a thinking habit of the mind that is important to choosing and using informatics, and it is augmented by informatics. Here we focus on the choosing and using part: If you are the person choosing computer applications for your office or unit, for example, you need to think about the whole picture. Who will be using them? What will they cost? How easy is it to use the hardware? How easy is it to access program information, such as patient records, student records, and so forth? How much training will staff need? What information technology support is available? Is the support available 24/7? Is the support a living, breathing person in your facility, or will it be in the form of a phone call to who knows where? Will your computer system be able to talk to other computers (programs) in the system to share information, or will they each work in silos? What security systems are needed to protect information? What will computers and technology add to or subtract from your resources? Take time to explore all these possibilities. Better yet, get a knowledgeable information technology person to help examine the full *contextual perspective;* we can't think of it all alone.

Keep in mind that, just as they aren't intuitive, computers and their programs are noncontextual; we, however, have to use them with our *contextual perspective.* If you are using a staffing program that says you need a staff of 10 people for Saturday, it will not tell you to think about the forecasted sunny day and the big party someone is having (factors that might very well influence how many call-ins you have). If the computer tells you that each practitioner should be able to see four patients every hour, you can't be a slave to that; you must look at the context of who those patients are (sometimes older people take 5 of their 15 minutes just to walk back to the exam room).

Discriminating

Another thinking dimension that will be augmented by informatics is also needed for choosing and using informatics: it is *discrimination.* One of the biggest drawbacks to information technology is the issue of reliability. Anyone can post anything on the Internet. People can identify themselves by any title. There is very little *discrimination* as to quality. This is a problem for all of us, but particularly for patients, who may make health decisions based on indiscriminate information, and students, who are quick to accept written information as authoritative.

Some attempts are being made to help consumers *discriminate* quality information today. For example, the National Library of Medicine has lists of reliable health-related resources (http://medlineplus.gov). For students and other library users, criteria for judging the quality (*discriminating*) of information can increasingly be found. Such guidelines have become standards in the library world (E. Bucciarelli, personal communication, May 15, 2013). Our library has posted A^3BCD; this acronym represents six categories of criteria, the details of which are easily available on our library website (Stanger, n.d.). A summary of the six criteria is as follows:

- **A**uthority of source (judging information about the organization or author)
- **A**ccuracy (documentation of facts)
- **A**udience (appropriateness of information for the intended audience)
- **B**ias/point of view (purpose of document, distinguishing fact from opinion)
- **C**urrency (creation date and updates)
- **D**esign/site navigation (ease of site navigation)

For healthcare providers looking for evidence-based clinical guidelines, we suggest using evaluation criteria for *discriminating* quality. Keeping such things in mind is very important as you exercise your *discrimination* thinking skills. You must constantly question what you see and read. You must also educate patients to be discriminatory in their thinking. People who have limited knowledge of a subject have more difficulty *discriminating* the relative importance or validity of information. Walji and colleagues (2004) made a startling discovery when they analyzed 150 websites on alternative medicine: 38 sites (25%) had statements that could cause harm if acted upon, and 145 sites (97%) had omitted information. Walji and colleagues cautioned consumers to use other means of validating information found on websites.

In another example, a clinician recently told this story: A depressed patient was started on Lexapro and stopped taking it within 2 days because she felt worse. When the clinician questioned this, the patient said, "Well, I went on their website, and it said this drug may worsen depression, so I figured that's what was happening to me." What the patient didn't do was read further to see the remainder of the explanation of how this drug's action builds over time.

Analyzing and *Logical Reasoning*

The last two CT dimensions on both sides of Figure 9-1, *analyzing* and *logical reasoning*, are augmented by informatics and are used for the nitty-gritty work of choosing and using informatics. Get away from looking at informatics as a whole—a scary, big field—and break things down (*analyze*) into manageable units. If you're in a position to choose a new information technology, ask these types of questions:

- What is it you are trying to accomplish?
- How are you doing it now?
- What's available as an alternative?
- What resources are needed to get something new?
- How will it work? What will the surrounding issues be? How long will a transition take?
- What are the external support systems I may need after the fact (e.g., software or hardware customer support and troubleshooting)?
- What are the costs and benefits?

If a new technology is thrust upon you, ask these questions:

- What is the goal of this change?
- What do I need to know?
- What do I already know that I can use during this change?
- How long will this take?
- Why am I angry?
- How anxiety producing is this?
- What about it is making me anxious?
- How can I deal with my anxiety?
- Who and what do I have as resources?

Logical reasoning will help you make the best decisions, ones based on evidence rather than emotional responses alone. If you've come to a conclusion that a new technology forced on you by your manager is a bad idea, on what have you based that conclusion? If you're gung ho to have a particular email system in your institution, on what is your enthusiasm based? It's easy to be critical or overly enamored of new technology if we don't know much about it. Knowledge is power; not having knowledge about something that is thrust upon us makes us feel powerless and potentially frustrated in our actions. (Should we start looking for a new entry in the DSM-V: Informatics Rage?)

How Informatics Augments Critical Thinking

There is no question that when it is used well, informatics can significantly help our thinking. Let's look at the CT dimensions listed on the right side of Figure 9-1. We'll start with the four we just discussed, which are listed on both the left and the right sides—those that are both augmented by, and necessary to choose and use, informatics (*contextual perspective, discriminating, analyzing,* and *logical reasoning*). Then we'll discuss the four listed at the top (*information seeking, predicting, applying standards,* and *creativity*).

Contextual Perspective

The communication ability that is afforded by informatics has broadened our *contextual perspective* enormously. For example, websites such as the Mayo Clinic's (http://www.mayoclinic.com/health-information/) give online users quick guides to a myriad of conditions. The Medical Library Association has excellent guidelines to help consumers access and determine the quality of healthcare information (http://www.mlanet.org/resources/userguide.html).

According to the Pew Research Center's survey of 3,000 adults, "59% of US adults have looked online for health information in the past year" (Fox & Duggan, 2013, p. 4). Almost half of the people who accessed such information followed through with visits to medical professionals and had their Internet findings confirmed. They also found value in online interactions with people who have similar conditions. A small percentage even wrote reviews of their experience with healthcare providers. The *contextual perspective* is big and getting bigger as the World Wide Web expands. How big that expansion will be is anybody's guess—the galaxy?

Discriminating

Not only does informatics broaden our *contextual perspectives* and those of patients, but it also helps us with our *discrimination* of information. Remember, as we discussed in the preceding section, you also need sharp *discrimination* skills to use informatics. Now we're focused on how informatics can help that cognitive skill. We can access much more information and broaden our field so much that we can begin to see patterns and differences in information. We can begin to distinguish and differentiate the information to make decisions that are the best fit for the situation. There's more *contextual perspective* here too! We can have computers link information for us to see if patterns exist; as educators, we can predict where our students will have trouble on the National Council Licensure Examination by looking at patterns in their other tests. We can *discriminate* any list of things according to rank with the touch of one button. As an example, the National Guideline Clearinghouse (n.d.) has a way to compare multiple clinical practice guidelines with the click of a mouse.

Analyzing

It is easy to miss the forest for the trees, and vice versa, with our natural cognitive abilities and emotions. Informatics allows for ease of *analyzing*—breaking things down into manageable units.

We're going to veer off a bit here and look at *analyzing* relative to standardized language. For computer programming, we must have information broken down and described in standardized descriptors—but there are still many challenges to standardizing healthcare and nursing terminology. Hannah saw us as having a long way to go with standard language; according to her, "we have built our profession's own Tower of Babel" (2007, p. 19). According to Androwich, "Nursing has not, to date, adopted one, single uniform language to reflect all aspects of nursing care" (2013, p. 40).

To standardize anything, one must break it down (*analyze* it) and give it a consistent designation (name, number, and so forth). Informatics has forced and helped nursing to define itself—to *analyze* the parts of our profession and standardize our nomenclature. These taxonomies, among others, have become standard in the United States and in many countries around the world: nursing diagnoses (NANDA International, 2012), nursing interventions (Nursing Interventions Classification) (Bulechek, Butcher, & Dochterman, 2013), and nursing outcomes (Nursing Outcomes Classification) (Moorhead, Johnson, Maas, & Swanson, 2013).

Back in the 1970s, when the first talk of describing components of nursing according to nursing diagnoses began, it was triggered by the need for us to keep up with informatics. The first conference to classify nursing diagnosis was called in 1973 by two nurses from St. Louis, Gebbie and Lavin, for two reasons. One reason was related to clinical issues, and the other was that they had been "offered space on a computerized record-keeping system" (Gordon, 1982, p. 2). You can't put something that has several names and definitions into a computer, it must be specific and broken down clearly. This need to specifically define our profession in terms of our diagnoses, interventions, and outcomes has already benefitted nursing practice, education, and research, and it will continue to do so. We transform data into nursing knowledge and build our theoretical frameworks in the field (Bakken & Constantino, 2001).

Although the work on standardizing languages in nursing has been extensive, when it comes to computer language, such as in electronic health records, there continues to be a need for refinement. "While standardized nursing languages can facilitate planning care . . . they also interfere with communication because of inaccuracies of patient information and lack of semantic understanding" (Carrington, 2012, p. 87).

Logical Reasoning

Just as *analyzing* is both necessary for choosing and using informatics and augmented by it, so too is *logical reasoning* used on both sides of the picture in Figure 9-1. Remember, *logical reasoning* requires that conclusions be clearly supported by raw data or evidence. Human logic, of course, is always influenced by emotions. We see things that don't necessarily exist because we want to see them. We ignore things in front of us because we don't want them to influence our decisions. Computers don't have that emotional component (except in some movies, like HAL in *2001: A Space Odyssey*). A computer can deal only with what's been put into it. Any conclusion reached by the computer is less likely to be influenced by human bias (taking into account the programmer); it has a logical progression back to the raw data put into it. Although we must acknowledge the value of *contextual perspective* and *intuition*, those cannot stand alone if we are to be safe, effective, and efficient providers. The logic that informatics promotes is the balance for our human biases.

We are seeing much more in the literature about clinical decision support systems (CDSSs). These are programs that help us make *logical* decisions. These systems, which are often joint ventures between medical librarians and healthcare providers, are at various levels of development, implementation, and evaluation (Moore & Loper, 2011). CDSSs range in form from older knowledge bases, such as PubMed, to expert systems, such as clinical guidelines, and, more recently, to predictive algorithms that may be used as decision trees (Eberhardt, Bilchik, & Stojadinovic, 2012). The Agency for Healthcare Research and Quality (2013; Berner, 2009) has launched an initiative to promote such systems. Systems to assist clinicians make decisions are used in many aspects of health care, but they are in relative infancy and need to be studied systematically; this is an area of research to watch closely in future years.

Information Seeking

Probably the easiest benefit to see from informatics is in *information seeking*. It's hard to imagine how we wrote papers and books before electronic searches, isn't it? You can find something about almost any subject on the Internet; you can access libraries around the world, and you can ask a question of someone in Taiwan as easily as you can ask it of the person in the office next door—sometimes more easily. With a PDA, one can carry virtually a whole library in one's pocket. Think of how electronic health records will ease our *information seeking* in patient care situations. According to MacDonald (2008), we will know our patients better and more quickly. We will have, at the click of a mouse, health histories, lab results, and so forth. In terms of *information seeking* and access, people in their 50s are frequently in awe of this new ability. Of course, as we discussed earlier, *information seeking* without *discriminating* skills can be very problematic and even dangerous.

Predicting

Because of the help we can get with our *information seeking* and *discriminating*, we are also better at the cognitive skill of *predicting*. Because informatics allows us to see patterns, it is easier to predict how patterns will continue. Think about the move to prospective reimbursement (Beyers, 1985) if you need an in-your-face example of the predictive capabilities of informatics. Using diagnosis-related groups for prospective reimbursement was a method of *predicting* how long patients would stay in the hospital, based on certain diagnosis-related data that were analyzed by a computer program. Budget programs help us predict what we'll need for the future. Computer scheduling applications help us *predict* how many nurses we'll need for the Saturday shifts in the summer. Tracking medication errors with adverse event documents and seminal event data helps *predict* problem medications and things like acuity or time of year associated with those medication errors. Remember, also, that CDSSs, discussed earlier, may be predictive algorithms that healthcare providers can use daily.

Applying Standards

Applying standards is sort of related to the earlier discussion of standardized language. In the same way that labels for nursing diagnoses, interventions, and outcomes are specified in information systems so that we're all on the same wavelength, so, too, can professional standards be unified and easily available.

Our ability to access evidence-based clinical guidelines is justification enough that informatics helps with *applying standards*. We can practice with the best, most current standards because technology allows for their availability to all clinicians. Joining an email list gives us nearly immediate updates without even having to search. Faculty can apply standards in their teaching by accessing the most current and accurate information on their teaching topics. We can find all kinds of help with teaching methodologies in informatics. Standards to protect human subjects in research situations can be accessed easily through government websites.

Imagine yourself as a clinician on a hospital unit, and you have to use an intervention you haven't used in a long time. In the old days, you could ask other nurses and possibly get the best standard of care, or you could go through the policy and procedure manual—that dog-eared book in the conference room whose updates were often nebulous. In most institutions today, you can pull up a computer program and find just what you need.

Creativity

Because we have tools such as computers at our fingertips, informatics can help our *creativity* thinking habits. Ask artists how their tools affect *creativity*, and most will say that those tools augment their *creativity*. It is easier to be creative and individualize your patient teaching, for example, if you have videotapes, computer-based learning modules, and written materials to work with. If you are an educator, are you using technology and assignments designed to get students to embrace the Internet to be the most creative thinkers and teacher? (See **TACTICS 9-4**.)

TACTICS 9-4: Using Informatics to Improve Teaching Creativity

Educators

Reflect on your teaching methods. When was the last time you updated them? Do an inventory of the available informatics that you may not be using to spice up your teaching. Have you considered any of these?

- Teleconferencing with nursing experts and leaders to engage students in critical dialogue on a particular topic
- In-class activities that require students to search the Internet
- Demonstrations of searching techniques on the Internet with the help of liquid crystal display projectors
- Mannequin simulations in the clinical laboratory to demonstrate the effects of medications on blood pressure
- Enhancement of your classroom activities with e-learning, podcasts, YouTube videos, and threaded discussions

Clinicians

Do a mental inventory of the things you repeatedly teach patients. Are you using standardized materials? Is it the most current information? How many options are available to you to teach that material? Are you using the most efficient teaching methods? The most creative ones? Have you used informatics to help you with this? Have you downloaded pictures or diagrams from the Internet to help illustrate concepts for patients? Has your hospital or organization developed a telehealth system for patient information?

Discussion

Creativity is not something we think of as a companion to informatics because one seems so right-brain and the other so left-brain. However, when you think of informatics as a tool, what it has to offer is boundless. Sometimes just using the tools forces a fresh look at content and how we teach. Magnussen (2008) noted that when she moved from face-to-face instruction to e-courses, she became less content centered and more learning centered. This was our realization also as we moved to online teaching last year. Creating meaningful e-learning experiences forced us to think about ways to help students engage in critical dialogue, reflect, justify their thinking, and teach themselves and others (real learning); we couldn't rely on the old-fashioned content-laden lecture.

Reflection *on Critical Thinking and Health Informatics*

We have now covered all the CT dimensions on the left and right sides of Figure 9-1. Obviously, dividing CT dimensions is somewhat false and awkward. However, keep in mind that you have to use CT with informatics, and you also augment CT with informatics. It is time now to reflect on how it all fits together.

Reflection is the big arrow at the bottom of Figure 9-1. It's down there to remind you that there's nothing static about thinking when it comes to incorporating informatics in health care. You will constantly need to reflect on where you're going. As we have said many times, informatics is constantly changing. While using the same 17 dimensions repeatedly, you will need to keep all the doors and windows of your mind open to let in the new ideas and seize the new opportunities that informatics has to offer. You will always use *logical reasoning*, for example, but the data you have available to make decisions will certainly change. You will always need *perseverance* because unfamiliar pieces of informatics that you have to slog through will keep cropping up. A friend of ours likes to say "get over it" when people voice disgruntled opinions about the rapid change of technology. Your thinking will *persevere* because it will have to if you are to achieve the quality level of nursing care you want to provide.

An overarching *reflection* focus involves being open to the future of informatics. According to Ball and Lillis (2000), whose trends we cited at the start of this chapter, new technology goes through three phases: replication, innovation, and transformation. Health care is lagging behind other systems—such as those used by banks and airlines—in that its informatics is still between the first and second phases. The first, replication, occurs when a manual job is replaced by a machine; and the second, innovation, is a new way of doing something. The last phase, transformation, in which an industry is completely transformed by informatics, has not yet occurred in health care. Ball and Lillis projected the three most important emerging technologies in health care to be "the computer-based patient record (CPR), Internet/intranet/extranet applications, and clinical decision support (CDS) systems" (p. 389).

Since the publication of the Ball and Lillis article (2000), great strides have been made in CPR, but we are still a distance away from the full implementation of CPRs that can be used at the bedside with voice activation. Most institutions use Internet and intranet communication applications; however, many issues, such as patient privacy, must be dealt with before these applications are widely used by patients and providers. CDSSs are also not yet widely used. As those of us who live and breathe topics like CT are quick to point out, the nuances and complexities of human decision making can be augmented by computers, but we don't see how computers will replace that thinking. We might have telephone, email, voice mail, or video mail available, but we still need a caring, thinking person to decide which one is best to use.

Challenges of Informatics

There are many challenges facing us in health care, and many of them can be helped with informatics. Critically thinking clinicians and educators must try to *predict* those challenges and use *creativity* along with the other CT dimensions to overcome the challenges. The overarching challenge, of course, is dealing with change and the magnitude of the change. Embracing informatics in health care qualifies for the high end on any change adaptation scale; this change requires not only that individuals change but that two huge systems change as well. Those two systems are, of course, the healthcare system and the educational system that prepares future healthcare providers.

A frequently cited challenge is the cost of innovative technologies. Even though many of the changes will ultimately save large amounts of money, an enormous outlay of resources is still required to get new and better systems going.

The politics of informatics can be a barrier for nursing. Some nurses want to avoid dealing with informatics; others wish they were more in the loop when it comes to choosing and planning for information technology (Simpson, 2007). McBride (2005) echoed these issues and added the challenges of an ill-prepared academia responsible for teaching future nurses. As cited earlier, the NLN, among other educational organizations, is keenly aware of the need to better prepare the 21st century nursing workforce when it comes to technology and informatics.

Politics overlaps human factors that affect accepting, choosing, and using informatics. We have several times touched on the difficulties folks in our age group have with informatics. Ironically, because of our age, we are leaders in our professions, and therefore we are making decisions about informatics. Kaminski pointed out the need to address the culture of nursing when addressing informatics:

> The professional nurse is now expected to function well within a technologically advanced healthcare environment, carry out higher-level, complex activities, and are held responsible and accountable for . . . humanistic nursing care . . . This is expected to occur within a system plagued by a nursing shortage, heavy workloads and long shiftwork hours . . . Technology does not function in a vacuum but within a social matrix. (2005, para 13)

This *contextual thinking* reminds us that there are no simple answers to choices about informatics. That's why we must constantly rely on our CT.

The human factor context must also be considered as we look to healthcare consumers. Repeatedly, we see the need to work on quality evaluation tools for consumers of electronic information. Health search improvements, especially consumer-directed tools, are strong themes in Greenberg, Andrea, and Lorence's (2004) online health action agenda. We need research in these areas, but we also need to develop education models for finding and intelligently using information.

These larger-scale challenges—money, politics, and human factors—are sometimes not the headaches that nurses are quick to point out as they deal with informatics in the form of electronic medical records and other new technologies. As examples, consider a few issues identified in recent literature. For starters, nursing is still struggling with standardized language issues: "Nursing has not, to date, adopted one, single uniform language to reflect all aspects of nursing care" (Androwich, 2013, p. 40). Related to standardized language are poorly defined electronic pick lists: "These lists are designed to be checked by the nurse upon completion. However, what behaviors or set of behaviors and patient responses actually constitutes completion . . . is not clearly identified" (Androwich, 2013, p. 40). Farri and colleagues qualitatively studied the cognitive processes and barriers involved in synthesizing electronic health record documents. The barriers they identified included "difficulty searching for patient data, poor readability, redundancy, and unfamiliar specialized terms" (2012, p. 1211).

Ultimately, many of the challenges faced by nurses relate to the complexity of nursing actions and thinking. Roberts pointed out the difficulties of capturing in electronic health records "the multifaceted art of nursing, which is arguably the most labor-intensive part of nursing practice" (2012, p. 12). Such activities do not lend themselves to simple check boxes.

Health professions are moving to meet the challenges of informatics. Specialists in informatics are increasing rapidly. The American Nursing Informatics Association (ANIA) has over 3,000 members (n.d.). Canada's Health Informatics Association (COACH) has more than 1,500 members from many health disciplines, including nursing (2013).

Before we leave our challenges behind, we'd like you to hear from a nurse who is, on a daily basis, facing the challenges of leading other nurses in a move toward electronic medical records in a large healthcare system that includes several geographically dispersed centers. Kate Kimmet is, in our minds, a very brave and resilient RN clinical liaison for this massive project. We talked to Kate twice, once when we were writing the second edition of this text and again when we wrote this third edition. Originally we asked her to talk about some of the challenges, and recently we asked her to tell us about the progress during the past 3 years. We've included excerpts from our fascinating conversations with her. We'd like you to actively think while you read her story.

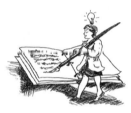

TACTICS 9-5: Finding Kate's Critical Thinking

Clinicians and Educators

After reading Kate's story, make a table similar to **Table 9-1** and fill in each column. (Those of us who are more linear thinkers appreciate this style of organizing our thinking.)

Kate's Original Story

Time has been a big issue. We started this project several years ago. It was to have been in place in 2006, but there was a long pause, and now going live is to be in 2009. It's hard to keep people excited and moving when there's a gap like this. I've had to adapt what I was meant to do; other duties were added to my job description, so I've had to deal with a larger area. Time is also a factor for the nurses. I wish I could take back all the minutes of people saying, "I don't have the time to do this . . ." ["this" being learning and practice sessions for the new system]. Nurses are so busy; they have to do these things on top of their usual duties.

TABLE 9-1 Critiquing Kate's Critical Thinking

The CT dimension that Kate used.	What did Kate do that demonstrated this CT dimension?	What would you have done differently to demonstrate this CT dimension?

Anxiety is also an issue. This is a new set of skills; nurses are used to being experts in their practice areas, but they are beginners with the electronic system. Basically, everyone feels incompetent, and that's scary. There is daily uncertainty. Another challenge is communication. We have teams of nurses set up, but it is difficult dealing with lots of groups. It is hard to get information. I ask a question and someone says, "We'll find out," and then they don't get back to you. Then there's a whole new language to learn. It was very difficult for me at first. I asked why I was in this position since I really didn't know anything about computer systems or even the language. They told me it was important to have nurses who have been taking care of patients using their critical thinking to be in on the planning phase of this project. Once I learned the language, I was more comfortable; it was a metamorphosis. I had to have confidence in my thinking; I could learn this.

Then, of course, there's the issue of change. It is huge and very complex; every part is a domino that bumps into something else. The staff mix is different from site to site, and each site has a different reputation for strengths and weaknesses. We have to come up with a transition system that can work for each unit. Also, things haven't shut down while this is going on; there are many other mandates that must be implemented at the same time. The go live date looms its huge and scary head.

Kate's Update

Three and a half years after the activation of the electronic medical records there is pride in what has been accomplished and anticipation of changes still to come. The activation was well planned and coordinated. Staff nurse end users adjusted well and were soon offering ideas for improvement. One such suggestion was to sort the menu of the contents by frequency of use by the staff. Now there is a different order to the menu depending on if you are in the Emergency Department, Surgery, Pediatrics, or ICU.

I would say that communication is still the biggest issue as changes to the application come monthly. Getting the news and training of changes to come out to everyone is a permanent job. Some changes have streamlined the nurses' work, such as the activation of a form that integrates all the sections needed to prepare the patient for surgery. Others have slowed them down, such as the documentation required for each patient medication. But all of them need to be incorporated into their daily workflow.

At a higher level, changes have allowed our parent organization to collect data to drive change, demonstrate meaningful use to the government and third-party payers, and support compliance to regulatory bodies.

Discussion

How many CT dimensions were you able to identify? Many of you probably realized how some of the dimensions overlap, merge, and work together. That is how CT works in real life and real nursing, so don't be distressed that things don't always fit into nice, neat boxes. If you want some additional challenges, compare your thinking about this task with that of a nurse colleague or a fellow nursing student; discuss differences and similarities and your reasoning behind your thinking. Talk about how you might combine your thinking to create some new ideas that neither of you thought about originally but that might help Kate's organization achieve its transition to an electronic medical record system.

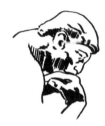

© Jesse Rubenfeld

PAUSE and Ponder

Health Informatics and the Future

The whole field of informatics, not just as it relates to health care, is an unknown future for most of us. Has technology changed the way we think? For sure! Is that a good or a bad thing? Carr (2011) cautioned that the new information age is changing our brains and producing a generation of "shallows." Citing various studies of neuroplasticity, Carr noted that the brain is actually changing in relation to today's access to and method of using information. "We become, neurologically, what we think" (p. 33). "The world of the screen, as we're already coming to understand, is a very different place from the world of the page. A new intellectual ethic is taking hold. The pathways in our brains are once again being rerouted" (p. 77). "We don't see the forest when we search the Web. We don't even see the trees. We see twigs and leaves" (p. 91).

Carr noted that the online environment "promotes cursory reading, hurried and distracted thinking, and superficial learning" (2011, p. 116). Browsing, rather than reading, is becoming the norm, and this does not lend itself to synthesis and deep thought. We are reading faster but we may not be understanding as well. "The strip-mining of 'relevant content' replaces the slow excavation of meaning" (p. 166). "The price we pay to assume technology's power is alienation. The toll can be particularly high with our intellectual technologies. The tools of the mind amplify and in turn numb the most intimate, the most human, of our natural capacities—those for reason, perception, memory, emotion" (p. 211).

We'll leave you with one parting challenge to consider: Dare we even envision a healthcare future without a wholehearted embrace of informatics? Of course not. Just what that future will look like we're not able to fathom yet. Will we someday see healthcare information managed as it was by Dr. McCoy in his *Star Trek* infirmary or with his tricorder? Cox (2007) envisioned 2050 as a time when we may never meet a patient face to face to provide care, robots will do surgery, and patients will have embedded computer chips and will be housed in virtual reality pods. Turley, Murray, Saranto, Ehnfors, and Seomun allowed that "the future will be stranger than we think" (2007, p. 55). Whatever emerges as the future of informatics, we should not embrace it without sharp thinking in order to determine the best technology and the best uses of it. Kleiman and Kleiman expressed these cautionary steps best: "Technology is not a neutral phenomenon and as such requires attention in our world of radical technologization" (2007, p. 158). They warn us about using terms like "the computer says" and about "the extent to which our reliance on computers has disenfranchised us from our status as . . . unique beings capable of rational thought who make choices" (p. 160). For a sobering consideration, read Eysenbach's 2003 article on severe acute respiratory syndrome and population health technology. This physician from Toronto General Hospital outlined the many technologies used that both helped the crisis and negatively fueled fear during the 2002–2003 outbreak of this scary new deadly disease. Eysenbach cautioned us to learn lessons for future public health emergencies: "Population health technology clearly has a vast potential to increase our preparedness for the next public-health emergency, but it also raises many questions related to ethics, libertarian values, and privacy, and has the potential to fuel an epidemic of fear and collective mass hysteria" (last para).

Reflection Cues

- Informatics has to do with managing information and knowledge, communicating, and making decisions.
- There are clear links between CT and health informatics.
- Healthcare technology is a vast, constantly changing force to be reckoned with.
- For baby boom generation healthcare workers, informatics does not come as easily as it does, and will, for generations who grew up with computers.
- Healthcare informatics has been defined by discipline—for example, medicine and nursing—but today there is a move toward the interdisciplinary idea of health informatics.
- Almost anything said to describe the current state of informatics in a textbook is out of date by the time the book is published; that's how fast things are changing.
- Having a futuristic perspective is helpful when considering informatics and the thinking surrounding it.
- Informatics is moving from data to decisions, communication to collaboration, information to knowledge, networking to ubiquitous computing, graphical to cognitive user interfaces, situated to mobile, physical to virtual, and business to consumer.
- The relationship between thinking and informatics comes from two directions; one's thinking will be augmented by informatics, but one needs CT to choose and use informatics.
- Informatics is a process of *transforming knowledge*.

- The primary CT dimensions needed for choosing and using informatics are *open-mindedness, flexibility, intellectual integrity, inquisitiveness, contextual perspective, intuition, perseverance, confidence, logical reasoning, analyzing,* and *discriminating.*
- Informatics particularly augments these CT dimensions: *information seeking, contextual perspective, discrimination, predicting, logical reasoning, analyzing, applying standards,* and *creativity.*
- *Reflection* is the CT dimension that must always be used to study where we are and where we're going with informatics.
- CPRs, Internet and intranet applications, and CDSSs are three areas where emerging technologies are particularly active today.
- Challenges of informatics today include the magnitude of the change in the healthcare and academic systems; costs; human acceptance factors; and the need for better tools to judge quality of information.
- We have organizations, such as ANIA and COACH, to meet some challenges.
- One nurse's story illustrates the challenges of implementing a new technology in her healthcare institution.
- An important challenge is to embrace the rapid advances of informatics without doing it blindly and without ignoring quality, ethics, and values.

References

Agency for Healthcare Research and Quality. (2013). *Clinical decision support initiative.* Retrieved from http://healthit.ahrq.gov/ahrq-funded-projects/clinical-decision-support-initiative

American Nurses Association. (2008). *Nursing informatics: Scope and standards of practice.* Silver Spring, MD: Author.

American Nursing Informatics Association. (n.d.). *About us.* Retrieved from https://www.ania.org/about-us

Androwich, I. M. (2013). Nursing as a learning discipline: A call to action. *Nursing Science Quarterly,* 26(1), 37–41. doi: 10.1177/08943184124667-46

Bakken, S., & Constantino, M. (2001). Standardized terminologies and integrated information systems: Building blocks for transforming data into nursing knowledge. In J. M. Dochterman & H. K. Grace, *Current issues in nursing* (6th ed., pp. 52–59). St. Louis, MO: Mosby.

Ball, M. J., & Lillis, J. C. (2000). Health information systems: Challenges for the 21st century. *AACN Clinical Issues, 11,* 386–395.

Berner, E. S. (2009). *Clinical decision support systems: State of the art.* AHRQ Publication No. 09-0069-EF. Rockville, MD: Agency for Healthcare Research and Quality.

Beyers, M. (Ed.). (1985). *Perspectives on prospective payment: Challenges and opportunities for nurses.* Rockville, MD: Aspen.

Bulechek, G. M., Butcher, H. K., & Dochterman, J. M. (Eds.). (2013). *Nursing interventions classification (NIC)* (6th ed.). St. Louis, MO: Elsevier.

Calabretta, N. (2002). Consumer-driven, patient-centered health care in the age of electronic information. *Journal of the Medical Library Association, 90,* 32–37.

Canada's Health Informatics Association. (2013). *About us.* Retrieved from http://www.coachorg.com /en/membership/About-Us.asp

Canadian Nurses Association. (2006). *E-nursing strategy for Canada.* Retrieved from http://www.cna-aiic .ca/sitecore%20modules/web/~/media/cna/page%20content/pdf%20en/2013/07/30/13/14/e-nursing -strategy-2006-e.pdf

Carr, N. (2011). *What the Internet is doing to our brains: The shallows.* New York, NY: W. W. Norton.

Carrington, J. M. (2012). The usefulness of nursing languages to communicate a clinical event. *CIN: Computers, Informatics, Nursing, 30*(2), 82–88. doi: 10.1097/NCN.0b013e318224b338

Coiera, E. (1999). 10 essential clinical informatics skills. *Journal of the Royal College of Surgeons of Edinburgh, 44,* 269–270. Retrieved from http://www.rcsed.ac.uk/RCSEDBackIssues/journal /vol44_4/4440042.htm

Cox, T. (2007). Nursing research in 2050. *Nursing Science Quarterly, 20,* 206–208. doi:10.1177 /0894318497303437

Crumley, E., & Koufogiannakis, D. (2002). Developing evidence-based librarianship: Practical steps for implementation. *Health Information and Libraries Journal, 19,* 61–70.

Duffy, M. (2012). Tablet technology for nurses. *American Journal of Nursing, 112*(9), 59–64. doi: 10.1097 /01.naj.0000418927.60847.44

Eberhardt, J., Bilchik, A., & Stojadinovic, A. (2012). Clinical decision support systems: Potential with pitfalls. *Journal of Surgical Oncology, 105,* 502–510. doi:10.1002/jso.23053

Effken, J. A. (2001). Informational basis for expert intuition. *Journal of Advanced Nursing, 34,* 246–255.

Eysenbach, G. (2003). SARS and population health technology. *Journal of Medical Internet Research, 5*(2), e14. Retrieved from http://www.jmir.org/2003/2/e14/HTML

Farri, O., Pieckiewicz, D. S., Rahman, A. S., Adam, T. J., Pakhomov, S. V., & Melton, G. B. (2012). A qualitative analysis of EHR clinical document synthesis by clinicians. *AMIA Annual Symposium Proceedings Archive 2012, 1211–1220.* Retrieved from www.ncbi.nlm.nih.gov/pmc/articles/PMC3540510/

Fetter, M. S. (2008). Enhancing baccalaureate nursing information technology outcomes: Faculty perspectives. *International Journal of Nursing Education Scholarship, 5*(1), Article 3. Retrieved from http://www.bepress.com/ijnes/vol5/iss1/art3/

Fox, S., & Duggan, M. (2013, January 15). *Health online 2013.* Retrieved from http://pewinternet.org /Reports/2013/Health-online.aspx

Gordon, M. (1982). Historical perspective: The national conference group for classification of nursing diagnoses (1978, 1980). In M. J. Kim & D. A. Moritz (Eds.), *Classification of nursing diagnoses: Proceedings of the third and fourth national conferences* (pp. 2–8). New York, NY: McGraw-Hill.

Greenberg, L., Andrea, G. D., & Lorence, D. (2004). Setting the public agenda for online health search: A white paper and action agenda. *Journal of Medical Internet Research, 6*(2), e8. Retrieved from http://www .jmir.org/2004/2/e18/HTML

Hannah, K. J. (2007). The state of nursing informatics in Canada. *The Canadian Nurse, 103*(5), 18–19, 22.

Health Information Technology. (2013). *About HealthIT.* Retrieved from http://www.healthit.gov/

Institute of Medicine. (2003). *Health professions education: A bridge to quality.* Washington, DC: National Academies Press.

Institute of Medicine. (2004). *Patient safety: Achieving a new standard for care.* Washington, DC: National Academies Press.

Institute of Medicine. (2011). *The future of nursing: Leading change, advancing health.* Washington, DC: National Academies Press.

Kaminski, J. (2005). Editorial: Nursing informatics and nursing culture. Is there a fit? *Online Journal of Nursing Informatics, 9*(3). Retrieved from http:ojni.org/9_3/june.htm

Kleiman, S., & Kleiman, A. (2007). Technicity in nursing and the dispensation of thinking. *Nursing Economics, 25,* 157–161.

Koeniger-Donohue, R. (2008). Handheld computers in nursing education: A PDA pilot project. *Journal of Nursing Education, 47,* 74–77.

Lasater, K. (2007). Clinical judgment development: Using simulation to create an assessment rubric. *Journal of Nursing Education, 46*(11), 496–503.

Leigh, G., & Hurst, H. (2008). We have a high-fidelity simulator, now what? Making the most of simulators. *International Journal of Nursing Education Scholarship, 5*(1), 1–9. Retrieved from http://www .bepress.com/ijnes/vol5/iss1/art33/

Logan, R. (2012). Using YouTube in perioperative nursing education. *AORN Journal, 95*(4), 474–481. doi:10.1016/j.aorn.2012.01,023

MacDonald, M. (2008). Technology and its effect on knowing the patient. *Clinical Nurse Specialist, 22,* 149–155.

Magnussen, L. (2008). Applying the principles of significant learning in the e-learning environment. *Journal of Nursing Education, 47*, 82–86.

Maneval, R., Fowler, K. A., Kays, J. A., Boyd, T. M., Shuey, J., Harne-Britner, S., & Mastrine, C. (2012). The effect of high-fidelity patient simulation on the critical thinking and clinical decision-making skills of new graduate nurses. *The Journal of Continuing Education in Nursing, 43*(3), 125–134. doi: 10.3928/00220124-20111101-02

Mastrian, K. (2008). Invited editorial: Cognitive informatics and nursing practice. *Online Journal of Nursing Informatics, 12*(1). Retrieved from http://ojni.org/12_1/kathy.html

McBride, A. (2005). Nursing and the informatics revolution. *Nursing Outlook, 53*(4), 183–191. doi:10.1016/j.outlook.2005.02.006

McGonigle, D. (2006). Editorial: Abbreviation frenzy. *Online Journal of Nursing Informatics, 10*(2). Retrieved from http://ojni.org/10_2/dee.htm

Mitchell, M. B. (2012). How mobile is your technology? *Nursing Management, 43*(9), 26–30. doi: 10.1097/01.NUMA.0000418776.69056.be

Moore, M., & Loper, K. A. (2011). An introduction to clinical decision support systems. *Journal of Electronic Resources in Medical Libraries, 8*(4), 348–366. doi:10.1080/15424065.2011.626345

Moorhead, S., Johnson, M., Maas, M. L., & Swanson, E. (Eds.). (2013). *Nursing outcomes classification (NOC)* (5th ed.). St. Louis, MO: Elsevier.

NANDA International. (2012). *Nursing diagnoses definitions and classification 2012–2014*. Ames, IA: Wiley-Blackwell.

National Guideline Clearinghouse. (n.d.). *Guideline comparison template.* Retrieved from http://www.guideline.gov/compare/comparison-template.aspx

National League for Nursing. (2008, May 9). *Position statement: Preparing the next generation of nurses to practice in a technology-rich environment: An informatics agenda.* Retrieved from http://www.nln.org/aboutnln/PositionStatements/informatics_052808.pdf

Newland, J. (2012). Celebrating medical librarians. *The Nurse Practitioner, 37*(10), 5. doi:10.1097/01.NPR.0000419301.77137.1a

Onda, E. L. (2012). Situated cognition: Its relationship to simulation in nursing education. *Clinical Simulation in Nursing, 8*(7), e273–e280. doi:10.1016/j.ecns.2010.11.004

Ornes, L. L., & Gassert, C. (2007). Computer competencies in a BSN program. *Journal of Nursing Education, 46*, 75–78.

Roberts, D. W. (2012). Representing nursing knowledge in electronic health records. *Nursing Management, 43*(8), 12–14. doi: 10.1097/01.NUMA.0000416411.06474.2f

Saba, V. K. (2001). Nursing informatics: Yesterday, today and tomorrow. *International Nursing Review, 48*, 177–187.

Saba, V. K., & McCormick, K. A. (Eds.). (2001). *Essentials of computers for nurses: Informatics in the next millennium.* New York, NY: McGraw-Hill.

Scheffer, B. K., & Rubenfeld, M. G. (2000). A consensus statement on critical thinking in nursing. *Journal of Nursing Education, 39*, 352–359.

Simpson, R. L. (2007). The politics of information technology. *Nursing Administration Quarterly, 31*, 354–358.

Stanger, K. (n.d.). *Criteria for evaluating resources (Internet and print based).* Retrieved from http://www.emich.edu/library/help/a3bcd/index.php

Tennant, R. (2008, May). *Virtual libraries/virtual learners: A matter of perspective.* Keynote address at the Michigan Library Association's Academic Libraries Day, Central Michigan University, Kalamazoo.

Technology Informatics Guiding Educational Reform Initiative. (2013). *About TIGER.* Retrieved from http://www.tigersummit.com/About_Us.html

Turley, J. P. (1996). Toward a model for nursing informatics. *IMAGE: Journal of Nursing Scholarship, 28*, 309–313.

Turley, J. P., Murray, P. J., Saranto, K., Ehnfors, M., & Seomun, G-A. (2007). What if nurses get what they have always sought: Totally personalized care? Trends affecting nursing informatics. In P. J. Murray, H. Park, W. S. Erdley, & J. Kim (Eds.), *Nursing informatics 2020: Towards defining our own future* (pp. 55–72). Fairfax, VA: IOS Press.

U.S. Department of Health and Human Services Health Resources and Services Administration. (2010, September). *The registered nurse population: Findings from the 2008 national sample survey of registered nurses.* Retrieved from bhpr.hrsa.gov/healthworkforce/rnsurveys/rnsurveyfinal.pdf

Walji, M., Sagaram, S., Sagaram, D., Meric-Bernstam, F., Johnson, C., Mirza, N. Q., ... Bernstam, E. V. (2004). Efficacy of quality criteria to identify potentially harmful information: A cross sectional survey of complementary and alternative medicine web sites. *Journal of Medical Internet Research, 6*(2), e9. Retrieved from http://www.jmir.org/2004/2/e21/HTML

Wang, Y. (2003). Cognitive informatics: A new transdisciplinary research field. *Brain and Mind, 4,* 115–127.

Williams, L-M., Hubbard, K. E., Daye, O., & Barden, C. (2012). Telenursing in the intensive care unit: Transforming nursing practice. *Critical Care Nurse, 32*(6), 62–69. Retrieved from http://dx.doi.org/10.4037/ccn2012525

CHAPTER 10

Assessing Critical Thinking

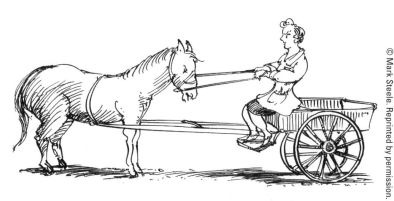

© Mark Steele. Reprinted by permission.

Now for the million-dollar question: How do we measure critical thinking (CT)? You might think that such a question has a neat answer, such as a list of exams or test questions that provide a picture of thinking. However, the answers are anything but simple. A big complication is the assumption that CT can be measured, or assessed, without a clear understanding of what CT is. The cart before the horse cartoon is meant as a visual reminder of this backward thinking. This chapter focuses on the terminology of measuring/ assessing CT; the rationale for discussing measurement/assessment at the end of the book; the challenges of measuring/assessing, including who does the assessing; the linkages among CT teaching, learning, and assessing in both academic and clinical settings; and finally, examples of both evidence-based and practical teaching/learning/assessing tools of CT.

Terminology of Measuring/Assessing Critical Thinking

Before we launch into the details of determining if CT is occurring, we'd like to discuss why we've used the word *assessing* instead of *evaluating* in our title and why we're going to use the term *assessment* from here on as we discuss measuring CT. First of all, what we call *evaluation* in nursing is often referred to as *assessment* in other fields—education and business in particular. *Evaluation* has a connotation of right or wrong; *assessment* implies data collection or measurement followed by interpretation, but the interpretation is not necessarily a judgment of right or wrong.

The nursing profession may have gone over to the word *evaluation* because of the established description of the nursing process, in which *assessment* means collecting data and interpreting patients' needs, and *evaluation* means determining if the patient has met the goals outlined in our plans of care after the implementation of planned interventions. In reality, our nursing process evaluation phase is really another assessment, with goals as a standard of comparison.

CT is not a right or wrong thing—it just is. Everyone thinks; granted, some do it better and more critically than others, but we rarely come to conclusions that someone's totality of thinking was wrong. Because most healthcare professionals are still discussing what CT actually is, we're a long way from being able to say that this thinking is right and that thinking is wrong. Most people would be hard pressed to even describe how one person's thinking is better than another's. At this point, we basically see the outcomes of thinking, but not the actual thinking that led to those outcomes. We're hard pressed to say whether the thinking that led to those outcomes was poor, mediocre, good, or top notch.

OK, can we live with *assessment* being the better word for now? We'll assume that you all nodded your heads, so we'll move on to a discussion of the points we laid out in the introduction to this chapter.

Rationale for Discussing Assessing Last

First and foremost, it is essential to understand the vocabulary and the complexity of CT—how difficult it is to talk about CT without a vocabulary for the components of CT; how the dynamic context of health care affects, and is affected by, CT; how it fits with current desired competencies in health care, such as those advocated by the Institute of Medicine (2003); and how it plays out in real life—before we discuss how it might be assessed. We believe that many of the existing approaches to the evaluation of CT have imposed a very reductionist view of CT in nursing; educators and clinicians have been led to believe that CT can be put into boxes to be dichotomously checked off. They have been using instruments that have little validity for nursing because they weren't based on descriptions of CT in nursing.

Second, we believe that nurses (especially in nursing education) jumped on the bandwagon of evaluating CT in the early 1990s, largely in response to accreditation standards, before they really understood what CT was all about. They started evaluating (assessing) something that they probably weren't overtly teaching. At the very least, there was incongruence between what was being taught and what was being assessed. We want to make sure that the horse (understanding and teaching CT) gets in front of and is ready to lead the cart (assessing/evaluating), not the other way around.

These issues—understanding CT complexity and pressures to evaluate CT—are interrelated. Quantitative measuring instruments do not do well at capturing the complexity of CT, but they are popular because of their ease of use. Qualitative processes can capture the complexity, but they are cumbersome and require more resources to use properly. Outside pressures to measure CT have pushed educators to find measurement instruments quickly. No objective measures accurately reflect what anecdotal reports from clinicians and educators show. Finding a suitable measure has been the most difficult problem in meeting the CT accreditation criterion (Stone, Davidson, Evans, & Hansen, 2001). The literature still documents the lack of valid and reliable tools to measure CT (Britton & Wissing, 2006; Romeo, 2010; Walsh & Seldomridge, 2006a, 2006b). Hold your horses! It appears that many authors have not found our research that does exactly that. Shortly we will show you a valid and reliable tool/protocol for assessing CT.

Finally, the third reason we saved assessing CT for the end is that we want you to have a solid foundation from which you can view our suggestions for valid and reliable CT assessment processes—processes with a real-life view of CT in nursing.

After completing the research to find a consensus on CT in nursing, we found that although there were many similarities between our statement and other definitions of CT, there were also unique components. Whether these are unique to nursing or characteristic of healthcare disciplines and applied sciences remains to be seen. Because we are convinced that CT in nursing has some discipline-specific characteristics, we don't believe it can adequately be assessed with nonnursing instruments or instruments that are not based on a nursing definition of CT.

The Challenges of Assessing Critical Thinking

Just how did we get the cart in front of the horse? There are several ways. CT is much more complex than most people realize. When it comes to testing, we like standardization and simplicity, and we are apt to grab instruments that are quick and easy to use. We also see assessment as something done only by others, not by thinkers themselves.

The Impact of the Complexity of Critical Thinking on Its Assessment

Whew! That subheading alone is complex, isn't it? As Walsh and Seldomridge noted, "Critical thinking is not one, monolithic thing . . . We have come to appreciate that the term critical thinking is a shorthand 'umbrella term' . . . to connote the many activities pertinent to good thinking, and specifically here, to the provision of high-quality nursing care" (2006a, p. 216).

So how do you assess something complex? First of all, you need to articulate what that complex phenomenon is. Then you must break it down (*analyzing*) into understandable parts without losing track of the whole (*contextual perspective*).

As you have probably figured out by now, that's no easy task with CT. Our research gave you a set of 17 dimensions that an international panel of nurses arrived at through a long process of consensus (Scheffer & Rubenfeld, 2000). That research-based description is only now starting to be cited in nursing literature by clinicians,

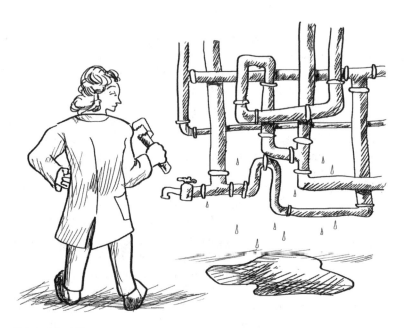

© Jesse Rubenfeld

researchers, and educators (e.g., Ali, Bantz, & Siktberg, 2005; Allen, Rubenfeld, & Scheffer, 2004; Lunney, 2003; Romeo, 2010; Staib, 2003; Tanner, 2005; Twibell, Ryan, & Hermiz, 2005; Walsh & Seldomridge, 2006a, 2006b).

Rush, Dyches, Waldrop, and Davis (2008) used our nursing Delphi conceptualization of CT in their qualitative study of distance learning for registered nurse (RN)-to-bachelor of science in nursing (BSN) degree students. They demonstrated that simulations via distance learning cultivated the CT of their subjects. Dickieson, Carter, and Walsh (2008) incorporated the 17 dimensions of our nursing Delphi study in a scenario-testing rubric when studying three approaches to integrative thinking and learning. Lunney (2008, 2010) reaffirmed the importance of using the 17 dimensions of the nursing Delphi study if nurses want to achieve accurate interpretation of data when making nursing diagnoses.

Things are improving, but it does not negate the issue of complexity. So if we accept the complexity of CT in nursing, what does this mean in terms of assessing CT of clinicians and students? To have any validity, assessment instruments must measure (assess) what they purport to measure (remember Research 101!). Multiple-choice tests are very popular because they provide objective numerical data that can be analyzed in varying configurations to show results for individuals and groups. They can be used easily and require very few personnel resources, so they are very desirable in fields such as nursing, which require lots of resources anyway. However, measuring/assessing something as complex as CT via quantitative measures is very difficult; items have to be cleaned up enough so the instrument has reliability, and in that process of cleanup, it is easy to lose what is important. In the process of reducing a complex concept to achieve reliability, validity can very easily go out the window.

Romeo (2010) came to a conclusion about questionable reliability and validity of CT instruments. While searching for research showing the relationship between CT and the NCLEX-RN performance, Romeo found only eight studies meeting her criteria, which included only quantitative research. "Some of the major limitations identified were related to the lack of a theoretical or conceptual framework, sampling issues, the definition of critical thinking, and measurement tools" (p. 380). Romeo further observed:

> Interestingly, neither of the current nursing specific definitions of critical thinking—the one developed by the NLN [National League for Nursing] for clinical nursing practice or the definition from the work of Scheffer and Rubenfeld (2000)—were used as the theoretical definition for critical thinking in any of the studies that were analyzed. Because the theoretical definition of critical thinking is directly related to a critical thinking theory, the exploration of these two factors needs to be conducted simultaneously. (p. 381)

Standardized Instruments

Even though there has been little consistency in the definitions of CT used by nursing over the years, and descriptions of CT have varied across nursing programs (Dickieson et al., 2008; Romeo, 2010; Scheffer, 2001; Walsh & Seldomridge, 2006a; Zygmont & Schaefer, 2006), attempts at assessment have been made. Nurse educators have traditionally gravitated to assessing CT with standardized multiple-choice tests for quite some time. Staib (2003) provided a concise review of these commonly used multiple-choice instruments: the Watson-Glaser Critical Thinking Appraisal, the California Critical Thinking Skills Test, the California Critical Thinking Dispositions Inventory, and the Minnesota Test of Critical Thinking. See **Table 10-1** for further descriptions of selected CT instruments.

Standardized tests for CT, however, are frequently not based on descriptions of nursing CT; rather, they are based on more general descriptions of CT. They also have another problem, as noted by Walsh and Seldomridge: "The use of standardized instruments to measure critical thinking skills is not particularly useful because such tools assess the skills of classic logic, as opposed to the critical thinking skills of clinical practice . . . [They] do not target such skills as clinical problem solving or decision making" (2006a, p. 216). Many of these standardized tests are still used today despite inconsistent research findings as to their value in assessing students' CT ability (Adams, 1999; Dulski, Kelly, & Carrol, 2006; Staib, 2003). The need for discipline-specific CT instruments continues to be addressed (e.g., Allen et al., 2004; Beckie, Lowry, & Barnett, 2001; Britton & Wissing, 2006; Dulski et al., 2006; Romeo, 2010; Stone et al., 2001; Walsh & Seldomridge, 2006a; Worrell & Profetto-McGrath, 2007).

TABLE 10-1 Selected Examples of CT Assessment Instruments

Name of Instrument	Source	Description of Instrument	Theoretical Basis for Defining Critical Thinking	Comments
CT Inventory	Rubenfeld & Scheffer (2006). See Appendix A	List of 3 reflective questions for each of the 17 dimensions from the Scheffer and Rubenfeld (2000) Delphi study. Questions are designed to stimulate awareness of existing and potential critical thinking skills and habits of the mind. Can be used in practice or educational settings at any point throughout a program.	Delphi study of 52 national and international nurse experts from education, administration, research, and practice who identified and defined 17 dimensions (10 habits of the mind and 7 cognitive skills) of critical thinking in nursing (Scheffer & Rubenfeld, 2000).	Research related to application with RN-BSN students located in Appendix A. The authors have used this throughout BSN programs and in national and international workshops.
Rubrics Assessing Critical Thinking (ACT)	Allen et al. (2004). See Appendix B	Fifteen critical thinking free-response items and vignette-response items based on the CT dimensions identified in the Scheffer and Rubenfeld Delphi study. Each free response and vignette response can be scored in 2–4 minutes. Items or groups of items can be used at any point throughout a course, a semester, or a program.	Delphi study of 52 national and international nurse experts from education, administration, research, and practice who identified and defined 17 dimensions (10 habits of the mind and 7 cognitive skills) of critical thinking in nursing (Scheffer & Rubenfeld, 2000).	Validity and reliability data cited in Allen et al. (2004). The authors have used this throughout BSN programs and in national and international workshops.

		Description		Notes
Lasater Clinical Judgment Rubric (LCJR)	Lasater (2007, 2011)	Quantitative instrument used in conjunction with a simulation activity in which groups of 12 students participate together. The patient care team students include the primary nurse and two team members. Other students in the group observe and debrief the 2.5 hour activity. The roles of the students are rotated along with patient scenarios. Can be used as a one-time event or throughout the semester.	Tanner's Clinical Judgment Model (2006) that focused on the ways nurses understand, address relevant information, and respond. Those phases are labeled as noticing, interpreting, responding, and reflecting.	Used in multiple studies (Davis & Kimble, 2011; Lasater, 2007, 2011).
Assessment Technologies Institute (ATI) Critical Thinking Assessment	Assessment Technologies Institute (n.d.)	Generic 40-item multiple-choice test of 6 cognitive CT skills: analysis, evaluation, explanation, inference, interpretation, and self-regulation.	CT assessment was "designed and developed by a collaborative team of experts in the field of critical thinking," some of whom were nurses (p. 1).	Used in many schools of nursing as part of a package of tests to assess competencies throughout programs.
California Critical Thinking Tests	California Critical Thinking Dispositions Inventory (CCTDI)	Insight Assessment (2013a, 2013b, 2013c)	CCTDI is a multiple-choice test that surveys dispositions needed to "engage problems and make decisions using critical thinking" (2013a, p. 1). CCTDI measures seven attributes: truth seeking, *open-mindedness*, anticipating consequences, proceeding systematically, *confidence* in reasoning, *inquisitiveness*, and mature judgment.	American Psychological Association (APA) Delphi expert consensus report on critical thinking (Facione, 1990).	Used extensively in research studies and educational settings across disciplines internationally.

(continues)

TABLE 10-1 Selected Examples of CT Assessment Instruments (continued)

Name of Instrument	Source	Description of Instrument	Theoretical Basis for Defining Critical Thinking	Comments
California Critical Thinking Skills Test (CCTST)		CCTST is a multiple-choice test that surveys "the critical thinking skills required to succeed in educational or workplace settings where solving problems and making decisions by forming reasoned judgments are important" (2013b, p. 1). It contains six scales: analysis, evaluation, inference, deduction, induction, and overall reasoning skills.	APA Delphi expert consensus report on critical thinking (Facione, 1990).	Used extensively in the United States and worldwide. It has been translated multiple times.
Health Sciences Reasoning Test (HSRT)		HSRT is a multiple-choice test developed as a version of the CCTST for use with students in the health sciences and for hiring and staff development in health settings (Facione, 2013; Insight Assessment, 2013c). It contains five scales: analysis, inference, evaluation, induction, and deduction.	APA Delphi expert consensus report on critical thinking (Facione, 1990).	Available in several languages. The literature is just beginning to report on the use of this test. See Huhn, Black, Jensen, & Deutsch (2011) for a report on construct validity.

HESI Critical Thinking Exam	Elsevier (n.d.)	Twenty-five health-oriented scenario items are included. Each item uses a Likert scale with four correct choices. The best of the four correct choices is designed to demonstrate the highest level of analysis and critical thinking.	Multiple authors, both within nursing and outside of nursing who have espoused the importance of critical thinking in nursing, are cited as the framework used for the foundation of the HESI exam.	Estimated reliability coefficients ranged from 0.87–0.99 using the Kuder Richardson Formula 20. Validity data are focused on predicting success on the NCLEX.
National League for Nursing (NLN) Critical Thinking in Clinical Nursing Practice/RN Examination	National League for Nursing (n.d.)	Multiple-choice exam with 120 items that assesses five CT skills: interpretation, analysis, evaluation, inference, and explanation.	Based on feedback from 14 nursing experts during an NLN Critical Thinking Think Tank in September 2000.	Nursing specific, based on a framework of the nursing process.

Other reasons have been postulated for the inability of standardized tests to show objectively that students learn CT while in nursing school. A major reason for this inability is that these standardized tests lack validity for nursing because they are not based on definitions of CT in the field. When we conduct workshops on CT around the world, we are frequently asked questions about CT assessment instruments. Academic-based educators are particularly frustrated with their present instruments. Practice-based educators haven't been using these instruments but are interested in how they can assess the CT of their staff. Clinicians want to know how they can see if their CT is on track.

One final concern regarding the use of standardized tests to assess CT is the potential language barrier for students and nurses who are not native-English speakers. This is particularly important as we move toward a more diverse nursing workforce. Whitehead (2006), the director of research at Assessment Technologies Institute (ATI), tested for potential language barriers with ATI's Critical Thinking Assessment test. She compared a sample of 192 native-English-speaking nursing students with 17 non-native-English-speaking nursing students from 21 universities who took the test at entry to and exit from their nursing program. Although the non-native-English-speaking students scored lower than the native-English speakers upon entry into the program, on exit they scored 72%, compared with 73% for the native-English speakers. This led the researcher to conclude that the ATI test was language neutral. Other researchers have explored similar issues; for example, Guttman (2004) studied the cultural and linguistic competence of nurses immigrating to the United States. The California Critical Thinking tests (CCTDI, CCTST, and HSRT, described in Table 10-1) described their testing with multiple test populations, and their tests are available in multiple languages (Insight Assessment, 2013a, 2013b, 2013c). It will be important to monitor results of other studies and to always consider language as one of the challenges in accurately assessing CT.

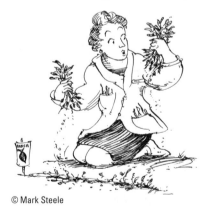

© Mark Steele

The Cart before the Horse Challenge with Assessing Critical Thinking

"Incomplete or premature assessment destroys learning" (Senge, 1998, section 4, para. 2). This should probably be posted in meeting rooms as academic-based educators contemplate accreditation visits, and it should appear in front of clinicians who look at their colleagues and conclude that there is little CT going on. In the same section of the document just cited, Senge quoted Bill O'Brien, retired chief executive officer of Hanover Insurance, as saying that "managers are always pulling up the radishes to see how they're growing."

This is what we've been doing—pulling up the radishes (that is, premature assessment). Some of the push for CT assessment came from accrediting bodies early in the 1990s. These days, there continues to be an expectation that nursing students be evaluated on their ability to think critically. The Commission on Collegiate Nursing Education (2013) requires that *The Essentials of Baccalaureate Education for Professional Nursing Practice* (American Association of Colleges of Nursing, 2008) be used to guide programs; that document lists CT as an assumed outcome for baccalaureate nursing graduates.

We started, at least in academic settings, assessing CT before we articulated what it was, how best to teach it, and indeed, whether we were teaching it at all. We valued CT and have been quite sure that nurses use CT. However, we mistook our valuing of the idea and assumptions about CT; we thought that meant we were teaching it, and we thought that students were learning it. In reality, we were assessing things that we didn't understand well, that we had difficulty articulating, and that we probably were not teaching.

Who Does the Assessing of Critical Thinking?

Based on the previous discussion, one could assume that assessing CT is a function of education coordinators, nurse managers (in the practice setting), and nurse educators (in the academic setting). For the most part, that is true, but we can't leave out one equally important assessor—you!

Your ability to self-assess—or, as we say in the language of CT, *reflection*—is as essential to your growth in CT as feedback from authority figures. The definition of *reflection* is "Contemplation upon a subject, especially one's assumptions and thinking for the purposes of deeper understanding and self-evaluation" (Scheffer & Rubenfeld, 2000, p. 358). This kind of assessment does not require purchased materials or even another person—just you. But it does require time, *open-mindedness*, and *intellectual integrity*.

Harris (2007) addressed the value of critical *reflection* in a 3-year qualitative study with nurses in South Africa. Scaffolding reflective journal writing was the focus of the study. The project included several support structures for *reflection*, such as feedback, mutually developed evaluation strategies, and planned dialogue between the reflector and the reviewer of the *reflection*. Question prompts were developed. Guidelines for reflective writing, feedback, and critique were established, and a self-evaluation rubric was developed. The nurses who participated found reflective writing quite challenging, but it was worth it for the "transformative learning" (moving to a level of *confidence* in your decision making and learning) that resulted. Harris concluded that the best self-reflection requires preparation, critique, feedback, reinforcement, and assessors/educators who are willing to "develop their own reflexive and facilitative skills" (p. 326).

In preparing this chapter on assessment of thinking, we were inspired by the writings of a nurse from New Zealand (Pothan, 2008). She described how she, an advanced-practice nurse, was taking a postgraduate nursing practicum course that required reflective writing. At the beginning of the course, she was skeptical about its value because she already possessed a strong knowledge base and could multitask from strategic planning to safe patient care with no problem. She could not imagine how reflective writing would make her a better nurse. By the end of the course, however, she had what she labeled as her "eureka" moment. She described the value of reflecting on both the positive and negative aspects of her practice. She acknowledged that the skill of *reflection* could be taught and learned. Her closing words best describe the transformation she experienced:

> Reflective writing has enabled me to produce some of my best nursing work to date. I describe this new awareness of my own personal/practice development as the final piece of the straight edged, outside frame of a jigsaw [puzzle]. Now this is complete, I feel confident to advance to complete the bigger picture, knowing there is a sturdy frame holding it all together. (p. 23)

Now, not all *reflection* requires writing. Much is done in a less formal way—for example, by simply taking the time to think about your day, a specific incident, a challenging situation, the outcome of a meeting, a grade on a paper assignment, or an interaction with a peer, teacher, or friend. For those who take CT seriously, *reflection* becomes a strong habit of the mind. You are teacher/learner/assessor all rolled into one, and *reflection* becomes a part of your being.

To summarize before moving on to the linkages among teaching, learning, and assessment, there are some challenges related to assessing CT. Its complexity cannot be ignored if we want valid and reliable assessments. We need to be aware of the advantages and disadvantages of standardized tests that purport to assess CT. We should not assess CT if we haven't first defined it and taught folks about it. And we must acknowledge that we ourselves are one of the key assessors of CT through *reflection*.

Linking Teaching, Learning, and Assessing Critical Thinking

Figure 10-1 is something we've used in workshops with academic-based educators who struggle to link CT with assessment. It's a simple idea but one that is easily overlooked. We ask educators to look at their expected program outcomes and follow the various steps along the way toward evaluation mechanisms; the steps in between are theoretical and operational definitions of CT, course objectives, CT course content and teaching strategies, and, finally, evaluation. Educators often express surprise when they see that they have gaps or inconsistencies in that sequence; they have course objectives related to CT but no real definition of it. Often, they have CT in the evaluation mechanisms box but nowhere else. They know that it is important and that accreditors are looking for it. CT is tacked on instead of being integrated into programs.

We see the same tacking on happening in textbooks. CT exercises have become the norm in most of the big undergraduate texts for adult health, obstetrical, pediatric, and community health nursing. However, if you look closely at many of those texts, you might wonder why those particular exercises are characterized as CT and how the authors are defining CT. There is often an assumption that everyone knows what CT is and that everyone defines it the same way. In reality, if you ask many

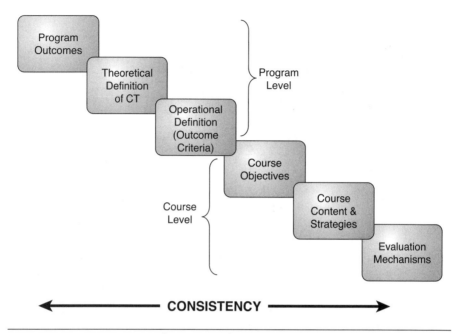

Figure 10-1   Consistency of CT in academic programs.

faculty how they are defining CT in their programs, they will have trouble answering (Scheffer, 2001). Faculty who teach CT have concerns about their CT skills (Blondy, 2010). And most respondents in a randomized sample of 300 full-time nurse educators answered no when asked if they have had any education on CT (Zygmont & Schaefer, 2006).

There is some danger that clinicians will be subjected to the same faulty means of assessment that have occurred in academic settings because increasingly there are messages that nurses must be good critical thinkers to promote safety and increase quality. Administrators and managers will look for quick assessment instruments to give a numerical value, or thinking number, to nurses. We are sometimes asked if we have remedial CT courses for nurses who have made serious mistakes and who need to improve their thinking. (We don't.) That kind of simplistic approach to CT makes it seem like any other tacked-on skill that can be fixed with a refresher course.

Because of our concerns about making the same mistakes in practice settings as in academic settings, we have included **Figure 10-2**, which shows organizational tracking points to look for consistency in CT. If personnel in practice settings value CT enough to evaluate it, they must be careful to consistently define it in mission statements, aims, objectives, expectations, and so forth.

CT must be integrated throughout clinical and educational programs. All the other things we teach, learn, and practice provide the context for CT. It can't be separated or tacked on. It must be defined, described, taught, and practiced. Clinicians and learners must have time to describe their thinking, and practice and demonstrate

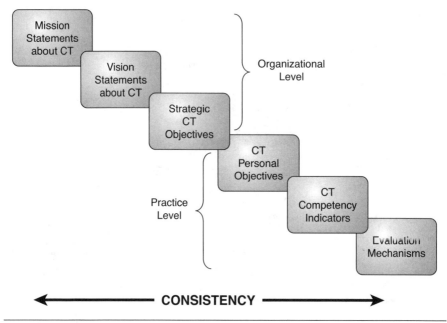

Figure 10-2 Consistency of CT in practice settings.

it, before being assessed on how well they've learned it. Assessment of CT must be linked to expectations and behaviors.

Facilitating the Linkages

If we accept that healthcare delivery and education occur in complex, adaptive learning environments, we want to make sure we assess what is being learned using methods that address complexity and that are also adaptive. Trying to take the complexity out of CT for the purpose of having clean, quantitative tools won't provide a picture of how we, and the people around us, are doing with CT. Likewise, we won't get a picture of CT if our assessment procedures are so vague that no one understands what is being assessed. In **Box 10-1**, we have outlined some considerations for your journey toward valid assessment of CT.

First, have a clear idea of what CT is for your organization. Is it defined as a complex collection of cognitive skills and affective habits of the mind, or is it overly simplified? Beware if it is defined very simply. The definition may have been driven by the assessment method: defined after the fact to fit with an instrument. That's the tail wagging the dog. If there's no description to be found anywhere, then consider if you need one. Is CT important in your organization? It should be in today's complex healthcare delivery and education. You may be the person who needs to develop, adopt, or adapt a description of your organization's thinking model.

If you find a very complex description of CT, is it broken down into manageable components or presented as an operational definition so it can be assessed? If it

---

Box 10-1 What Do You Need before You Actually Assess Critical
Thinking?

---

1. Find, create, adapt, or adopt a description of CT—the whole and the
   components:
   a. Does it exist?
   b. Is it in writing?
   c. Who knows about it?
   d. Is it too simple?
   e. Is it too complex?
2. Accept the complexity but make it workable.
3. Plan an assessment that fits with the CT description.
4. Think about how the assessment will be used:
   a. Self-evaluation
   b. Peer evaluation
   c. Career placement
   d. Program or course evaluation
   e. Accreditation purposes
   f. Other
5. Consider the overall methods of assessment:
   a. Actions are not enough
   b. Verbal
   c. Written
6. How will the assessment be scored?
   a. Check marks
   b. Yes, no, or partial
   c. Numbers
7. Pick specific methods to try.
8. Develop clear instructions for those being assessed.
9. Develop clear, specific scoring criteria and distribute them to those who
   are being assessed.

---

hasn't been broken down, beware; the chances are that CT is not being assessed, or
there is a misfit between the definition and the assessment process.

If there is no assessment plan in place, should there be one? If your answer is yes,
then, as with finding a description, it may be up to you to develop, adapt, or adopt one.
If there is a description and an operational working model of CT, you can make a list of
what should be assessed. Now you have to consider what the assessment results will be
used for. Will they be for staff performance evaluations? Self-evaluations? Peer evaluations? Career advancement? Program evaluation? Course grades? Accreditation justification? Obviously, those questions and answers will be largely specific to the institution.

Once you have those answers, you're ready to consider various methods of assessment. We have some suggestions, but first we'd like to address a question that often emerges at this point. Maybe you haven't considered this, but many nurses ask, Isn't what I do (or my students or staff do) proof enough of CT—that is, isn't it all about actions anyway? The answer to that is, it depends. Sometimes actions can show CT, sometimes not. You might see the same actions from two people, but the first one just happened to see the second one doing something and mimicked the behavior. The second one might have spent hours thinking to come up with that approach. It's only when you start asking them to describe why they're doing what they're doing that you begin to see the thinking. The mimic will likely have trouble adapting the action to a different set of circumstances because the background thinking hasn't occurred. To assess thinking, we need the person's descriptions of his or her thinking to judge it.

You need to either hear or read a person's description of thinking to assess that thinking. Now comes the harder part. How can you do that in ways that will meet all of your needs? Does it always have to be set up like an interview or an essay? No. Do you have to spend hours reading or listening to these answers to make a judgment about how someone is thinking? No. Can you ever get numerical data from such seemingly qualitative assessment processes? Yes.

Much of the challenge in these assessment methods is setting up the criteria for judging quality. We're so conditioned to the right-or-wrong mentality that is implicit in multiple-choice questions that it's hard to see alternatives. First, be very clear in your directions for assignments used to assess CT. If the directions are fuzzy, the person being assessed will waste valuable thinking time trying to figure out what is expected. Next, set up the scoring ahead of time and tell the person how he or she is being assessed. Is it going to be a yes or no score (the thinking dimension was demonstrated, or not)? Will there be a middle ground (the dimension was partially demonstrated)? Will you assign numbers or letters to those criteria? Remember, to set up specific criteria, you, as the assessor, must know what you are assessing. Once again, you must know what CT is and how you and your organization define it and its parameters.

In the next two sections of this chapter, we will suggest methods to assess CT. In the first section, we will report briefly on our latest research, in which we studied a quantitative approach. We assessed all dimensions of CT, assigned numbers, and checked out the reliability of that method. In the final section, we have descriptions of other strategies that we have used in workshops and classes (for these, we have only anecdotal evidence of their success).

An Evidence-Based Quantitative Method to Assess Critical Thinking in Nursing without Losing Its Complexity

As soon as we finished the Delphi study to find a consensus on CT in nursing, people started asking us if we had an instrument based on that description of CT. Initially we raised our forefingers in front of our faces, crossed them, and said, "No way are we doing psychometric research!" Most of you probably understand our aversion to the long process of developing an instrument. In addition, the more we studied CT, the more we realized that an objective multiple-choice-type test could never test all dimensions of CT. We also realized that essay-type tests, such as the Ennis-Weir Critical Thinking Essay Test (Ennis & Weir, 1985), would be very time consuming and not helpful in tracking aggregate data.

In our courses, we started giving students *reflection* assignments to show their CT and to help them learn the vocabulary necessary to articulate their abstract thinking processes. Sometimes we gave them vignettes and asked them to do something to show their thinking. At other times, especially in clinical courses, we asked them to reflect on events from their clinical time to show their thinking. We used the 17 dimensions of CT from our research to give direction so that students could zero in on specific parts of the thinking processes. They wrote about one or two dimensions at a time, not all 17. Over the course of a semester or year, they addressed all dimensions of CT.

As any educator will tell you, grading essays can be extremely time consuming. To save ourselves time, we developed scoring rubrics to give to students ahead of time so they would know what a 3 or a 2 meant. Then we could just put numerical scores on their papers. After we tried this for a few years, we thought it might work as a more formal means of assessing CT. We knew that we had some validity going for us because we were basing this work on a research-derived description of CT in nursing. However, we weren't sure if our assessment procedure could be done reliably by others. We decided it was time for help from someone more knowledgeable about psychometrics and statistics than we were. Enter Dr. George Allen from Michigan State University, up the road from us at Eastern Michigan University. We teamed up with George and told him about our consideration of *reflection* assignments graded with a scoring rubric as a means to reliably assess CT in nursing students.

We developed a plan and piloted it at four schools with undergraduate nursing students. Because we knew that assessment must be linked with teaching and learning, we conducted workshops for those faculty and described the procedure for assessment. The faculty who agreed to try this in a course assigned the *reflections*, scored them using the rubric, and sent them to George, who sent them blind to the two of us. We scored them independently and sent them back to George to analyze the results for reliability. We were happy to see that our coefficient alphas for inter-rater reliability were between 0.70 and 0.80, which, according to most authorities, is quite satisfactory for educational purposes (e.g., Nunnally, 2002). For a detailed report of this research, see Allen et al. (2004).

We learned from this process that short-essay-type CT *reflection* assignments may be scored quite quickly using a rubric. It took us between 1 and 2 minutes to score each assignment after doing the first few. Remember, we weren't grading things like grammar and writing style, so we did not have to insert written comments as we read; we just used the rubric and assigned numbers. We need to keep that in mind; nursing faculty often feel the need to grade all written projects for writing style. If that is your aim, do it with other assignments, not those for which you primarily want to assess CT. In this third edition of this text, we have added Appendix B, which includes the materials used in this "Assessing Critical Thinking" (ACT) project: 16 vignettes, and directions for students and evaluators for both the vignette approach and the free response approach. We are hoping our readers will want to try using these valid and reliable approaches to assessing CT.

The final section of this chapter expands on the two lists of practical teaching/learning/assessing tools for CT listed in **Box 10-2**. List A includes strategies to assess all or selected dimensions of CT, including more details on the Free Response and Vignette protocols researched in the Allen et al. (2004) study. List B contains strategies that fit better with some dimensions than with others. In keeping with our view that assessment must be closely linked with teaching, learning, and practicing CT, all these methods may be used for teaching, learning, or assessment purposes.

Examples of Practical Teaching/Learning/Assessing Tools of Critical Thinking from List A in Box 10-2

Free Responses and Vignettes

Both types of *reflections* are written projects that focus on one or two CT dimensions at a time. In a free response, students are asked to reflect on an activity, such as a clinical encounter, and describe three things: (1) how they demonstrated one or two of the dimensions, such as *creativity* and *intuition*, (2) justification of why that description represents those dimensions, and (3) expansion—projecting how they could better use those dimensions the next time. For more details on this scoring, see ACT materials in Appendix B.

Box 10-3 is an example of a junior student's free-response *reflection* on a clinical situation in which the CT dimension of *flexibility* was used. This was scored as 8. The description clearly identified thinking *flexibility* (Identification = 2); the student justified this as *flexibility* at the end of the second paragraph (Justification = 1); and the expansion was very sophisticated, beyond what we'd expect for a second-semester junior (Expansion = 5).

With vignette responses, students are given a short patient situation/case study and are asked to describe how they would do something to demonstrate specified CT dimensions. They are also asked to justify why their description represents those dimensions. These vignette responses are scored with the same scale used for free responses. The expansion (third) part in this case judges the level of detail of the descriptions according to the students' class level. **Box 10-4** has an example of a vignette assignment. You might want to try responding to the assignment in Box 10-4.

Obviously, vignettes could be specific to units, levels, or courses. They could be used as a means of assessment (our focus here) or as a teaching/learning focus. Service-based educators could use unit-specific vignettes to help new staff get used to the thinking needed on that unit, for example. Clinicians could write vignettes and prepare a bank of them for others to use.

Both free responses and vignettes can be used as a way to cover all dimensions of CT but allow for a detailed assessment of each dimension one at a time. These

---

Box 10-2 Practical Teaching/Learning/Assessing Tools of Critical Thinking

---

LIST A: TOOLS FOR ALL OR SELECTED DIMENSIONS

- Written or verbal free-response *reflections* (ACT) (See also Appendix B.)
- Written or verbal *reflections* on vignettes (ACT) (See also Appendix B.)
- CT Inventory (See also Appendix A.)
- Mind maps
- My Understanding through Dialogue and Debate (MUDD) mapping
- Rubrics

LIST B: TOOLS FOR SPECIFIC DIMENSIONS

- Developing a new approach to something (*creativity, inquisitiveness, transforming knowledge*)
- Debate from an opposite perspective (*intellectual integrity, open-mindedness*)
- Differential diagnosing (*discriminating, logical reasoning, confidence, contextual perspective, intellectual integrity, intuition*)
- Listing hunches (*intuition*)
- Answering "But, what if . . . ?" questions (*transforming knowledge, flexibility*)
- What is likely to happen to this patient? (*predicting, contextual perspective*)
- What would you assess next? (*information seeking, discriminating, contextual perspective*)
- What is the principle? (*applying standards*)
- Calling the physician (*discriminating, analyzing, contextual perspective*)
- What's wrong with this picture? (*discriminating*)
- Critique of literature (*applying standards, discriminating, analyzing, logical reasoning*)
- Moral dilemmas (*analyzing, intellectual integrity, flexibility*)

Box 10-3 Example of a Junior BSN Student Free-Response *Reflection*

One critical thinking reflection *dimension that I used during clinical was* flexibility, *the capacity to adapt, accommodate, modify, or change thoughts, ideas, and behaviors. During an interaction with a patient, several times I had to adapt my approaches to her. She was bipolar, having psychosis, and was in a severely manic acute phase of the disorder, delusional and hearing voices. In my attempts to interact and interview the patient, she displayed disorganized and illogical thought processes.*

(continues)

Box 10-3 Example of a Junior BSN Student Free-Response *Reflection* (continued)

She would jump from one topic to the next and even tried to get me to witness her hallucinations. My attempts to obtain information were constantly being hampered, and it was difficult to keep her oriented and focused. With every attempt at keeping the patient focused, I had to adapt to her various replies. I tried to change my approach and posture in order to find a way to connect with her. When she seemed to be overstimulated by her environment, I moved to the less stimulating atmosphere of the back lounge area. I changed directions in my mind over and over again. I had to appraise the situation and interactions with the patient in my mind.

At first I was at a loss as to how to make the interaction successful. Next, I was overly determined to make it work and even felt frustration starting. Consequently, I thought about stopping and trying again later. Something clicked in my mind that made me realize that silence, a break, and maybe just some time and patience would be beneficial. I realized that maybe my thinking of getting goals accomplished was hampering my thought processes and thus my interviewing abilities. I thought about waiting for a time when her antipsychotic medication was peaking and then implementing this plan of approach. This approach worked much better, and I was able to obtain more information and interact more effectively with my client. Thus, I used flexibility in my ability to constantly reevaluate, adapt, and accommodate to the situation by changing my plan of action.

In this kind of situation again, I'd still need to consider many different alternatives until one worked, but I'd remember from this experience that I always have to be flexible in my thinking and actions with these kinds of patients. I would probably not be so fixated on the goals, and I'd be less frustrated because I'd turn on my flexible thinking right away.

Box 10-4 Example of a Vignette with Student Directions

DIRECTIONS

1. Read the clinical vignette that follows.
2. Read the definition of the CT skill or habit that accompanies the vignette.
3. Describe how you would use the designated CT habit or skill to accomplish the proposed nursing intervention. Include the following in your description:
   a. What you would do, including enough detail of your thinking to show someone who was not there how you demonstrated the designated habit or skill.

Box 10-4   Example of a Vignette with Student Directions (continued)

---

        b. Why you believe your actions illustrate the designated habit or skill.

     (You will be assessed for your ability to accurately represent the CT skill or habit, your justification of how your actions demonstrate the skill or habit, and the specificity of the description.)

VIGNETTE: CHARLOTTE AND MARY'S ADOPTION PLANS

Critical thinking habit of the mind: *intellectual integrity* (defined as seeking the truth through a sincere, honest process, even if the results are contrary to one's assumptions and beliefs)

    Charlotte Jones and Mary Kelly are partners who have lived together for 2 years. They are considering adopting a child. They are patients in the obstetrics/gynecology practice where another patient, Susan Simone, is 11 weeks pregnant. Susan is unmarried and wishes to carry her child to term and consider adoption even though her partner, Tom, would rather she had an abortion. Susan, a sophomore in college, is very close to her mother, who is supportive of the plan to offer the child for adoption. Susan has no health insurance and has income only from her part-time job as a waitress. When Susan was told that Charlotte and Mary were interested in adopting her baby, she immediately told the nurse that she wanted to go ahead with whatever was necessary to arrange the adoption.

    Describe how you, as the nurse in this situation, would use the *intellectual integrity* habit of the mind to help Susan, Charlotte, and Mary **prepare for and interact** during their first meeting.

---

can be used to identify areas of strength and weakness; they allow for individual interpretations but require that persons be able to justify why they believe their statements represent the particular dimensions. That justification part is important because it demonstrates *logical reasoning*. Students must be able to articulate why their described thinking logically demonstrates the dimensions. It's not enough to say that they do; such statements must be justified.

    If you want a numerical assessment of CT so you can track aggregate data, you can use scoring rubrics, which allow you to maintain the complexity of CT with a time-efficient, manageable tool. **Box 10-5** provides several examples of tracking forms for individual and aggregate data.

CT Inventory

The CT Inventory in Appendix A is another way to assess all dimensions of CT. This inventory has been updated since the first edition of this text. The updated version, which consists of fewer questions with more clarity for each of the dimensions, was based on feedback and its use in multiple nursing courses. The inventory is especially

---

Box 10-5 Examples of Methods of Tracking Critical Thinking
Dimensions

EXAMPLE 1

Compiling *Individual* Student Data on CT Skills and Habits of the Mind

Student name _____ ID# _____
Undergraduate ❑   Graduate ❑

	Scores		
Dimension	**Course** _____	**Course** _____	**Course** _____
Confidence	_____	_____	_____
Contextual perspective	_____	_____	_____
Creativity	_____	_____	_____
Flexibility	_____	_____	_____

(and so forth for all dimensions)

EXAMPLE 2

Aggregate *Course* Data on Critical Thinking Skills and Habits of the Mind

Undergraduate ❑   Graduate ❑   Semester/year _____
# of students   _____   _____   _____

	Averages of Scores for All Students		
Dimension	**Course** _____	**Course** _____	**Course** _____
Confidence	_____	_____	_____
Contextual perspective	_____	_____	_____
Creativity	_____	_____	_____

(and so forth for all dimensions)

EXAMPLE 3

Aggregate Entry/Exit Year Data on Critical Thinking Skills and Habits of the Mind

Undergraduate ❑   Graduate ❑

	Year _____	**Year** _____	
# of students	_____	_____	
Dimensions: Average scores for all students in year			
Confidence	_____	_____	_____
Contextual perspective	_____	_____	_____
Creativity	_____	_____	_____
Flexibility	_____	_____	_____

(and so forth for all dimensions)

valuable as a self-assessment guide and as a teaching/learning tool to open up minds to the complexities of CT. This is a qualitative approach to assessment; it is difficult to assign numerical points except in terms of clarity, precision, or depth of description. We have used similar instruments for many years, starting with a THINK Inventory in our textbook for beginning-level students (Rubenfeld & Scheffer, 2006). It works best for self-evaluation and peer sharing.

Our colleague, Dr. Sandra Hines, conducted a research study, "RN Reflections on the Critical Thinking Inventory," with RN-to-BSN students. Students completing the CT Inventory reflected on which dimensions of CT had changed throughout their education. These students also reflected on their experience with CT in practice. Her report can be found in Appendix A, following the inventory itself.

TACTICS 10-1: Practice with the CT Inventory

Part I

1. Read Appendix A, including the research study report demonstrating the use of the CT Inventory with RN-to-BSN students.
2. Share with a peer the three most important things you gleaned (what you learned, what surprised you, what made you wonder, what you disagreed with, etc.).

Part II

1. Select one of the 17 dimensions of CT in nursing (7 cognitive skills and 10 habits of the mind) that are listed and defined in the CT Inventory in Appendix A.
2. On the top of a piece of paper, copy the name of the dimension you selected and write out, word for word, the name of the dimension *and* the definition.
3. Answer the three questions listed under the dimension you selected.
4. Describe or share your rationale for *why* you selected to write about that particular dimension.
5. Think about how you might use this CT Inventory with your students or peers to increase their awareness of their CT.

Discussion

Part I: How different or similar was your response compared to that of your peer? What insights did you have about your thinking after doing part I?

Part II: How difficult was completing number 3 of this task (answering the three questions)? How difficult was completing number 4 of this task (why you selected that dimension)? Why do you think providing your rationale might be challenging? If you had to select a different dimension, which one would it be? How will you use this to help students or peers to increase their awareness of CT?

Mind Mapping

Mind maps can be used to assess CT. Most health professions' literature on mind mapping, or its close cousin, concept mapping, describes its value in teaching and learning CT (e.g., Mueller, Johnston, & Bligh, 2002; Pudelko, Young, Vincent-Lamarre, & Charlin, 2012; Spencer, Anderson, & Ellis, 2013; Wheeler & Collins, 2003). However, others spoke directly to assessing. For example, Daley, Shaw, Balistrieri, Glasenapp, and Placentine (1999) outlined a method of assigning points for connecting links in concept maps that had good reliability between two scorers. Taylor and Wros (2007) provided examples of concept mapping grading criteria.

MUDD Mapping

My Understanding through Dialogue and Debate (MUDD) is an active learning strategy designed by two nurse educators from Newfoundland and Prince Edward Island, Canada (Barringon & Campbell, 2008). It is essentially a form of group mind mapping that is done in stages and that requires ongoing interaction among the participants as the map emerges. The instructor or facilitator considers course objectives and provides the central concept of the map, such as computer-based patient record intervention, and draws a number of spokes extending out from the center concept. This can be done on a whiteboard or flip chart. The learners take turns adding one piece of information at a time, with time given for collaborative discussion of all aspects of that piece of information before moving to the next student's contribution. The authors described the thinking required as "collective . . . corrective . . . improved . . . expanded . . . and supported" (p. 161). The dialogue continues to focus on both new concepts and relationships among the added data. The activity finishes with a debate in which learners are able to state their position and support that position related to the overall components or issues that need to be addressed when considering the concept or intervention.

Rubrics

Have you ever struggled when deciding what grade to assign a student paper or a clinician's project? How do you differentiate between an A– and a B+? Or worse yet, between a C– and a D+? Have your assessments ever been challenged? Are students achieving the learning you want them to achieve on the assignments you give? These questions are more prevalent when we are assessing processes, such as CT, as opposed to more concrete issues, such as administering a subcutaneous injection.

One way to address those questions is with the use of a rubric. Rubrics are assessment scoring tools, and much more (Stevens & Levi, 2005). Designing a rubric requires several aspects of CT on the part of the assessor/educator. Assessors must *analyze* an assignment or project and break it into its component parts. Each component is further *analyzed* for what represents various levels of performance, from acceptable to unacceptable. *Discriminating* and *applying standards* are necessary to separate and level performance variables.

Britton and Wissing (2006), both respiratory care educators, described two kinds of rubrics—holistic and analytic—to achieve "authentic assessment." They cited authentic assessment as a strategy for helping students "develop desirable traits such as critical thinking, problem solving and life-long learning" (p. 21). Holistic rubrics are exactly that: looking at the whole. They examine an overall process or outcome without dissecting the parts. Analytic rubrics analyze the components in detail and score the details. **Tables 10-2** and **10-3** provide examples of each type of rubric as they would apply to learning in nursing.

A major advantage of rubrics is that they serve the teaching, learning, and assessment roles all at once. They do this because they provide clear guidance for nurses or nursing students to achieve the learning goals you have identified. Nurses or students can see ahead of time how they will be assessed and work toward achieving those criteria. Rubrics have also been found to work well with both face-to-face and online coursework (Blood-Siegfried et al., 2008). The work by Lasater (2007, 2011) is particularly promising and practical to those who want to measure CT in the form of clinical judgment. Lasater developed a rubric for evaluating clinical judgment using Tanner's 2006 model of clinical judgment. What is especially refreshing in

---

TABLE 10-2 Example of a Holistic Rubric

The assignment is a 10-page paper designed to engage students' critical thinking regarding the current nursing shortage. Students are advised to (1) compare and contrast the current nursing shortage with shortages in the past, (2) address the impact of this shortage on the quality of patient care, and (3) discuss at least five of the critical thinking dimensions needed to help resolve the problem. Proper American Psychological Association (APA) format is required.

Criteria	*Score*
All three components of the assignment are clearly addressed and supported with literature.	95
Two of the three components of the assignment are clearly addressed and supported with literature.	80
One of the three components of the assignment is clearly addressed and supported with literature.	70
None of the three components of the assignment are addressed.	0
APA format is accurate.	5
Minor errors in APA format.	3
Significant errors in APA format.	0
Total Score (Maximum possible score = 100 points)	

TABLE 10-3 Example of an Analytic Rubric: Grading the Assessment Phase of the Nursing Process

This type of rubric can be used to assess some of the critical thinking dimensions (*contextual perspective, inquisitiveness, intellectual integrity, perseverance, analyzing, applying standards, discriminating, information seeking, logical reasoning, and transforming knowledge*).

	Exemplary (5)	Competent (3)	Needs Work (1)	Score
Data Collection	Included data from interaction, observation, and measurement, as well as multiple sources (patient, family, chart, and other healthcare providers)	Included data from two of the following: interaction, observation, and measurement.	Included data primarily from patient's chart.	
Data Analysis	Identified all relevant data. Compared data with population norms as well as personal norms to support conclusions. Listed data gaps.	Identified most relevant data. Compared data with only population norms to support conclusions. Listed some data gaps.	Identified some relevant data. Did not compare data with norms to support conclusions. No data gaps noted.	
Identification of Patient's Strengths	Addressed all strengths re: biopsychosocial-spiritual & environmental issues.	Addressed most of strengths.	Limited determination of strengths.	
Interdisciplinary Problems	Identified all	Identified some	Identified none	
Problems for Referral	Identified all	Identified some	Identified none	
Nursing Diagnoses (N. Dx.)	Identified all N. Dx. using proper NANDA terms. Included all related factors for each N. Dx. and provided defining characteristics for each N. Dx. Described all CT dimensions used during assessment.	Identified most N. Dx. using proper NANDA terms. Included most related factors for each N. Dx. and provided most defining characteristics. Described some of CT dimensions used in assessment.	Identified some N. Dx. using proper NANDA terms. Included some related factors for each N. Dx. & provided some defining characteristics. No CT dimensions ID'd.	

reading Lasater's work is her acknowledgment that thinking in nursing situations is not linear and very context bound, factors that often are lost in traditional multiple-choice instruments that purport to measure CT.

Lasater's rubric was used by Mann to study the effectiveness of a grand rounds "strategy to develop critical thinking and clinical judgment skills in baccalaureate nursing students" (2012, p. 27). The results showed "no significant relationship between critical thinking and clinical judgment, no significant difference between critical thinking scores at the beginning of the nursing program or at the conclusion of the study" (p. 26). However, there was a significant difference in clinical judgment scores between the intervention (grand rounds) and comparison groups, suggesting that the group work helped with clinical judgment.

Six rubrics to evaluate outcomes in simulation situations were identified by Davis and Kimble (2011). A link was made by these authors to how these rubrics could be used to evaluate the American Association of Colleges of Nursing's *The Essentials of Baccalaureate Education for Professional Nursing Practice* (2008). Lasater's rubric was among those six.

For more information on rubrics, do a Google search with just the term *rubric*, and you might be pleasantly surprised at how much helpful knowledge you gain.

Examples of Practical Teaching/Learning/Assessing Tools of Critical Thinking from List B in Box 10-2

The remainder of the teaching/learning/assessment tools from list B in Box 10-2 are a very useful and practical means of assessing parts of CT. We provide a brief explanation of how these might be used, but keep in mind that these methods work best when they are adapted to fit the *contextual perspective* of your teaching/learning/assessment situation.

Developing a new approach to something to show *creativity, inquisitiveness,* or *transforming knowledge* may be used to evaluate staff nurses, for example. A career placement assessment could include an innovation criterion. Points could be assigned in accordance with the whole assessment plan when a nurse improves a practice on the unit. This works well with moves toward evidence-based practice to reward staff who are innovative in using the best evidence to improve practice.

Debating from an opposite perspective to demonstrate *intellectual integrity* and *open-mindedness* is a valuable exercise for learning and assessment of CT. It is very difficult to debate a controversial issue from a viewpoint opposite your own. Assigning a *reflection* at the end of this exercise can help show the debater's thinking processes. This could be accompanied by a checklist or rubric and scored. For example, one could assess the number of issues addressed, the depth of study of those issues, the distance of the viewpoints from the debater's true beliefs, strength of expression, and so forth.

Differential diagnosing is a great mechanism to see *discriminating* and *logical reasoning* cognitive skills, as well as *confidence, contextual perspective,* *intellectual integrity*, and *intuition* habits of the mind. A case could be made for using all 17 dimensions in this activity. Using case studies and comparing staff nurses' and clinical experts' diagnosing, Lunney (2001) reported wide variability in the accuracy of nurses' diagnosing. Lunney (2003) proposed 10 CT strategies to promote diagnostic accuracy. A strong case could be made for using her methods and Scale for Degrees of Accuracy (2001, p. 36) as a means to assess CT. Making her point especially poignant, Lunney (2003) shared case examples in which achieving accuracy of nursing diagnoses was particularly challenging and in need of CT.

Listing hunches is related to differential diagnosing as part of the diagnostic process. Taken alone, it can be a good measure of *intuition*. Again, case studies could be used; these could be unit specific if this method is used by clinicians, and they could be class specific in academic settings. Experts in those areas could list their hunches, and those lists could be used as a standard for comparison while assessing nurses. Prematurely shutting down one's thinking relative to hunches often leads clinicians to inaccurate conclusions.

Asking and answering "But, what if . . . ?" questions is a good way to test for *transforming knowledge* and *flexibility*. At our school, we have been trying this as a component of our skills check-off procedures to add assessment of CT to that process. To use a simple example, think about teaching beginning students to make an occupied bed. Checking their ability to do this merely by watching a demonstration of the classic procedure—turning the patient, pushing the old sheets under him or her, placing new bedding on that side and pushing them under, turning the patient, and pulling everything through to the other side and tucking—does little to show you the students' thinking. What if you add, "The patient has had a right hip replacement"? That allows you to assess CT. The students should, of course, answer with something that indicates they know not to turn the patient on the unaffected hip, therefore internally rotating the replaced hip and causing problems. You want to hear that they can visualize changing the bed from the top of the bed to the bottom, or some other plan that maintains hip precautions.

Using case scenarios and **asking what is likely to happen to this patient** is a method to assess *predicting* and *contextual perspective*. Again, as with many of these assessment examples, this could be made unit specific if used in practice settings. We often encourage practice-based educators to record case studies for thinking purposes. This is a good thing to have experienced nurses do. In addition, as a way of checking their CT, have them develop the answers to whatever questions you'll want to attach to that case study; novice nurses can then benefit from their collective wisdom. In addition, relevant setting-specific cases are available for future assessments.

Similar to *predicting* what is likely to happen to this patient is asking the question, What would you assess next? This can be used to assess *information seeking, discriminating*, and *contextual perspective* dimensions. We have tried this out with RN-to-BSN students to see what kinds of responses we get. This is a very simple exercise and one that would work well for practice-based educators who want a quick assessment of CT abilities of new nurses. In our trials, we've done this two ways. In the first method, we ask nurses to list the five most important and common patient signs and symptoms found on their units and then to list the parameters that they immediately check upon finding those signs and symptoms. In the second method, we give them a list of signs and symptoms and ask them what they think of right away to check. See **Box 10-6** for some examples. This exercise could easily be scored numerically using expected assessment standards established by setting-specific experts. A rubric could be developed for consistency.

What is the principle? This is a question that promotes *applying standards*. It is also an old assessment technique that was used when we were undergraduates in the 1960s. Asking for standards behind behaviors reveals why someone is doing something and therefore affords the listener a partial picture of that person's thinking. This is an easy assessment method adaptable to almost any setting; it quickly separates

---

Box 10-6 Sample Answers to the Question, What Would You Assess Next?

Confusion: Check medications, pulse oximetry, blood pressure, arterial blood gasses, specific neurological signs, temperature, blood glucose, previous mental status patterns, urinalysis, heart rate, headache, weakness

General complaint of pain or discomfort: Check pain rating, intensity, description, onset, location, duration, history of similar pain, factors that affect pain, last pain medication time, temperature, pulse oximetry, any surgical/dressing sites

Increased blood pressure: Check pain, medications, pulse, cardiac rhythm, anxiety, temperature, past history of hypertension, patterns since admission, headache, IV status, recent patient activity; recheck blood pressure manually

Complaint of constipation: Check bowel sounds, abdominal distention, tenderness or pain, last bowel movement, duration of constipation, past history, links to medical diagnosis, nausea and vomiting, eating pattern, fluid intake, recent GI tests, medications

Decreased urine output: Check intake and output balance, urine color, blood pressure, pulse, temperature, intravenous fluids, weight change, urinalysis, medications such as diuretics, history of renal problems, edema, bladder distention, BUN, creatinine lab values

Request for darkened room: Check depression, headache, history of headaches, fatigue, light sensitivity, privacy issue, drug use

Angry responses to staff: Check what is wrong, pain, fear, anxiety, stress, loss of personal control, family or significant other issue, conflict with specific staff

those who do tasks without much thought from those who know why they are doing something. The latter group is engaged in thinking.

Calling the physician shows *discriminating, contextual perspective,* and *analyzing* in particular. Incidentally, it also shows communication skills. This could be applied to calling any other healthcare professional; because nurses often have to call physicians, this is a familiar situation. Ask physicians about nurse phone calls, and they will immediately tell you that one of their pet peeves is a nurse who does not seem to have thought through the situation before picking up the phone.

Nurse Smith:	Oh, hi, Dr. Jones; thanks for calling back. Mrs. Frank has only had 100 cc of urine out in the past 6 hours. [Pause . . .]
Dr. Jones:	She has heart failure, right?
Nurse Smith:	Yes, she's been on Lasix
Dr. Jones:	What was her last dose and when?
Nurse Smith:	Oh, let me get the med list and check; I just floated down from 700, so I don't know these patients very well.

You get the picture, right? We don't mean to be critical of nurses, and being floated to an unfamiliar unit is all too common in the world of hospital-based nurses. Nevertheless, this kind of conversation is very time consuming and not very helpful because the nurse has not been using much CT.

If you were the educator for that unit, you'd probably want to have an in-service on communication and CT. You could use a phone call to a physician as a way of assessing the nurse's level of thinking. Start with a simple situation: Mrs. Frank's urine output has been 100 cc for 6 hours. "Nurse Smith, would you demonstrate your thinking as you prepare for a call to Dr. Jones?" Once you do this a few times, you can come up with a list of connections that you expect thinking nurses to have made, and you would have your assessment standard.

By the way, you might also invite physicians to your in-service, making it an interdisciplinary session. Communication is a two-way street, requiring CT on both sides.

What's wrong with this picture? Asking this question after showing a videotape or presenting a written or verbal case situation is another simple assessment technique that is especially helpful in showing a person's ability to *discriminate*. Our brains are funny things; it is often easier to see when something is wrong than to figure out how to do it right. But if we can identify what's wrong, we can avoid making that same mistake. Be careful with the right-or-wrong messages, though. A better question might be, How can I do this better?

A critique of literature is a common assessment method used in academic research classes that shows students' abilities to *apply standards, discriminate, analyze,* and *reason logically*. Unfortunately, literature critiques are less commonplace in practice settings. However, evidence-based practice requires that all clinicians critique articles, guidelines, Internet reports, and so forth. With the indiscriminate glut of information out there, all healthcare providers have to be able to respond critically to that information, and that response requires CT. It is important to know how well those providers can judge the relative merit of that information, so assessing their abilities is becoming more of an issue. Using words like *critique of a report* can be daunting to clinicians who probably see this as an academic exercise, so we recommend that you stay away from those words. If you want to assess a person's ability to read something critically, use an article or report that you know has some flaws. (It's harder to find one that doesn't.) Use that article as a measure of CT.

The last suggestion we have from list B in Box 10-2 is to **use moral dilemmas** to assess *analyzing, intellectual integrity,* and *flexibility.* Moving to a relativistic thinking perspective and dealing with the realities of ambiguity in health care these days is vital. There are many moral dilemmas for which there are no easy answers. How long should we keep a baby alive who has a severe brain problem? Should people older than 90 have expensive medical diagnostic tests? How far should we go with stem cell research? Asking individuals to respond to a moral dilemma gives important clues as to how well they analyze situations to see the various perspectives, what they are willing to see that might go against conventional answers, and how flexible they are with their possibilities.

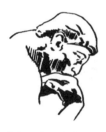

© Jesse Rubenfeld

PAUSE and Ponder

Assessment Is Not an End unto Itself

There are no simple answers to the challenges in assessing CT. Each approach to judging someone's CT must be scrutinized closely. Remember, this is not something that can be assessed with the same methods that we use to assess skills such as giving an injection. CT is not a set of linear steps, but a process that is adapted in various contexts. Because it is complex and dynamic, it calls for assessment methods that are equally dynamic. It is not an end point with specific criteria that can be judged as right or wrong. We must give credit for pieces of CT—for the process, not just the results of thinking. We all have periods when our CT is sharp, and periods when it waxes and wanes. Assessment parameters should give credit for the CT waxing and allow for coaching when waning.

However, engaging in the whole of teaching/learning/assessing CT is the key to achieving the core competencies of the Institute of Medicine—patient-centered care, interdisciplinary teamwork, evidence-based practice, informatics, and quality care—addressed throughout this text. The processes of teaching/learning/assessing are essential to the changes necessary in both healthcare practice and healthcare education. We are at a crossroads; CT and managing change will set us in a positive direction.

REFLECTION CUES

- The words *evaluation* and *assessment* are often used interchangeably; we have chosen *assessment*, which has less of a right-or-wrong connotation.
- Premature assessment, ahead of clear definitions of CT and teaching CT, is problematic.
- The complexity of CT does not easily lend itself to simple, quantitative means of assessing, such as with standardized tests.
- Nursing education in particular has been prone to premature assessment, largely driven by accreditation expectations.
- Many approaches to assessing CT in nursing have been reductionistic.
- Because of CT's complexity, measurement instruments that aim for simplicity of scoring often compromise validity and are incomplete measures of CT.
- Many methods to assess CT, for the most part, are unable to show the changes in thinking that are reported anecdotally.
- Teaching/learning/assessing CT must be linked.
- *Reflection* is an essential aspect of assessing CT.
- One method to assess CT (short essays based on free responses and vignettes) is (1) based on a valid nursing definition of CT; (2) supported by interrater reliability; and (3) quantifiable using a scoring rubric.
- Various methods to combine teaching/learning/assessing CT can be adapted to numerous learning environments.

REFERENCES

Adams, B. L. (1999). Nursing education for critical thinking: An integrative review. *Journal of Nursing Education, 38,* 111–119.

Ali, N. S., Bantz, D., & Siktberg, L. (2005). Validation of critical thinking skills in online responses. *Journal of Nursing Education, 44,* 90–94.

Allen, G. D., Rubenfeld, M. G., & Scheffer, B. K. (2004). Reliability of assessment of critical thinking. *Journal of Professional Nursing, 20,* 15–22.

American Association of Colleges of Nursing. (2008). *The essentials of baccalaureate education for professional nursing practice.* Washington, DC: Author.

Assessment Technologies Institute. (n.d.). ATI critical thinking assessment. Retrieved from http://www.atitesting.com

Barringon, K., & Campbell, B. (2008). MUDD mapping: An interactive teaching-learning strategy. *Nurse Educator, 33,* 159–163.

Beckie, T. M., Lowry, L. W., & Barnett, S. (2001). Assessing critical thinking in baccalaureate nursing students: A longitudinal study. *Holistic Nursing Practice, 15*(3), 18–26.

Blondy, L. C. (2010). Measurement and comparison of nursing faculty members' critical thinking skills. *Western Journal of Nursing Research, 33*(2), 180–195. doi: 10.1177/0193945910381596

Blood-Siegfried, J. E., Short, N. M., Rapp, C. G., Hill, E., Talbert, S., Skinner, J., ... Goodwin, L. (2008). A rubric for improving the quality of online courses. *International Journal of Nursing Education Scholarship, 5*(1), Article 34, 1–13.

Britton, L. A., & Wissing, D. (2006). Authentic assessment of learning outcomes. *Respiratory Care Education Annual, 15,* 21–30.

Commission on Collegiate Nursing Education. (2013). *Standards for accreditation of baccalaureate and graduate nursing programs.* Retrieved from http://www.aacn.nche.edu/ccne-accreditation/standards-procedures-resources/baccalaureate-graduate/standards

Daley, B. J., Shaw, C. R., Balistrieri, T., Glasenapp, I., & Placentine, L. (1999). Concept maps: A strategy to teach and evaluate critical thinking. *Journal of Nursing Education, 38,* 42–47.

Davis, A. H., & Kimble, L. P. (2011). Human patient simulation evaluation rubrics for nursing education: Measuring the essentials of baccalaureate education for professional nursing practice. *Journal of Nursing Education, 5*(11), 605–611. doi: 10.3928/01484834-20110715-01

Dickieson, P., Carter, L. M., & Walsh, M. (2008). Integrative thinking and learning in undergraduate nursing education: Three strategies. *International Journal of Nursing Education Scholarship, 5*(1), Article 39, 1–15.

Dulski, L., Kelly, M., & Carrol, V. S. (2006). Program outcome data: What do we measure? What does it mean? How does it lead to improvement? *Quality Management in Health Care, 15,* 296–299.

Elsevier. (n.d.). *HESI critical thinking specialty exam* [Product description]. St. Louis, MO: Author.

Ennis, R. H., & Weir, E. (1985). *The Ennis-Weir critical thinking essay test.* Pacific Grove, CA: Midwest.

Facione, N. (Ed.). (2013). *Health sciences reasoning test manual.* Millbrae, CA: Insight Assessment.

Facione, P. A. (1990). *Critical thinking: A statement of expert consensus for purposes of educational assessment and instruction.* Millbrae, CA: California Academic Press. Retrieved from ERIC database. (ED315423)

Guttman, M. S. (2004). Increasing the linguistic competence of the nurse with limited English proficiency. *Journal of Continuing Education in Nursing, 35,* 264–269.

Harris, M. (2007). Scaffolding reflective journal writing—negotiating power, play and position. *Nurse Education Today, 28,* 314–326.

Huhn, K., Black, L., Jensen, G. M., & Deutsch, J. E. (2011). Construct validity of the health science reasoning test. *Journal of Applied Health, 40*(4), 181–186. Retrieved from http://ezproxy.emich.edu/login?url=http://search.proquest.com.ezproxy.emich.edu/docview/917627899?accountid=10650

Insight Assessment. (2013a). *California Critical Thinking Disposition Inventory (CCTDI).* Retrieved from http://www.insightassessment.com/Products/Products-Summary/Critical-Thinking-Attributes-Tests/California-Critical-Thinking-Disposition-Inventory-CCTDI/%28language%29/eng-US

Insight Assessment. (2013b). *California Critical Thinking Skills Test (CCTST).* Retrieved from http://www.insightassessment.com/Products/Products-Summary/Critical-Thinking-Skills-Tests/California-Critical-Thinking-Skills-Test-CCTST

Insight Assessment. (2013c). *Health sciences reasoning test: Selected sections from the HSRT test manual.* Milbrae, CA: California Academic Press. Retrieved from www.insightassessment.com

Institute of Medicine. (2003). *Health professions education: A bridge to quality.* Washington, DC: National Academies Press.

Lasater, K. (2007). Clinical judgment development: Using simulation to create an assessment rubric. *Journal of Nursing Education, 46*(11), 496–503.

Lasater, K. (2011). Clinical judgment: The last frontier for evaluation. *Nurse Education in Practice, 11,* 86–92. doi: 10.1016/j.nepr.2010.11.013

Lunney, M. (2001). *Critical thinking and nursing diagnosis: Case studies and analysis.* Philadelphia, PA: North American Nursing Diagnosis Association.

Lunney, M. (2003). Critical thinking and accuracy of nurses' diagnoses. *International Journal of Nursing Terminologies and Classifications, 14*(3), 96–107.

Lunney, M. (2008). Critical need to address accuracy of nurses' diagnoses. *The Online Journal of Issues in Nursing, 13*(1). doi: 10.3912/OJIN,Vol13No01PPT06

Lunney, M. (2010). Use of critical thinking in the diagnostic process. *International Journal of Nursing Terminologies and Classifications, 21*(2), 82–88. doi: 10.1111/j.1744-618X.2010.01150.x

Mann, J. (2012). Critical thinking and clinical judgment skill development in baccalaureate nursing students. *The Kansas Nurse, 87*(1), 26–31.

Mueller, A., Johnston, M., & Bligh, D. (2002). Joining mind mapping and care planning to enhance student critical thinking and achieve holistic nursing care. *Nursing Diagnosis, 13,* 24–27.

National League for Nursing. (n.d.). *Test products catalog.* Retrieved from http://www.nln.org/testingservices/test_catalog.htm

Nunnally, J. C. (2002). *Psychometric theory.* New York, NY: McGraw-Hill.

Pothan, Z. (2008). Reflective practice aids critical thinking. *Kai Tiaki Nursing New Zealand, 14*(8), 23.

Pudelko, B., Young, M., Vincent-Lamarre, P., & Charlin, B. (2012). Mapping as a learning strategy in health professions education: A critical analysis. *Medical Education, 46,* 1215–1225. doi: 10.1111/medu.12032

Romeo, E. M. (2010). Quantitative research on critical thinking and predicting nursing students' NCLEX-RN performance. *Journal of Nursing Education, 49*(7), 378–386. doi: 10.3928/01484834-20100331-05

Rubenfeld, M. G., & Scheffer, B. K. (2006). *Critical thinking in nursing: An interactive approach* (2nd ed.). Ann Arbor, MI: Dollar Bill Copying.

Rush, K. L., Dyches, C. E., Waldrop, S., & Davis, A. (2008). Critical thinking among RN-to-BSN distance students participating in human patient simulation. *Journal of Nursing Education, 47,* 501–507.

Scheffer, B. K. (2001). Nurse educators' perspectives on their critical thinking. *Dissertation Abstracts International, 62/2B,* 786. (ProQuest C, No. 3003400)

Scheffer, B. K., & Rubenfeld, M. G. (2000). A consensus statement on critical thinking in nursing. *Journal of Nursing Education, 39,* 352–359.

Senge, P. M. (1998, Summer). The practice of innovation. *Leader to Leader, 9,* 16–22. Retrieved from http://www.leadertoleader.org/knowledgecenter/journal.aspx?ArticleID=159

Spencer, J. R., Anderson, K. M., & Ellis, K. K. (2013). Radiant thinking and the use of the mind map in nurse practitioner education. *Journal of Nursing Education, 52*(5), 291–293. doi: 10.3928/01484834-20130328-03

Staib, S. (2003). Teaching and measuring critical thinking. *Journal of Nursing Education, 42,* 498–508.

Stevens, D. D., & Levi, A. J. (2005). *Introduction to rubrics: An assessment tool to save grading time, convey effective feedback and promote student learning.* Sterling, VA: Stylus.

Stone, C. A., Davidson, L. J., Evans, J. L., & Hansen, M. A. (2001). Validity evidence for using a general critical thinking test to measure nursing students' critical thinking. *Holistic Nursing Practice, 15*(4), 65–74.

Tanner, C. A. (2005). What have we learned about critical thinking in nursing? *Journal of Nursing Education, 44,* 47–48.

Tanner, C. A. (2006). Thinking like a nurse: A research-based model of clinical judgment in nursing. *Journal of Nursing Education, 45,* 204–211.

Taylor, J., & Wros, P. (2007). Concept mapping: A nursing model for care planning. *Journal of Nursing Education, 46,* 211–216.

Twibell, R., Ryan, M., & Hermiz, M. (2005). Faculty perceptions of critical thinking in student clinical experiences. *Journal of Nursing Education, 44,* 71–79.

Walsh, C. M., & Seldomridge, L. A. (2006a). Critical thinking: Back to square two. *Journal of Nursing Education, 45,* 212–219.

Walsh, C. M., & Seldomridge, L. A. (2006b). Measuring critical thinking: One step forward, one step back. *Nurse Educator, 31,* 159–162.

Wheeler, L. A., & Collins, S. K. R. (2003). The influence of concept mapping on critical thinking in baccalaureate nursing students. *Journal of Professional Nursing, 19,* 339–345.

Whitehead, T. D. (2006). Comparison of native versus nonnative English-speaking nurses on critical thinking assessments at entry and exit. *Nursing Administration Quarterly, 30,* 285–290.

Worrell, J. A., & Profetto-McGrath, J. (2007). Critical thinking as an outcome of context-based learning among post RN students: A literature review. *Nurse Education Today, 27,* 420–426. doi:10.1016/j.nedt.2006.07.004

Zygmont, D. M., & Schaefer, K. M. (2006). Assessing the critical thinking skills of faculty: What do the findings mean for nursing education? *Nursing Education Perspectives, 27,* 260–267.

CHAPTER 11

Thinking Realities of Yesterday, Today, and Tomorrow

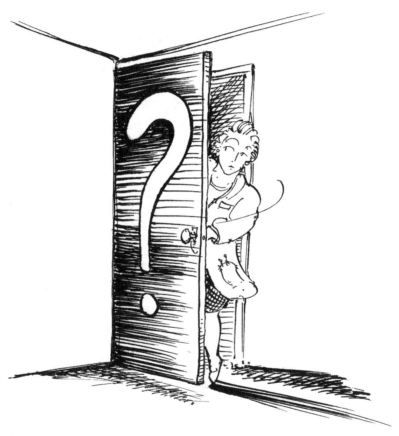

© Mark Steele. Reprinted by permission.

Now we step back to look at what all this means to our day-to-day existence as healthcare providers and educators. This existence is certainly not what it used to be 10, or even 5, years ago. We are working in a different world today. Change is an overwhelming theme, which is summarized in **Box 11-1**.

The inevitability of change in health care right now is a timely topic. Statements like these abound: "The U.S. healthcare system requires radical,

---

Box 11-1 Evolving Themes of Change in Health Care

From . . . Provider-centered care	to . . .	Patient-centered care
From . . . Giving patients information	to . . .	Coaching patients to find information
From . . . Present patient needs/tasks	to . . .	Future patient needs/tasks
From . . . Multidisciplinary work	to . . .	Interdisciplinary teamwork
From . . . Individual perspective	to . . .	*Contextual perspective*
From . . . Individual CT	to . . .	Team/system CT
From . . . Dichotomous thinking	to . . .	Relativistic thinking
From . . . Tradition-based practice	to . . .	Evidence-based practice
From . . . Change based on anecdotes	to . . .	Change based on strong evidence
From . . . Paper and pens	to . . .	Informatics
From . . . Information	to . . .	Knowledge
From . . . Quality assurance	to . . .	Quality improvement
From . . . Culture of blame for errors	to . . .	Culture of safety
From . . . Status quo	to . . .	Innovation
From . . . Hierarchical power	to . . .	Empowerment of all professionals

---

not incremental, change" (Waldman, Smith, & Hood, 2003, p. 5). "It's the end of an era. The type of nursing learned by the average, 47-year-old nurse is ending" (Porter-O'Grady, 2003, p. 4). We will discuss the thinking needed to deal with these changes shortly, but first let's reflect on why change is so necessary in health care right now, and the implications of that constant, complex change to our daily existence.

Why Is Change So Necessary?

The answers to why change is necessary right now are all around us. Read any newspaper, and you'll see articles on problems with healthcare systems and the health of people around us—our ill-prepared plans to deal with the increased numbers of elderly patients with multiple health conditions, the huge increase in Type 2 diabetes in young people, the high rate of obesity, our ability to keep people alive without quality of life, potential deadly outbreaks of new and mutated microorganisms, the imbalance between infinite needs and finite resources, the shortage of nurses and nurse educators, the high rates of medical errors, the rapid growth of new medications and treatment possibilities, genetic research, antibiotic resistance—shall we keep going?

By the way, as an aside for you educators, we'll share a strategy that we use in many of our courses—assignments to increase students' awareness of local to global health issues that are in the news. We have students find articles from the popular media and discuss their implications for nurses. It is always an eye-opening project because many students perceive nurses as dealing with one patient at a time. We are trying to get them better socialized to the many issues that will force them to be changeable and adaptable in their careers.

The examples we just listed are areas that need change specifically in healthcare delivery, but remember that according to the Institute of Medicine (IOM), those changes need to start in the health education arena. We are talking not only about the complex changes in health care; we are also talking about complex educational change. Changes in educational systems may be even harder to realize because of the traditions. As Senge, Scharmer, Jaworski, and Flowers (2004) noted, our present educational system is based on industrial-age assembly-line principles that will not prepare people to deal with tomorrow's realities. Likewise, Gardner had this to say:

> At the start of the third millennium, we lie at a time of vast changes—changes seemingly so epochal that they may well dwarf those experienced in earlier eras . . . These changes call for new educational forms and processes. The minds of learners must be fashioned and stretched in . . . ways that have not been crucial—or not as crucial—until now . . . We must recognize what is called for in this new world—even as we hold on to certain perennial skills and values that may be at risk. (2006, p. 11)

We health educators have a double whammy to deal with; we cannot escape change either in the classroom or in clinical settings.

What Kinds of Change Are We Talking About?

There have been zillions of books, articles, monographs, and so forth written on the change process and strategies to implement and deal with change. Those that are relevant to healthcare delivery and education start with descriptions of change that depict the confounding complexity of systems such as ours. Paul Plsek (2003) presented a thoughtful, practical perspective for a conference convened in Washington, DC, by the National Institute for Health Care Management Foundation and the National Committee for Quality Health Care. Plsek focused on change in health care as a complex issue, making a distinction among complex, complicated, and simple issues. Change in health care is complex because the healthcare system is a complex adaptive system. "A complex adaptive system is a collection of individual agents who have the freedom to act in ways that are not always totally predictable, and whose actions are interconnected such that one agent's actions change the context for other agents" (Plsek, 2003).

Models for complex adaptive systems are organic systems such as the human body—in which a change in one part will affect a change in another—and the body must always be viewed as a whole, not a collection of parts. In these systems, although there are feedback mechanisms to maintain the status quo, there is always something changing; there are contradictions and lots of unknowns. Think of what happens with a sore knee. To ease the knee pain, a person changes his or her gait and gets hip or foot pain, takes medications such as nonsteroidal anti-inflammatory drugs for the pain, and has side effects of edema that aggravate hypertension. A simple sore knee now presents a potential cardiac problem. We would do well to keep that image in mind when we start to consider complex system changes.

Other authors have made distinctions between types of complexity: detailed, dynamic, or both (Senge, 1990). Dynamic complexity is what we see in health care—the very nature of the complexity is focused on change. Senge et al. (2004) discussed this as transformational change, which is highly focused on the people involved in the change, not just on what change is made and how. It must focus on who we are. "The changes in which we will be called upon to participate in the future will be both deeply personal and inherently systemic" (2004, p. 2). People transform systems; systems don't transform themselves.

Educational systems and change are equally complex, according to Fullan: "Complexity, dynamism, and unpredictability . . . are not merely things that get in the way. They are normal" (1993, p. 20). Many processes are unknowable in advance, and there is nothing linear about the complexities of educational systems and their change. Making educational change more paradoxical in that change is a continuous theme, but the educational system is essentially conservative. Change in these circumstances cannot occur through isolated reforms; the whole educational system needs to become a "learning organization—expert at dealing with change as a normal part of its work" (p. 4).

Linear thinking about change as going from data to conclusions, mandates to coercion, chaos to order, and so forth is facile, revealing unrealistic thinking processes for today's changes in these complex systems. Fullan advocated better thinking as a solution: "The solution lies in better ways of thinking about, and dealing with, inherently unpredictable processes" (1993, p. 19). Among his eight basic lessons for this new paradigm of change are three of our favorites: "You can't mandate what matters . . . Connection with the wider environment is critical for success . . . [and] every person is a change agent" (pp. 21–22). These lessons emphasize the involvement of everyone in this thinking journey.

Senge (2003) echoed these ideas, reminding us that systems thinking must be a priority when considering change; we live in a global society and must use collective creating. He made a distinction between problem solving and creating. "In problem solving we seek to make something we do not like go away. In creating, we seek to make what we truly care about exist" (p. 4). It will require a radical change in our thinking to go beyond the old-fashioned problem solving and take on a creative stance.

In a little while, we'll discuss the changes in thinking that need to accompany the changes in healthcare delivery and education. First, however, we must consider the reactions of people involved in change.

Implications of Living with Constant, Complex Change

What about the implications of living with constant, let alone complex, change? With change comes the certainty of uncertainty, messiness, excitement, challenges, learning, refining self, redefining positions, more interactions among people, and calls for *creativity*. With change comes the possibility (probability?) of coercion, increased work, fatigue, anger, anxiety, judgments, feelings of inadequacy, and a desire to run away. It's all pretty scary stuff, right? How can we survive with our wits intact in this kind of changing day-to-day reality? For starters, we have to reflect on how we view change and the kinds of experiences we've had with change in the past. Then we have to look at how that view fits with the thinking needed today.

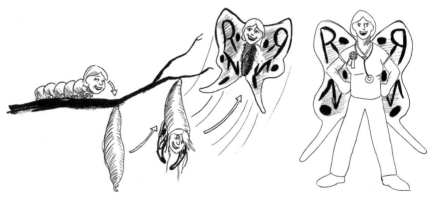

© Jesse Rubenfeld

What have your experiences been with change? Many (most?) clinicians and educators have had negative experiences. Changes have been handed down from upper-level administration and management. Before we can settle into one change, another comes along to take its place. Sometimes that happens even before we've settled into the first change! People far removed from the day-to-day implementation of the change developed the plan without our input. Before we feel comfortable with the change, we are being evaluated on how well we are doing with it. The focus is on the end point of the change rather than the process of change. Many changes are instigated to save money. Money-saving changes often have a short-term rather than long-term goal. Many changes seem irrelevant or were tried and found ineffective in other situations. Every time we hear from our manager that something is about to change we feel anxious!

This hierarchical system, with rapidly increasing frequency of episodic change, has been the norm for nurses for a long time. We need to acknowledge that, reflect on it, think about the feelings it brings up, then think about how we can deal with it successfully in the future. Maybe we can see ourselves within a metamorphosis frame of mind; we are moving toward an image of nurses as safety champions.

Thinking for Effective Change

The old ways of thinking about change won't work any longer. "As long as our thinking is governed by habit—notably by industrial, 'machine age' concepts such as control, predictability, standardization, and 'faster is better'—we will continue to re-create institutions as they have been, despite their increasing disharmony with the larger world" (Senge et al., 2004, p. 5).

As we consider the critical thinking (CT) dimensions that are our model in this text, we can look at all 17 of them and see how integral they are to the change process. However, here we'd like to examine six dimensions that are especially important in dealing with the complex, dynamic change that is needed and inevitable. We will focus on *contextual perspective, creativity, intuition, inquisitiveness, reflection,* and *transforming knowledge.* It's not that the others aren't used or important; it's just that these six are particularly useful in helping us initiate and deal with change.

We aren't going to separate these six dimensions very much because they are so interrelated. What we've done instead, in **Box 11-2**, is list 15 patterns of change in thinking and learning that, from our review of the literature and our collective experience, require an amalgamation of these six dimensions.

Box 11-2   Emergent, Necessary Patterns of Change in Thinking and Learning

---

1. From . . . Passivity	to . . .	Engagement/presence
2. From . . . Answers	to . . .	Questions
3. From . . . Separate thinking and doing	to . . .	Thinking and doing together
4. From . . . Destinations	to . . .	Journeys
5. From . . . Reactive learning	to . . .	Proactive learning
6. From . . . Mechanistic models	to . . .	Living system models

Box 11-2	Emergent, Necessary Patterns of Change in Thinking and Learning (continued)		
7. From . . .	Dichotomous thinking	to . . .	Relativistic thinking
8. From . . .	Thinking of pieces	to . . .	Thinking of wholes
9. From . . .	Alone/separated	to . . .	Connected/systems
10. From . . .	Reduction	to . . .	Complexity
11. From . . .	Matching existing patterns	to . . .	New patterns
12. From . . .	Linear	to . . .	Maps/knots/shapes
13. From . . .	Constant success	to . . .	Failure possibilities
14. From . . .	Valuing only objectivity	to . . .	Being open to *intuition*
15. From . . .	Reviewing	to . . .	Reflecting

Sources: Fullan, 1993; Plsek, 2003; Plsek & Greenhalgh, 2001; Porter-O'Grady, 2003; Senge, 1998; Senge et al., 2004.

Emergent, Necessary Patterns of Change in Thinking and Learning

Today's reality just doesn't fit with yesterday's thinking patterns. We are not dealing with a machine; we are dealing with a complex system of human beings that is intertwined with many other systems, all in a state of constant flux. As Senge et al. (2004) and Plsek (2003) noted, much of our thinking about organizations has come from the industrial age and a mechanistic mentality that favors assembly lines. Modern systems like health care don't work that way; they are adaptive, with complex feedback mechanisms (**Figure 11-1**). If we want to successfully change health care, we have to approach it more like a living organism system than a machine. (Remember our knee example earlier in this chapter.) Of course, as soon as we move to the living system metaphor, we can see that, in contrast to machine systems, there is very little predictability and a whole lot of potential chaos. As clinicians and educators, not only do we need to initiate change ourselves, but we also must survive changes instigated by others. For that, we've developed the 15 patterns of change in thinking and learning in Box 11-2. We added learning because today's systems are learning environments, not just places to do things.

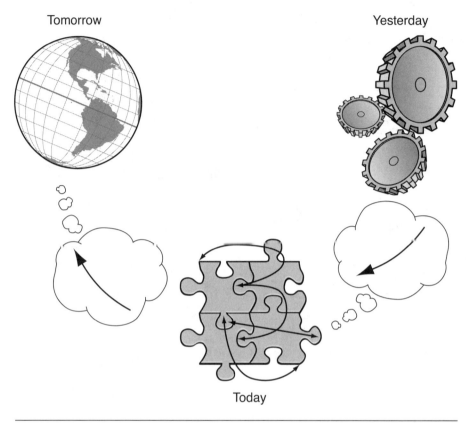

Figure 11-1 Realities of thinking.

From Passivity to Engagement and Presence

We have to see that this inevitable change will affect us, but we also have to see that we will affect that change as well. It is not a one-way street, but a two-way street. No longer can we sit back and let someone tell us what to do. We have a long tradition of learning and thinking in this passive mode. Educators keep presenting lectures; students keep reading, underlining, memorizing, and spitting back. If you don't already have an active approach to your job, think about what it would take to make you more engaged in thinking about changes that are necessary and how you might instigate those changes. If you're an educator, are you promoting passive or active learning? If you are continuing the passive tradition, you are not helping students prepare for the reality they will face. You have to risk getting some bad evaluations while trying different active strategies because students are pretty stuck in their passive learning modes. Most have come through passive educational systems in which they've been taught that there is one right answer.

From Answers to Questions

Because change is constant with many issues, unknown until they evolve, there are fewer answers, especially simple ones, and for sure, there is not just one right answer. Senge said, "Genuine inquiry starts when people ask questions to which they do not have an answer" (1998, section 4). Focusing on questions keeps the door to change open. Problem-based learning is starting with a problem or a question to guide learning (Rideout, 2001). Creative people ask questions: How can I represent the best aesthetic placement of these flowers? Why is this happening? What will this patient need to adapt at home?

We tend to focus more on answers because it's neater. Think of how much better most people feel after they've straightened up their homes, closets, workbenches, or desks. For a brief period, we have a sense of order in what is increasingly a disorderly world. Questioning takes us down a path of ambiguity because it allows for the possibility that the world isn't perfect. But, of course, the world isn't perfect, especially healthcare practice and education. We really do need to change things, so let's get rid of that desire for perfection, step out into uncertainty, and question everything, especially those things for which we don't already have answers.

From Separate Thinking and Doing to Thinking and Doing Together

A class activity that we have used for many years at the start of our CT course is to have students draw their thinking caps. You may want to try this strategy; it's a great CT discussion initiator. After the initial questions about what we want, students get enough reassurance to draw their caps. The results are quite interesting. Some talk about putting on a hat and going someplace quiet and peaceful to think. They tend to have neat hats with brims. Other students have pictures of things that could only be called hats by the most creative people; they have all kinds of things going on at once, and they discuss how everything is open and accessible. Secretly we think, "Ah, they'll be better able to adapt to thinking in nursing," but we never say that, of course; we wait for them to see that as the semester progresses, and they broaden their thinking as they see their peers' hats and hear them described.

Now, why do you think we see the latter group of students as being more adaptable to nurse thinking? It's because their thinking is all tied up with their doing, their emotions, things in their lives. They don't picture their thinking in neat, safe, clean spaces; therefore, thinking in the midst of the chaos of healthcare situations will not be a shock to them, and they will likely have an easier time doing *reflection* in practice.

You might want to reflect on when and how you do your thinking. Do you tend to sit back and do it after the fact, or while you're actively doing something?

From Destinations to Journeys

This is similar to moving from answers to questions because it's about uncertainty and ambiguity. We tend to think about our end points. *Things will be better once I get the kitchen fixed; we'll have more money once the kids have finished school; I'll get some order back in my life once the semester ends.* This kind of thinking actually sets us up for frustration because, of course, in today's complex world, almost nothing goes into a neat box on which we can write "finished." Just ask people about projects they have never finished; ask them how they feel about them. You'll find some who say, "This is just how life is; I always have things unfinished, and I've learned to live with it." Others are bothered by the lack of closure and try endlessly to close boxes.

Healthcare service and education will never be finished with their changes because every change will affect something else that will have to change. New technology will come along and redefine even the simple things that we have firmly in place, and we'll have to open boxes all too frequently. Accept that—start to look more at the journey than the destination—and you'll be less crazy in this world.

If you want a hard lesson in journey versus destination thinking, write an article or a book, and you'll realize how hard it is to let it go as a finished product. As soon as you send it off to the publisher, you read something that you wish you had addressed. That, of course, is why you should always cite authors in the past tense. There's a good chance they might not say today what they said last year!

From Reactive Learning to Proactive Learning

This, too, is related to the first patterns we discussed—to move from passivity to engagement and from answers to questions—but we feel that it's worth describing in these alternate terms to make sure this whole idea comes through. Senge and colleagues described reactive learning as "governed by 'downloading' habitual ways of thinking, of continuing to see the world within the familiar categories we're comfortable with . . . At best, we get better at what we have always done" (2004, p. 6). They made a distinction between reactive and deeper learning, but we've chosen to call the other end of the pattern proactive learning, which we think becomes deeper because learners are much more involved in seeking knowledge and putting it into a better workable frame for themselves.

How much of what you read is a result of someone telling you to read it or someone recommending it to you? How does that compare with what you read because you are curious enough to go digging something out yourself? How many of you, when you were students, read the recommended readings in addition to the required ones? Ahem, did we strike a nerve there?

When you meet new people, how much do you ask about what they do and try to learn from them? We have a friend, Connie, and everywhere she goes, she asks tons of questions of everyone she meets. If you happen to be tagging along, you might get antsy as she gets deeper and deeper into conversations, oblivious to time. She is very bright and knows a lot about a lot of things and has worked as a writer and reporter for many years. We're not sure if this is a chicken or egg thing—if she became a writer because she was so curious and wanted to share her knowledge, or if she became that way from being assigned to stories. It's probably a bit of both—just a good match.

What she is, without a doubt, is a proactive learner—so much so that she made a guilt-free decision not to finish her doctoral dissertation because it became too narrow a focus for her, and she didn't want to endorse that type of learning!

So where are you compared with Connie? Most of us are more reactive. We go along with the reactive-learning model of mainstream education, and many of us promote reactive learning in our students. It's tough to give up the power of the teacher's teaching to the power of the learner's learning, but we educators have to move more in that direction if we are to coach active, creative innovators in health care. Remember Fullan's (1993) lesson number 1: you can't mandate what matters. Learners need to come to their learning proactively to be invested in what they are learning and achieve deeper understanding as a result.

From Mechanistic Models to Living Systems Models

We discussed this earlier when we described the types of change needed today. What about the thinking involved in this change of perspective? You might think, "This is running like clockwork" or "We have a well-oiled machine here." Even though we use such metaphors, do we really believe that our healthcare and education systems fit that picture? Probably not. Senge (1999) repeatedly pointed out the need to consider living systems as our model of change in today's complex world. A most important lesson that we have learned from his writings is to consider the impact of compensating feedback mechanisms in living systems and how that differs from the workings of machines. If you've ever dieted to lose weight (and who hasn't?), you can relate. Initially you lose weight, and then you gain a bit or level off, even when you think you're eating the same way. Your body is hanging on to your survival fat and has a starvation feedback signal. Some of us try to reset that thermostat periodically, some with more success than others, by changing our eating and activity patterns. Much of the resistance to change that we observe is the system trying to conserve itself or something within itself. If we don't recognize the process or what it is trying to conserve, we will continue to be frustrated with resistance to change.

Senge (1990, 1998) used the example of a hot room with a thermostat. You enter, and, without knowledge of the thermostat, you open the windows to cool things off. Soon it gets warmer again. If you want change, you have to get to the thermostat and reset it or turn off the furnace. Think about that image the next time you wonder why your group is hanging on to something and doesn't want to change; figure out where the furnace is or figure out how to reset the thermostat. Translate that to what the group is hanging on to and what will change their value of that.

From Dichotomous Thinking to Relativistic Thinking

OK, this is all about *contextual perspective*, right? Is there anyone out there who still sees things clearly in terms of right or wrong, blue or yellow, yes or no? We'd like to think that all of you would say, "Well, that depends." And that's the answer that goes chi-ching on the relativistic side. Of course, we know that all clinicians and educators don't say that, and those who do say it acknowledge that they only do it sometimes. Have you taken a multiple-choice test lately? Better yet, have you given one? What do you do with a student who argues a what-if scenario?

One of the great education ironies in nursing is that we try and try to promote relativistic thinking in students so they'll look at the whole context of a clinical situation, but then we test them with dichotomous exams that have rigid right or wrong answers. Because we still have to prepare students for multiple-choice licensure exams, even those of us who hate such exams feel pressure to allow some practice with them. We've gotten around our discomfort with this dichotomous approach by allowing students to challenge questions and answers. "If you can show in writing that your answer is as good as mine, you get credit for that question." It's not the best lesson in relativistic thinking, but it lets us sleep at night.

It is very easy to forget context when looking at a problem or planning change. Foster-Fishman, Nowell, and Yang developed a model for changing systems. At the outset, they declared that "most systems change efforts have not fully attended to the dynamics and properties of the contexts they are attempting to shift" (2007, p. 198). We must look at issues from many perspectives—find out the view of multiple stakeholders—so we don't delude ourselves that a straight line from intervention to outcome is possible.

From Thinking of Pieces to Thinking of Wholes

It is very easy to focus on the tree in front of you and forget about the forest, but because living systems are so interconnected, it is folly to be too narrow in your view. Think about how short patient stays in the hospital are these days. Recently, in a class of registered nurses, we asked about patient teaching, and several students replied that they rarely do any patient teaching because they worked in intensive care units (ICUs)—that this was something done more by the nurses on the floors. Needless to say, I raised my eyebrows a bit and asked questions like this: *Don't your patients have family members sitting around? How often are your patients discharged home only a day or two after leaving the ICU? What constitutes patient teaching to you?* Ultimately, the students realized they were working in a very task-oriented way and were not seeing the whole picture of these patients' lives and how this episode of illness fit within it. They realized there were lots of little things that they could and should be teaching to patients and to family members.

How are we going to get past that task orientation that has been such a huge part of our history in nursing? Educators, how can we teach novices who are so focused on tasks to periodically look up and see the whole patient? One idea is to start teaching tasks with more focus on the absolute essential parts so that students can stop using up their RAM with unnecessary details and leave more of their hard drives open for bigger pictures. We can also pepper our check-off routines with what-if questions to get them thinking of this task in a large, constantly changing context.

Clinicians, look around you at things like end-of-shift reports and count how many times a larger view of patients' worlds is mentioned. Start modeling that yourself. Put something in your report room to remind nurses of the larger view—a globe or a picture of a family picnic.

From Thinking Alone to Systems Thinking

We need to hone our individual thinking skills, but we also have to focus on how we think as groups and the dynamics of systems thinking. In their systems change model, Foster-Fishman and colleagues noted the importance of thinking about system dynamics: "interaction characteristics . . . the role of feedback . . . delays between actions and consequences, and how unexpected consequences from actions can create new conditions or problems" (2007, p. 200). The complexity of subjectivity within systems cannot be ignored.

Carole Estabrooks (2003) presented a view of nurses within communities of practice. On first reading, we feared that we would have trouble getting nurses to move to new thinking approaches, such as evidence-based practice (EBP). However, her remarks proved worthy of *reflection* beyond our first reactions. Here's what she found: "Increasingly, we are aware that nurses rely more on knowledge generated within their communities of practice than on knowledge generated by research. In particular, we have found that 'social interactions' and 'experience' are the two most important sources of knowledge for nurses . . . learning is social" (pp. 60–61). From that perspective, group thinking is perhaps already in place in nursing practice. Estabrooks acknowledged that this social learning phenomenon needs to be studied more, and we agree with her.

If we assume that Estabrooks is on to something, maybe we're halfway there in increasing our group or systems thinking. Maybe we're closer to systems thinking in nursing than professionals in some other disciplines are. Perhaps we should put our energies into the type of learning and thinking that is occurring in those social interactions. To continue with our EBP example, if a group of nurses is using traditions as a basis for practice, then we need to target that group and encourage some of them to explore EBP. All it takes is an instigation of social interactions around a new evidence report or a question about a practice that all nurses can relate to. This is the place for a clinician who models CT, talks aloud about thinking, and asks lots of questions.

From Reduction to Complexity

We probably have our logical positivist tradition to thank for our penchant for reductionist thinking. Although analysis and reducing problems to discover and learn are definite assets to CT, we have to take care that we put things back together after we've done that reduction. This is an issue that comes up when trying to explain CT. It is so complex that we have to break it down to make it understandable; hence, the 17 dimensions. However, as you can probably see by now, each time we try to address each dimension separately, it is never clean. These dimensions work best in harmony, as a whole where they augment each other.

Educators need to be especially aware of complex new patterns of change; years ago, we were able to teach in a reductionist manner—break everything down so students could understand the pieces. However, students are left with skills that they can't put into use because nothing in the clinical world is reduced in that way. Educators must help students put the pieces back together to see the enormous complexity that is the setting for these reduced skills.

This putting the pieces together would occur in what Gardner (2006) called the "synthesizing mind." Anyone who has tried to write a scholarly paper can appreciate how difficult synthesis is. Pulling something together to create a new view acknowledges the complexity but attempts to make it clear. Gardner called synthesis a "considerable feat" but attempted to define four components of the synthesis process: "a goal . . . a starting point . . . selection of strategy, method and approach . . . and drafts and feedback" (pp. 51–52). Perhaps we can use these components to help deal with the complexity.

From Matching Existing Patterns to New Patterns

When we see something new, we tend to interpret and store it in the established patterns in our brains. It's easier to remember something when it's in the form of a familiar pattern (Hart, 1983). An old pattern might be used to process and store something you hear your manager say—"I want everyone to be involved in coming up with ideas for improvement." If the usual style of change on your unit is hierarchical, with edicts handed down from above, that old pattern for registering the manager's remark might be, "That means we should all be nice and go along with things." It is very hard to throw off old patterns and make new ones. It means standing back and looking at things with different eyes. It doesn't necessarily mean throwing away the old patterns; sometimes it might be easier to change the shape of the existing ones.

Plsek (2003) gave a great example of creative thinking in new connections of patterns to help us teach patients better. We know that repetition helps learning; we know that elderly patients and those under stress often forget things we teach them; we know that if we could tape record what we tell patients, they could go back and listen to it again; we know that most people have telephone answering machines. The new pattern, then, is to put all those existing patterns together and come up with a plan to record our teaching on patients' home answering machines while we teach them face to face. We just ask them if we can call their homes and record the teaching session. Then, when they get home, they can listen to it as often as needed.

These ideas are often called *thinking outside the box*; some people are better at it than others. In today's world of change, we all must get outside our boxes and open ourselves to new patterns. To tease your brain a bit, look at **Box 11-3**; see if you can figure out these puzzles. The first one was brought home from school by one of our sons, and we're not sure who created it. We both had trouble with it, even though it's very simple, because we have moved to thinking patterns in which numbers are things we count, add, subtract, multiply, and so forth. We don't look at numbers as words, and

---

Box 11-3 Brain Teasers to Help Develop and Use New Brain Patterns

---

THE FIRST EXAMPLE

1
11
21
1211
111221

What is the next line?

THE SECOND EXAMPLE (PERKINS, 1994)

$2 + 7 - 118 = 129$

Add one straight line to the mathematical statement to make it true instead of false. There are at least three solutions.

---

that's the key to figuring out that pattern. Have you figured it out yet? The next line is 312211—three 1s, two 2s, and one 1. Start at the top now and say the words instead of seeing the numbers; one 1—two 1s—one 2 and one 1, and so on.

The second example is from a wonderful book by Harvard's David Perkins (1994) on learning to think by looking at art. In a chapter called "Making Looking Broad and Adventurous," he presented the number puzzle shown in Box 11-3. Once again, you have to get away from usual patterns and assumptions to see the possible solutions. The first solution is to put a vertical line through the equal sign. The second solution is to put a line starting at the left end of the top part of the equal sign and extend it diagonally up to the right. This creates the sign meaning less than or equal to and makes the statement true. The third solution is different; with one line on the plus sign, you make it into a 4; then the equation becomes $247 - 118 = 129$. As Perkins explained, we tend not to cut across categories in our minds. We tend to see things in habitual patterns.

From Linear to Maps, Knots, or Shapes

There is nothing linear about the thinking necessary for initiating and dealing with change in complex adaptive systems. Looking for straight lines just sets us up for frustration. Linear thinking does not allow us to be contextual and see the whole. We don't even have neat circles and ovals with today's thinking; we have various shapes such as knots, where things are so interconnected that it's hard to separate the pieces.

There are many resources in nursing today advocating mind or concept maps as learning mechanisms (e.g., Mueller, Johnston, & Bligh, 2002; Novak, 1998; Wheeler

& Collins, 2003). We have been using them for many years in clinical courses (instead of columnar care plans), in CT classes to show nonlinear thinking, and in nursing research courses as a way to study. Increasingly, students are more accepting of them as a way to learn, but we still have students who balk at them. They want linear formats—columns and outlines—because that's what they've used for years. But for others, it has become very liberating because their brains can now focus more naturally on the whole along with the parts in a matrix pattern instead of straight lines.

From Constant Success to Failure Possibilities

If you are going to be innovative, you must risk failure, and that's that. Now, think about that in today's society, which values success over all else, and you'll see the difficulties in moving toward this kind of thinking. A decade ago, there was a news item about physicist Stephen Hawking admitting that he was wrong about black holes (Wardell, 2004). He has now revised his theory that had been considered flawless since the 1980s. It was great to see that news item, not because he failed, but because he was so matter-of-fact about his failure. He exhibited *intellectual integrity*. Great ideas don't just appear wrapped up neatly; they develop over time, with experimentation and repeated failures preceding their success. This is another area in which Senge (1998) is adamant: innovation is a process of failure, and true learning doesn't occur when we train people to avoid failure. There's a story about Thomas Edison, who, in response to a reporter who asked about his failed results while inventing the light bulb, replied, "Results? Why, man, I have gotten lots of results! If I find 10,000 ways something won't work, I haven't failed. I am not discouraged, because every wrong attempt discarded is often a step forward" (Brainy Quote, 2009).

Gardner saw those using their creative minds as being dissatisfied and different from others, and often failing. "Creators fail the most frequently and, often, the most dramatically. Only a person who is willing to pick herself up and 'try and try again' is likely to forge creative achievements" (2006, p. 83). This sounds like *perseverance* too, doesn't it?

Think about the last time you gave someone positive feedback for failing. Have you ever done that? Maybe it's time we started doing that so that our creative folks keep creating.

From Valuing Only Objectivity to Being Open to Intuition

You'll note that we have a qualifying adjective there: only. We don't want to imply that we shouldn't value objectivity, but we have to be careful that we don't ignore *intuition* in our attempts to overcome bias and be objective. *Intuition* was identified and defined in our consensus research on CT in nursing as an "insightful sense of knowing without conscious use of reason" (Scheffer & Rubenfeld, 2000, p. 358). Years ago Polanyi (1964) described it as "tacit knowing." It has been studied extensively in nursing, the most notable being Benner and Tanner's work (1987). Effken, after an extensive review of the literature, placed *intuition* in an ecological

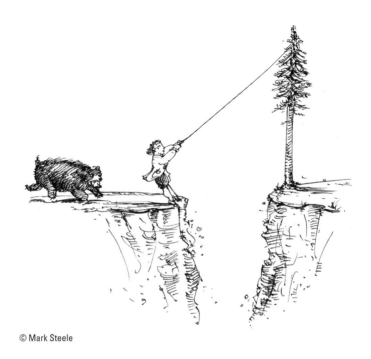

© Mark Steele

psychology framework, allowing us to look beyond cognitive or perceptual processes to "the information provided by the patient and the context of care" (2001, p. 252).

Viewing *intuition* in this way links it with *contextual perspective*, making it valuable in living systems environments. Intuitive responses take in a broader view of events, and that's what we need today. Rosanoff (1999) saw deeper intuitive responses as valuable in today's healthcare world, where quick decisions are called for. She suggested strategies to promote *intuition*—stop and look inside for your intuitive response, practice being attentive to intuitive responses, and keep a journal of your intuitive responses to see how accurate they are. She even suggested starting meetings by asking members to look at the agenda, record their thoughts and feelings, and then share them. This probably would enhance intuitive responses if those directions were couched in intuitive-sounding words, such as "your first gut reactions," "immediate hunches," and so forth. Senge (1996) suggested a similar process of meeting check-ins and check-outs focused on the thinking of participants.

From Reviewing to Reflection

The final pattern of change in thinking needed today is perhaps self-evident. If you have read the preceding pages in one sitting, go back now and review what you read. After you've done that, reflect on what you've read. How are reviewing and *reflection* different? Reviewing can be done fairly passively, but *reflection* can't. You have to put your personal self into *reflection* because it's deeper thinking. The Delphi study consensus group defined *reflection* as "contemplation upon a subject, especially one's assumptions and thinking for the purposes of deeper understanding and self-evaluation" (Scheffer & Rubenfeld, 2000, p. 358).

That deeper understanding and self-evaluation is where you need to be to prepare for the challenges of today's and tomorrow's healthcare delivery and education. The old thinking will not work; you need to evaluate yourself and your present thinking patterns and contemplate what you need to do to transform them to meet present and future needs. In the spirit of self-evaluation and *reflection*, we would like to conclude with some of our latest *reflections* on CT.

In the past years of our careers, we have been primarily educators. Our perspective has been to reflect on CT from many lenses so we can help others improve their thinking. We realize that the muddy waters of nursing practice are never as neat as the scenarios we develop in our minds, so we applaud nurses who are doing sound CT while providing quality care.

There are many healthcare providers who are trying to follow the recommendations of the IOM to increase quality of care through evidence-based, patient-centered, interdisciplinary care while optimizing the informatics revolution. As an example, consider Kaiser Permanente group in California, where we have been privileged to conduct several CT workshops. If you want some inspiration during this time of change and challenges, we recommend you pick up the book *Caring: Making a Difference One Story at a Time* (Bream & Johnson, 2009).

Besides being practicing nurses and educators, we have dabbled in research. We would like to leave you with a taste of our latest pet projects, one being a research study and the other being a compilation of some *reflections* on teaching CT from expert nurse educators.

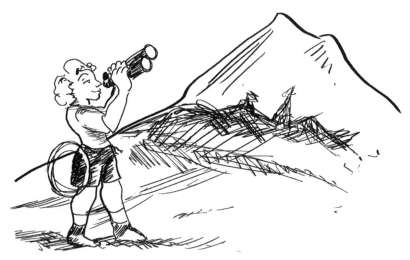

© Jesse Rubenfeld

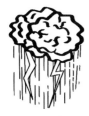

© Jesse Rubenfeld

Our Latest Research Reflection: Synthesis as Transforming Knowledge

After years of writing and thinking about, studying, and teaching CT we have decided that *transforming knowledge* may be the biggest challenge of all 17 dimensions. The definition of *transforming knowledge* is "changing or converting the condition, nature, form, or function of concepts among contexts" (Scheffer & Rubenfeld, 2000, p. 358). Of the seven CT skills, the first six—*analyzing, applying standards, discriminating, information seeking, logical reasoning,* and *predicting*—have fairly concrete approaches that can be described noncontextually but can be used in practice situations. *Transforming knowledge*, however, necessitates a context and is much more challenging to describe. There is no right way to transform knowledge. It all depends on the situational factors in play.

One could make a case that all of nursing today is predicated on the ability of nurses to transform knowledge. Consider this: "To be safe and effective practitioners nurses need to enter practice ready to draw on knowledge from a wide range of fields. Because practice will only become more complex over time, nurses must leave their formal programs prepared to be lifelong students, with the disposition and skills to be reflective practitioners and expert learners" (Benner, Sutphen, Leonard, & Day, 2010, p. 4).

Benner's group, calling for a transformation of nursing education, cited the dichotomy between how we teach in classrooms and the realities of nursing practice. "Classroom teachers must step out from behind the screen full of slides and engage students in clinic-like learning experiences that ask them to learn to use knowledge and practice thinking in changing situations, always for the good of the patient" (Benner et al., 2010, p. 14). They advocate "teaching for a sense of salience" to promote "situated learning" or "thinking in action" (p. 94). Such approaches are all about putting pieces together and transforming the collective into something usable in practice. With the constant, rapid change of health care and society, nurses, and, indeed, all people, need to be able to adapt their knowledge and thinking to multiple situations.

The challenges of *transforming knowledge* have led us to study the process of synthesis in particular. Whether one calls this process transformation, synthesis, or something else, the challenge to practicing nurses and nurse educators is how nurses can become better at pulling together huge amounts of information in messy contexts and form a synthesized outcome that promotes safe, effective care.

The idea of synthesis is not new. Most nurse educators are familiar with Bloom, Engelhard, Furst, Hill, and Krathwohl's famous taxonomy of cognitive objectives that ranks synthesis above knowledge, comprehension, application, and analysis and below only evaluation in terms of cognitive complexity (1956). In spite of years of using the term *synthesis*, we have not studied this cognitively challenging process very much.

Carl Hall (1995) defined synthesis as "a way of thinking and doing, of providing a vision, in which an idea or a thing, imagined or real, is seen as a coherent whole; often consisting of parts, from which a thought can be developed, action can be rejected or taken, and the thing made, assembled, or constructed; either as a new creation or activity or as a duplicate or substitute of known substances" (fly leaf). Hall directed his ideas to "those people interested in interdisciplinary, multidisciplinary, and crossdisciplinary studies and work in the professions and applied fields, policy development, and education. The objective is to show the increasing importance of synthesis in philosophical thinking and technological approaches to meet the needs of the 21st Century" (p. 1).

Hall made a specific point of comparing and contrasting synthesis with analysis (which is a separate CT skill in our description of the dimensions of CT): "The literature on synthesis is not nearly as extensive as that for analysis. Indexes, book contents, encyclopedias, and dictionaries often identify or list synthesis as part of analysis, providing a limiting approach" (1995, p. 1). "Analysis is very important and fundamental to synthesis. Analysis has provided information, data, and critical thinking without which there wouldn't be 'pieces' for synthesis" (p. 36). The challenge, therefore, is how to elucidate the slippery path of not just breaking apart a situation and making sure you have all the necessary information, but how to put that back together into something new and transformed to meet the needs of the situation.

It is easier to see synthesis as an outcome than as a process. Outcomes of synthesis are around us in, among others, art, music, books, theories, clinical guidelines, research reviews, and the news. In nursing, it looks like excellent patient care outcomes. Think of the best nurse you've ever worked with—that person who seems to have it all together and takes the best approaches in patient situations. That person exemplifies the outcome of synthesis. But what if you ask that nurse how he or she came to that outcome. Ask anyone how he or she came to that outcome and one usually is met with a quizzical look and answers like, "I don't know; I just came to it," "Well, let's see, what did I do first?" "It's in my head," or "I can't explain it."

Now let's talk about this new research study. Along with a group of faculty and graduate student colleagues (L. Blondy, A. Blakeslee, R. Luster-Turner, and B. Cronin), we decided to study the process of synthesis by asking people from a variety of disciplines (e.g., teachers from biology and English, financial analysts, an aerospace engineer, a musician, a librarian, a fitness entrepreneur, etc.), including nursing, open-ended questions about synthesis. In three focus groups of six or seven people each, we asked participants to describe the following:

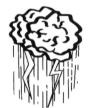
© Jesse Rubenfeld

- How they learned to use synthesis
- What were the most challenging aspects of doing it
- What were the essential elements of synthesis
- Which of the elements might cross disciplines
- How they taught others to synthesize

We are currently *analyzing* these data, but there seems to be commonalities across disciplines. We have included in **Table 11-1** examples of preliminary findings from this qualitative study. Look for a journal publication in the near future (we hope) for the final analysis report.

TABLE 11-1 Examples of Preliminary Findings of Interprofessional Synthesis Study

Preliminary Themes	Selected Examples of Theme Descriptors
Question 1: How did you learn how to achieve the skills and the thinking required for synthesis?	
Cognitive actions	Looking for patterns
	Seeing relationships
	Clarifying information
Situational influences	Directed learning
	Learning on the job
	Professional involvement and engagement
Dispositions	*Confidence*
	Being purposeful
	Collaboration
Preparation	Practice
	Expanding information
	Teaching
Question 2: What do you find to be the most challenging aspects of achieving synthesis?	
Assumptions	Adding/deleting information due to assumptions, prejudices, biases
	Thinking you know it all
Information-related challenges	Insufficient information
	High volume of information and difficulties filtering and prioritizing
	Having sufficient knowledge and experience
Situational influences	Time involved in being sure impression or conclusion is correct
	Rules and being able to go beyond them and break them; need for courage
	Difficulty moving out of comfort zone
Cognitive complexities	Being flexible and changing habits
	Having patterns for doing synthesis; connecting dots
	Keeping an open mind
Question 3: What do you see as the essential elements of synthesis in your individual professions?	
Cognitive processes and actions	Careful observation
	Probing and clarifying
	Predicting based on information
Information management	Keeping up with new information
	Translating and connecting knowledge
	Looking at multiple sources of information

(continues)

TABLE 11-1   Examples of Preliminary Findings of Interprofessional Synthesis
Study (continued)

Preliminary Themes	Selected Examples of Theme Descriptors
Question 3: What do you see as the essential elements of synthesis in your individual professions?	
Interactions	Communicating
	Gathering input from others
Dispositions	Fortitude
	Intuition
	Adaptability/*flexibility*/ability to change directions
Knowledge base	Understanding fundamental concepts
	Knowledge of subject matter
	Knowledge of audience
Question 4: What elements of synthesis might cross over disciplines and be shared across disciplines?	
Information-related elements	Collecting and sorting information
	Contextual awareness
	Probing experiences
Cognitive processes and actions	Reevaluating
	Prioritizing/determining relevance/weighting
	Recognition of biases
Interactions	Communication
	Sharing information
Dispositions	Curiosity
	Tolerance for risk and ability to judge it
	Introspection and *reflection* (asking why we think something)
Question 5: How do you teach others to synthesize?	
Methods	Leading by example/modeling
	Stories and case scenarios
	Providing labels and vocabulary
Characteristics of the teaching/ learning processes	Ongoing
	Learning from ambiguity
	Confidence
Desired learner characteristics	*Intuition*
	Confidence
	Engaged
Challenges of teaching others to synthesize	Learner lack of self-awareness (don't know what they don't know)
	Diverse learning backgrounds of students
	Getting beyond biases

Our Latest Teaching *Reflections*

In preparation for the third edition of this chapter, we informally assembled a group of expert nurse educators to find out how they were teaching critical thinking after a decade or so of critical thinking being identified as important in nursing. We fed them lunch and asked them the following questions:

1. What are the biggest challenges you have encountered when teaching critical thinking?
2. What are some of the key approaches you have found that work when teaching critical thinking? Why do you think they work?
3. What recommendations do you have as we continue to help faculty do a better job of teaching critical thinking?

We had a lively dialogue in which comments and ideas branched and expanded for several hours. Below is a distillation of key aspects of that dialogue. See if you agree with the thinking of these experts.

Biggest challenges:

- Working with other faculty who do not understand critical thinking or how to teach it.
- Using the term *critical thinking* that has either become out of date or has acquired a negative connotation.
- Multiple definitions and meanings of critical thinking among colleagues as well as in the literature.
- Students who want the right answer versus thinking of multiple possibilities.
- Demonstrating critical thinking. (It is harder to teach it than to demonstrate it.)
- Finding ways to test and measure critical thinking without using multiple-choice examinations.
- Learning how to be comfortable, as a faculty person, sharing your own mistakes and being open with students about your thinking processes.
- Helping students realize they already use many of the critical thinking dimensions in their lives and just need to become more aware so they can focus on enhancing those skills and habits of the mind.

Key approaches and recommendations:

- Provide students with time to think, debrief, and process information.
- Consider changing the label of critical thinking to something like *thinking threads*.
- Reserve time at the end of each semester for *reflection* on learning; this could be an online assignment.
- Keep asking branching questions, steering students to think more deeply.
- Have students develop care for two or more people with the same nursing diagnosis (for example, the president of the United States, an elderly grandmother with several chronic illnesses, and a 10-year-old boy, all with the diagnosis of impaired physical mobility).

- Promote a classroom culture in which it is safe to make mistakes. The goal in class is to share thinking, not provide the right answer immediately.
- Create or select situations in which students must identify poor, good, better, and best interventions to help them see that not every intervention is right or wrong.

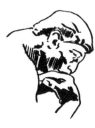

© Jesse Rubenfeld

PAUSE and Ponder

The Hard Work of Thinking

If we thought yesterday's thinking was hard, based on today's thinking, we can project tomorrow's thinking to be even harder.

Do you think that's true? Certainly the context is getting more and more complex. However, it could get easier. Remember when we tried to use CT in the context of yesterday's view of systems as mechanistic and it didn't fit? CT fits better with systems that are nonlinear and dynamic—complex adaptive systems. Today critical thinkers are still considered troublemakers in some systems; however, that is changing, and clinicians and educators with CT abilities are gaining acceptance and are being held up as people who have superior survival skills. If you're sitting there saying we've gone a bit wifty again, you might want to reconsider, because we think we're on track, and there are many who seem to agree.

REFLECTION CUES

- The overwhelming message in discussions of the five IOM (2003) competencies is change—change in healthcare delivery and education.
- New conceptualizations of change are needed for today's complex world.
- Realistic models for change in health care and education come from living, adaptive systems, not the older mechanistic models.
- Today's systems are dynamically complex; change is constant, and each part of the system that changes influences all other parts of the system.
- Old thinking patterns will not work with the reality of today and the near future.
- Fifteen patterns of change in thinking are described: passivity to engagement; answers to questions; separate thinking and doing to thinking and doing together; destinations to journeys; reactive to proactive learning; mechanistic to living system models; dichotomous to relativistic thinking; pieces to wholes; alone to systems; reduction to complexity; matching existing patterns to new patterns; linear to maps, knots, or shapes; constant success to failure possibilities; valuing only objectivity to being open to *intuition*; and reviewing to reflecting.
- Critical thinkers will fit better with systems that are complex and adaptive.
- Our final *reflections* on CT include a salute to nurses in practice and education.

- A preliminary report on synthesis research across disciplines reveals new insights on *transforming knowledge.*
- Nurse educators' insights about teaching CT illuminate challenges and suggestions for creative approaches.

REFERENCES

Benner, P., Sutphen, M., Leonard, V., & Day, L. (2010). *Educating nurses: A call for radical transformation.* San Francisco, CA: Jossey-Bass.

Benner, P., & Tanner, C. (1987). Clinical judgment: How expert nurses use intuition. *American Journal of Nursing, 87,* 23–31.

Bloom, B. S., Engelhart, M. D., Furst, E. J., Hill, W. H., & Krathwohl, D. R. (1956). *Taxonomy of educational objectives: The classification of educational goals handbook I: Cognitive domain.* New York, NY: David McKay.

Brainy Quote. (2009). *Thomas A. Edison quotes.* Retrieved from http://www.brainyquote.com/quotes/authors/t/thomas_a_edison.html

Bream, T. L., & Johnson, J. A. (2009). *Caring: Making a difference one story at a time.* Pasadena, CA: Kaiser Permanente.

Effken, J. A. (2001). Informational basis for expert intuition. *Journal of Advanced Nursing, 34,* 246–255.

Estabrooks, C. A. (2003). Translating research into practice: Implications for organizations and administrators. *Canadian Journal of Nursing Research, 35*(3), 53–68.

Foster-Fishman, P. G., Nowell, B., & Yang, H. (2007). Putting the system back into systems change: A framework for understanding and changing organizational and community systems. *American Journal of Psychology, 39,* 197–215. doi:10.1007/s10464-007-9109-0

Fullan, M. (1993). *Change forces: Probing the depths of educational reform.* Bristol, PA: Falmer Press.

Gardner, H. (2006). *Five minds for the future.* Boston, MA: Harvard Business School Press.

Hall, C. W. (1995). *The age of synthesis: A treatise and sourcebook.* New York, NY: Peter Lang.

Hart, L. A. (1983). *Human brain and human learning.* New York, NY: Longman.

Institute of Medicine. (2003). *Health professions education: A bridge to quality.* Washington, DC: National Academies Press.

Mueller, A., Johnston, M., & Bligh, D. (2002). Joining mind mapping and care planning to enhance student critical thinking and achieve holistic nursing care. *Nursing Diagnosis, 13*(1), 24–27.

Novak, J. D. (1998). *Learning, creating, and using knowledge: Concept maps as facilitative tools in schools and corporations.* Mahwah, NJ: Erlbaum.

Perkins, D. N. (1994). *The intelligent eye: Learning to think by looking at art.* Los Angeles, CA: J. Paul Getty Trust.

Plsek, P. (2003, January). *Complexity and the adoption of innovation in health care.* Paper presented at Accelerating Quality Improvement in Health Care Strategies to Speed the Diffusion of Evidence-based Innovations, by National Institute for Health Care Management Foundation and National Committee for Quality Health Care, Washington, DC. Retrieved from www.nihcm.org/pdf/Plsek.pdf

Plsek, P. E., & Greenhalgh, T. (2001). The challenge of complexity in health care. *British Medical Journal, 323,* 625–628. Retrieved from http://bmj.bmjjournals.com/cgi/content/full/323/7313/625

Polanyi, M. (1964). The logic of tacit inference. In M. Grene (Ed.), *Knowing and being: Essays by Michael Polanyi* (pp. 138–158). Chicago, IL: University of Chicago Press.

Porter-O'Grady, T. (2003). Innovation and creativity in a new age for health care. *Journal of the New York State Nurses Association, 34*(2), 4–8.

Rideout, E. (2001). *Transforming nursing education through problem-based learning.* Sudbury, MA: Jones and Bartlett.

Rosanoff, N. (1999). Intuition comes of age: Workplace applications of intuitive skill for occupational and environmental health nurses. *AAOHN Journal, 47,* 156–162.

Scheffer, B. K., & Rubenfeld, M. G. (2000). A consensus statement on critical thinking in nursing. *Journal of Nursing Education, 39,* 352–359.

Senge, P. M. (1990). *The fifth discipline: The art and practice of the learning organization.* New York, NY: Doubleday.

Senge, P. M. (1996, Fall). The ecology of leadership. *Leader to Leader, 2*, 18–23. Retrieved from http://www .leadertoleader.org/knowledgecenter/journal.aspx?ArticleID=137

Senge, P. M. (1998, Summer). The practice of innovation. *Leader to Leader, 9*, 16–22. Retrieved from http://www.leadertoleader.org/knowledgecenter/journal.aspx?ArticleID=159

Senge, P. M. (1999). Leadership in living organizations. In F. Hesselbein, M. Goldsmith, & I. Somerville, (Eds.), *Leading beyond the walls* (pp. 73-90). San Franscisco, CA: Jossey-Bass.

Senge, P. M. (2003). Creating desired futures in a global society. *Reflections, 5*(1). Retrieved from www .solonline.org/resource/resmgr/Docs/Reflections5-1.pdf

Senge, P. M., Scharmer, C. O., Jaworski, J., & Flowers, B. S. (2004). Awakening faith in an alternative future. *Reflections, 5*(7), 1–11. Retrieved from www.ottoscharmer.com/docs/articles/2004 _AwakeningFaith.pdf

Waldman, J. D., Smith, H. L., & Hood, J. N. (2003). Corporate culture: The missing piece of the healthcare puzzle. *Hospital Topics, 81*(1), 5–14.

Wardell, J. (2004, July 16). *Hawking changes his mind on black holes.* Associated Press. Retrieved from NBC News.com at http://www.nbcnews.com/id/5452537/ns/technology_and_science-space/t /hawking-changes-his-mind black holes/#.Us3Ii_uMaWg

Wheeler, L. A., & Collins, S. K. R. (2003). The influence of concept mapping on critical thinking in baccalaureate nursing students. *Journal of Professional Nursing, 19*(96), 339–346.

Critical Thinking (CT) Inventory

Critical Thinking Habits of the Mind

Confidence—**"Assurance of one's reasoning abilities."** (Scheffer & Rubenfeld, 2000, p. 358)[1]

1. How do you justify your thinking to someone who questions your conclusions?
2. Do you ever think aloud, or do you wait to speak until you have your ideas firmly in place? Why?
3. In what situations are you easily swayed from your thinking by someone else's opinion?

Contextual Perspective—**"Consideration of the whole situation, including the relationships, background, and environment that are relevant to some happening."**

1. Describe how you approach an ambiguous situation.
2. How often, and under what circumstances, do you ask questions that start with "But what if . . . ?" or "It depends . . ."?
3. When you tell a story, do you tend to include background information, or do you keep more strictly to the point? Why?

Creativity—**"Intellectual inventiveness used to generate, discover, or restructure ideas; imagining alternatives."**

1. Describe something you did in the past month that required innovative thinking. Why do you think it was innovative?
2. Do you tend to approach a situation the way other people do, or are your interpretations often different from theirs? Give an example.
3. If your boss told you to think outside the box, how would you change your usual thinking process?

Flexibility—**"Capacity to adapt, accommodate, modify, or change thoughts, ideas, and behaviors."**

1. When your practice routines are interrupted, how does your thinking help you adapt?

---

[1] All quoted material in the CT Inventory is from Scheffer & Rubenfeld, 2000, p. 358.

2. How much of your mind is open to change and how much is closed?
3. What has to occur for you to change your mind about something important?

Inquisitiveness—**"An eagerness to know by seeking knowledge and understanding through observation and thoughtful questioning in order to explore possibilities and alternatives."**

1. What is your motivation for questioning information provided by an authoritative source, such as a person, an article, or a book?
2. On a continuum from *extremely curious to not curious*, where would you place yourself and why?
3. How do you distinguish the thinking differences between information seeking and inquisitiveness?

Intellectual Integrity—**"Seeking the truth through sincere, honest processes, even if the results are contrary to one's assumptions and beliefs."**

1. How do you deal with ideas and information that conflict with your thinking?
2. How do you feel about debate on issues, as opposed to having everyone agree? Why?
3. When you feel strongly about something, do you also try to see the situation from the opposite point of view? How do you get your thinking to achieve that?

Intuition—**"Insightful sense of knowing without conscious use of reason."**

1. How often do you have gut feelings, a sixth sense, or a premonition? Describe how you respond to those feelings.
2. Describe how your hunches emerge in your thinking.
3. How do you explain your intuitive behavior to those who might question your choices?

Open-Mindedness—**"A viewpoint characterized by being receptive to divergent views and sensitive to one's biases."**

1. How do you recognize when you have made assumptions, as opposed to basing your conclusions on data collected with your five senses (sight, sound, touch, smell, and taste)?
2. What are your assumptions (about cultures, health, illness, time, eating, exercise, economic status, education, and so forth), and how do they affect the questions that you ask or don't ask, or the conclusions that you draw?
3. Why would others describe you as judgmental or nonjudgmental?

Perseverance—**"Pursuit of a course with determination to overcome obstacles."**

1. Describe a challenging situation, the obstacles involved, and how your thinking allowed you to stick with the task.

2. Describe your thinking when you have to decide whether to pursue a task or move on.
3. How would others describe your ability to persevere?

Reflection—**"Contemplation on a subject, especially one's assumptions and thinking for the purposes of deeper understanding and self-evaluation."**

1. Which of the 17 dimensions of critical thinking (CT) are your strongest? Your weakest? Why do think this?
2. What helps and what hinders your ability to reflect on your thinking before, during, and after an event or activity?
3. Describe how the following emotional states affect your thinking: love, hate, loneliness, frustration, sorrow, ecstasy, anxiety, and embarrassment.

Critical Thinking Skills

Analyzing—**"Separating or breaking a whole into parts to discover their nature, function, and relationships."**

1. Describe your thinking when you need to deal with a complex issue, such as writing a major research paper or presenting a staff development workshop.
2. How would you describe your thinking to a nursing student or a new nurse who needs to learn how to analyze a patient situation?
3. What goes on in your mind when situations seem overwhelming?

Applying Standards—**"Judging according to established personal, professional, or social rules or criteria."**

1. How do you decide if something is right or wrong?
2. When you are working with someone who is not doing his or her job as you think it should be done, what standards are you thinking about, and what do you usually do about it?
3. How do you decide which authority is the highest, and why?

Discriminating—**"Recognizing differences and similarities among things or situations and distinguishing carefully as to category or rank."**

1. How do you decide what information is missing when you are problem solving so you can better zero-in on the real problem?
2. How did you learn to distinguish the nuances of assessment that allow you to customize or individualize patient care?
3. Describe the thinking you use to help a nursing student or a new nurse make differential nursing diagnoses.

Information Seeking—**"Searching for evidence, facts, or knowledge by identifying relevant sources and gathering objective, subjective, historical, and current data from those sources."**

1. What are your five primary sources for finding accurate information? Have you changed those sources over the past year? If so, how?
2. What format do you prefer for information input—hearing, seeing, a combination of those, or another? How does your preferred method influence the accuracy of your data collection?
3. Describe a typical time frame and process that you used when you searched for information, such as an Internet search.

Logical Reasoning—**"Drawing inferences or conclusions that are supported in or justified by evidence."**

1. Describe how you have solved a problem using one or all of the following approaches: sequential, random, inspirational, or something different. How effective is your approach?
2. When someone asks, "Why did you conclude that?" how do you describe the thinking behind your conclusion?
3. How do you decide when you have enough information to draw a conclusion?

Predicting—**"Envisioning a plan and its consequences."**

1. Describe how you project potentially positive and negative consequences of your decisions or actions, and the decisions or actions of others.
2. How often during the day do you think, "What will happen if . . . ?" Under what circumstances do you ask yourself that question?
3. When caring for patients, how far into the future, on average, do you think? How does the healthcare setting (acute care, long-term care, home care, etc.) impact your thinking into the future?

Transforming Knowledge—**"Changing or converting the condition, nature, form, or function of concepts among contexts."**

1. Describe two situations, one in which you demonstrate abstract thinking and one in which you demonstrate concrete thinking. Which is your predominant mode of thinking? Why do you think that?
2. Describe a situation in which you learned something new and thought about how you would use that information in different situations.
3. Describe an event in which you have drawn on knowledge from several different sources and blended that knowledge to deal with a problem.

Using the CT Inventory

Our colleague at Eastern Michigan University has used the CT Inventory with students for several years and has done a qualitative research study looking at reflection patterns of RNs using the CT Inventory. Here is her report.

RN Reflections on the CT Inventory

Sandra Hines

In the first semester of the program, students in our school of nursing take a course named Essentials in Professional Nursing I. In this course they are introduced to the 17 dimensions of CT defined by Scheffer and Rubenfeld (2000). After reading numerous samples of the CT Inventory completed by students in this course, I became very interested in common ideas expressed in student papers and their awareness of their thinking processes in nursing. Many students in our program are registered nurses (RNs) returning to school to earn their bachelor of science in nursing (BSN) degree. During class discussions, these students talked at length about their use of CT skills. After learning about the 17 dimensions of CT in nursing and reflecting on the questions in the CT Inventory, they seemed to have a new appreciation for the importance of understanding CT using these new concepts of the habits of the mind and the CT skills. I decided to take a more formal approach toward understanding CT in this group of nurses and how the CT Inventory impacts it.

Brunt (2005) likened the 17 dimensions of CT in nursing to competencies that can be used as a measure against which to gauge one's nursing practice. Through a reflective process nurses or nursing students are able to evaluate their approach to nursing. The CT Inventory provides a selection of questions that allow students to reflect on and describe their application of each dimension. While previous studies have evaluated CT in nursing students, none have used the CT Inventory to stimulate reflection. Staib (2003) completed a literature search to identify teaching strategies used to increase CT in nursing students. The purpose of the current study was to learn which dimensions of CT the students self-identified as most changed and identify common themes these students described as they reflected on their responses to the CT Inventory and their own experience with the CT dimensions in their practice.

Study Participants

All students in this research project were RNs returning for a BSN. Fifty-two students were recruited, and 46 enrolled in this study, with 37 students completing all documents. Ten students were enrolled in an online section and 27 students in face-to-face sections of the course. Ages ranged from 26 to 54 years (mean 37 years); 34 students were female and 3 were male. Twenty students were African American; 12 were Anglo American, Caucasian; one was Hispanic, Latino, Mexican American; two were mixed/other racial groups; and two did not report their racial/ethnic group. The number of years in nursing as an RN ranged from 1 to 27 years (mean 7 years). Twenty-eight students worked as inpatient hospital staff nurses, three in home health care, two in administration, and one each in wound care, nursing education, insurance, and pain management.

As part of the coursework in Essentials in Professional Nursing I, the students learned about the habits of the mind and the CT skills. A number of the TACTICS recommended in *Critical Thinking TACTICS for Nurses* (Rubenfeld & Scheffer, 2009) were also completed as part of the class work. The students completed the CT Inventory, responding to two questions from each of the CT dimensions, and wrote a summary identifying their strengths and weaknesses based on the dimensions and what they learned about their own CT as they answered the 34 questions. Throughout the semester students discussed individual experiences, based on the 17 dimensions, in small groups or in reflective in-class writing. At the end of the semester, the students reviewed their CT Inventory and wrote a reflective paper on how their CT had changed over the semester. Approval was received from the university's Human Subjects Review Committee, and consent was received from the students to closely review their reflections. Some interesting trends were found, with meaningful examples provided by students.

Analyzing the Reflection on Critical Thinking

A phenomenologic approach was utilized to explore how the students perceived their CT skills and approaches at the end of this course designed to facilitate professional growth. "Nursing phenomenologic research perspectives aim to enhance understanding through reflective awareness, describing human experience fully, processing and interpreting experience, and explicating meaning(s) in experience" (Munhall, 2007, p. 217). This interpretive approach placed great importance on the students' experiences as they expanded their awareness of the nursing profession.

The student reflections on change in CT were initially read in total to identify common narrative themes across the papers. The papers were then reread to identify the individual dimensions discussed by the students in describing their CT. The papers were surveyed a third time to identify quotes representing the narrative themes that had been identified and exemplars.

Critical Thinking Dimensions Identified

Students identified change or growth in all 17 dimensions of CT in the consensus statement (Scheffer & Rubenfeld, 2000). The dimension identified by the largest number of participants was *confidence*, which was identified as an area of growth in 21 of the 37 participants. *Flexibility* and *open-mindedness* were each identified by 15 of the 37 participants. These dimensions most frequently discussed are classified as habits of the mind (affective dimensions). **Table A-1** lists the number of participants identifying a change in each of the dimensions. The students' reflections on their thinking in all of the dimensions provided clear evidence of their comprehension of the importance of each individual dimension identified by Scheffer and Rubenfeld (2000). This will become clearer as the common themes discussed by students are described.

TABLE A-1   Self-Evaluation of Change in Critical Thinking Dimensions

Critical Thinking Dimension	# Students Indicating Change*
Confidence	21
Flexibility	15
Open-mindedness	15
Analyzing	14
Applying standards	13
Creativity	13
Contextual perspective	12
Information seeking	12
Reflection	11
Inquisitiveness	10
Intuition	10
Logical reasoning	9
Predicting	9
Intellectual integrity	8
Discriminating	7
Perseverance	7
Transforming knowledge	5

*$n = 37$

Common Themes Identified by Student Reflections

Several themes were identified from the narratives of students. General comments about CT at the end of this course indicate a perceived difference in the students' approach to thinking. They indicated how learning about the dimensions of CT in nursing and completing the CT Inventory offered an opportunity for growth and self-awareness.

> I have to admit that prior to this class I really had not thought or learned about the CT process. However, upon learning more about it, I realized that everyone uses this process to some degree, and that like most things, knowledge and practice can improve one's skill. (Case 138)

> I began thinking about my thinking in everything I consider. I have gotten to know myself better because of this process. (Case 140)

The themes revealed through the end of the semester reflections were predominantly related to the students' professional activities, but at times other areas of their lives were also referenced. The themes and exemplars to illustrate the themes follow.

Awareness of Critical Thinking

Students described becoming more aware of their CT through an awareness of the 17 dimensions. Related subthemes included gaining a language to describe their thinking and the use of many CT dimensions. Some students pointed out that they had not changed but had become more attentive to their thinking process.

> *To say I am using the CT dimensions differently now than I did at the beginning of the semester would be an inaccurate statement. I attribute the growth I have achieved this semester to becoming more aware of the CT habits I have already been using. Recognizing my own CT has been an enlightening process.* (Case 109)

Some realized through reflection that they desired a change in their usual responses. Through an awareness of the dimensions of CT, they were able to identify specific areas in need of change or attention.

> *Although I try not to make assumptions about others, I did learn of some assumptions I used to make and how it affected my nursing practice . . . I realized that if there was a patient I perceived to be in the middle to upper socioeconomic class, I was less likely to inquire if they needed help paying for medical treatments or supplies. Now, I am more aware of my inclination to omit these questions and I make sure to include them in my assessment of every patient.* (Case 102)

> *I would still have to say that others would describe me as judgmental, although I have grown in my ability to base my conclusions on the facts of a situation. I can still catch myself being stubborn and dismissive with others. In the area of open-mindedness I could use a little work.* (Case 131)

Students were also able to identify how awareness contributed to growth in their practice providing an important bridge between content learned in the course and professional behavior.

> *I began to reflect on . . . why we do things the way we do in our department. I began to wonder if we were doing things because of routine and began to contemplate . . . what is best for the patients. Reflection of each thing I do is something new to me and has caused me to think more about the nursing process and how we could improve patient care in our department.* (Case 110)

> *Now whenever I leave work, either on my way home or while I'm at home, I analyze my actions during the day and wonder if I could have done something different to produce a more positive outcome.* (Case 146)

The manner in which the nurses described their increasing awareness of the relationship between what they practice and what their coursework suggests about approach to practice provided validation of their understanding and proficiency in the profession. These students expressed an enthusiasm about the potential of becoming even more aware for the purpose of improving outcomes. The increasing complexity in healthcare practice demands such motivation from clinicians.

Language to describe thinking. Learning the components of CT in nursing was described by some as providing a vocabulary to explain what they do; others were encouraged to value behaviors that may have been previously undervalued.

I have often been asked to describe what I do as a registered nurse. To me, my answer always seemed to minimize what I actually do and tended to focus on tasks or actions. Over the course of the semester I have come to realize that what I've actually been doing all these years is developing and exercising CT skills that enable me to deliver the best care I can to patients entrusted to me. Exposure to the 17 dimensions of CT has provided me with a vocabulary that I did not have. I am confident that this new vocabulary will allow me to effectively and intelligently describe the thinking that occurs prior to implementing the action. (Case 119)

Having been an RN for less than one year, I realize that since learning of the CT dimensions I use inquisitiveness more frequently due to my understanding that it is an actual component [of] CT and not just simply a lack of knowledge due to my inexperience. (Case 108)

Using many CT dimensions. The complexity of CT was described by students who expressed the many dimensions of CT they use or will be using more. The thinking behind nursing actions performed every day was revealed through both an awareness of the CT dimensions and the important role they play in patient care.

It's been exciting and informative to learn how I . . . think. I have great expectations that by expanding my CT I will become a more knowledgeable and rounded individual. I am going to spend more time seeking information, analyzing, logically thinking, and then reflecting on my decisions. I am also going to take that knowledge and use it in all areas of my life. (Case 139)

My confidence has increased because of my knowledge of flexibility and open-mindedness. These habits of the mind have helped me to adapt and modify my thought patterns and become more receptive and non-biased. (Case 143)

The general theme of awareness of CT may relate to the identification by many of an increase in confidence. Some students in this study are long-time practitioners and have likely developed expertise in the dimensions of CT; the language provided about CT can serve to validate abilities already developed. The realization of the important function of an aspect of their thinking that may have been viewed as a distraction (e.g., reflection, intuition, or contextual thinking) reframes it to be an essential component of safe practice and clinical judgment. Such reframing also focuses attention away from the tasks of practice and toward the thinking behind the tasks. This realization is important for nurses to be proficient in articulating the important role of the nursing profession in the provision of health care.

Better Patient Outcomes

Descriptions of better patient outcomes. Students were able to describe examples of improved outcomes for the patients they cared for. The dimensions of CT contributed to these improvements. Awareness of improved outcomes also contributed to confidence in practice.

> I have changed my use of predicting from an attempt to "see what happens" to analyzing the evidence and being prepared for what I predict to occur. I attempt to envision the outcomes of my actions as a proactive approach rather than a reactive approach. I gain confidence and a better understanding of the mechanisms at hand when I envision what the outcome should be, allowing me to be better prepared for the outcome, and able to anticipate any consequences. (Case 108)

> I have learned in a short time that being flexible is not always good. It is not beneficial if it compromises integrity or patient care. In the past, I have changed directions in my thinking and a patient died. Now, I redefine a situation that requires me to be flexible and consider another path if I think it is unsafe. (Case 115)

> Considering the whole picture, for example, the family dynamics and available resources help me to plan realistic and obtainable outcomes for the clients and their families. (Case 143)

Some improved outcomes went beyond the care provided by an individual nurse. Awareness of improved outcomes is important to allow RNs to articulate their role in improved patient care.

> A few weeks ago, I came up with a new format to write our 24-hour report for my unit. This was welcomed by everyone because the report is written as the day goes along rather than at the end of the shift. This new system has decreased gaps in our nursing care. (Case 141)

Exemplars of better patient outcomes. Students provided significant exemplar experiences to illustrate how CT improved patient care and outcomes.

Now I'm starting to become more inventive and discover new ideas and ways to make a situation better. For example some of the patients were complaining . . . there was too much light in the hallways at night and too much noise. I suggested maybe if the lights go down at the nursing station at night, that would help cut down or make the staff aware of the volume of their voices. Since then patients have had no complaints. (Case 112)

I have always been inquisitive, but I have rarely viewed myself as being intuitive or confident in my reasoning ability. We had a patient in the unit who had been neurologically intact during the night and developed a neurological change early in the morning. I used my intuitive skills along with the confidence in my reasoning skills to act quickly to improve the patient's outcome. I did this by contacting the appropriate health professionals and taking measures to protect the patient's airway and improve his neurological state. In the past I would have been frantic, yet in this situation I remained calm and collected my thoughts in order to act appropriately. (Case 129)

The relational component of the nurse–patient interaction was evident in the descriptions of better patient outcomes. Better patient outcomes were described by nurses who were often using the CT dimensions in the affective realm. The cognitive skills of predicting and analyzing were described, but more often the dimensions of flexibility, contextual perspective, creativity, inquisitiveness, intuition, and confidence were referenced. These affective domains are an important component of nursing care because nurses interact continuously with patients over the course of their workday.

Changes in Approach to Nursing

Descriptions of changes in approach to nursing. Changes in the students' overall approach to work and life situations were revealed through reflection. The number of possible approaches to problems was expanded by use of more dimensions of CT.

As I have learned the new vocabulary related to CT skills, I have thought more about the decisions that I make on a daily basis and how they relate to the different dimensions of CT. I also have thought about which dimensions I might not have used and how that might improve the decision-making process. (Case 110)

When a change in circumstance requires me to adapt, I analyze the new situation, identify my priorities, consider my options, and create a new plan with which I can accomplish what needs to be done. Since I am actually thinking about this whole process while doing it, I am considering each of these steps more comprehensively now. (Case 138)

Exemplars of changes in approach in nursing. Descriptions were provided of how approaches to practice changes were perceived. Recognition of the value of changes in CT by the nurses themselves and by others was described.

I attended a multi-disciplinary meeting today and asked several questions. My manager approached me after the meeting and stated that I asked excellent questions. I have been to meetings in the past and have asked questions, but she has never commended me for the type of questions that I asked. (Case 143)

I utilized my CT when dealing with a recent patient who was a constant complainer. Every time anyone went into the room, he complained that the whole hospital staff was incompetent and the hospital itself mismanaged. At face value we all took him as difficult to please and annoying. Upon review of his chart, I realized that he had recently been an independent and hardworking lawyer who was recently diagnosed with terminal lung cancer. This patient went from independent and healthy to completely dependent having a tracheostomy and [feeding] tube. He was suffering from pain, depression, marital problems, and loss of hope along with his recent loss of independence. After realizing this patient's use of poor coping skills, I was able to make an impact on him. I was told that I was the most helpful and inspiring nurse and actually gave him some hope for the future. If I had not researched the situation, I would have thought this patient to have a difficult personality and not realized that his demeanor was not his norm but instead his response to his disease. (Case 144)

The exemplars presented by the nurses indicating how their approach to nursing had changed were clear examples of improvement in nursing practice and patient care. The nurses described attention to the situation at hand and how their problem-solving skills had a positive impact on patient outcomes.

Self-Image as a Professional Nurse

Based on self-reflection both with the CT Inventory and the assessment of changes over the semester, the students identified professional behaviors they had developed. The language they used to describe these behaviors provided evidence of an understanding of the 17 CT dimensions and how they enhanced practice.

When speaking with other members of the healthcare team, I make an intelligent, well-thought-out case for my decisions, based on a thorough understanding of the path of my decision making from initial data to conclusion. The increased use of logical reasoning not only aids in my confidence but allows me to justify my conclusions with sound evidence for exactly how the conclusions I have made were reached. (Case 108)

I have learned to accept constructive criticism. I no longer become offended by criticism. I have learned to listen to the criticism and reevaluate myself. Most of the time, after looking at the criticism, I agree and change my ways. I feel reevaluating self is making me a better person and nurse. I look at constructive criticism as a tool of growth. (Case 113)

Working at an inner city hospital, I care for many types of patients, many [of] whom are homeless, mentally ill, or drug addicts. I try to remain open-minded, nonjudgmental, and take more interest in not only the care, but how I provide the care for these types of patients. I had to realize that there are standards I must uphold and as a professional I am to be consistent with care regardless of circumstance. (Case 142)

Interactions with Peers

Examples of changes in interaction patterns with colleagues were provided. These involved sharing information, rethinking communication approaches, gaining respect from, and forming bonds with others in their workplace. Their comments revealed the importance of consultation with other nurses and articulation of thinking for improved patient care.

I have learned to observe and explore more possibilities, ask more questions, and get more opinions from my peers in my nursing profession. (Case 101)

This has really helped my practice as a new nurse. I work with very open-minded nurses who are willing to examine the materials . . . from this course and weigh the pros and cons of each skill with skills that they have from their years of experience. This has allowed me to form closer bonds with them both professionally and personally. They respect my interest in improving my nursing skills and I respect their interest in learning new things as well. (Case 145)

I am definitely asking more questions. If I'm given a piece of information by my director or from the doctor, I ask why is that so? Why have we decided to do that? What does it mean for me? What does it mean for the patient? (Case 141)

When I would receive report from the previous shift nurse, my thoughts and feelings were based on her statements or emotions as to how her shift had gone. If she had a very busy shift and struggled with getting everything done, then my own thoughts would react to this and cause me to feel overwhelmed even before I had started my shift. In order to move myself away from these thoughts and feelings, I would focus on analyzing the whole situation to feel more confident in planning and implementing my goals for the day. (Case 136)

I have demonstrated confidence by thinking clearly and being decisive in my decision making. For example, doctors have begun to trust my judgment and ask me what I think in regards to patient care. (Case 115)

Gaining a sense of increased professionalism may be integrally related to the reported increase in confidence and terminology to describe the processes used to arrive at conclusions. The nurses have an expanded view of their ability to impact the situation in which they find themselves. The themes describing self-image as a professional nurse and interactions with peers demonstrate an increasing sense of collegiality, both within the circle of nursing associates and with members of other healthcare disciplines. These intradisciplinary and interdisciplinary approaches have been recognized by the Institute of Medicine (2003) as a basic competence for healthcare education. This competence contributes to an overall vision of meeting the needs of the patient.

Discussion of Findings and Comparison to Previous Studies

Critical Thinking Dimensions Identified

Confidence, flexibility, and open-mindedness were the dimensions of CT most commonly identified by nurses as undergoing a change. These three dimensions fall in the category of habits of the mind and represent affective dimensions of CT in nursing. Confidence, as defined by the Delphi study (Scheffer & Rubenfeld, 2000) is "assurance of one's reasoning abilities" (p. 358). Haffer and Raingruber (1998) similarly found confidence to be a significant aspect of improved reasoning skills identified by prelicensure undergraduate nursing students in a course focused on clinical reasoning and CT. Staib (2003) identified open-mindedness as one of the most common habits of the mind addressed in teaching strategies by nursing faculty. Flexibility, a "capacity to adapt, accommodate, modify or change thoughts, ideas, and behaviors" (Scheffer & Rubenfeld, 2000, p. 358) and open-mindedness, "a viewpoint characterized by being receptive to divergent views and sensitive to one's biases" (p. 358) are evident in a theme identified by Delaney and Piscopo (2007) labeled "envisioning the whole" (p. 172). In their study of RNs transitioning through a BSN program, nurses described their everyday practice as moving beyond old patterns to envision a patient as a whole person. Munhall (1993) described a state of "unknowing" in nursing that promotes a working relationship between the nurse and the patient. This state of conscious unknowing allows a nurse to establish a working relationship with patients through active listening that allows the nurse to view the experience from a patient's perspective. The dimensions of open-mindedness and flexibility exemplify this state of unknowing.

The concept of nursing as both an art and a science is foundational to the educational preparation of nursing students. The American Nurses Association (ANA) recognized both the art and science of nursing. The scientific aspect is embedded in the use of scholarly research to guide competence in use of the nursing process and the art of nursing expressed through a tenet of care, respect for the individual, and use of a holistic approach (American Nurses Association, 2010). In the face of increased use of technology in the provision of patient care, the art of nursing may become less visible. Positioning the affective domains (e.g., confidence, open-mindedness, and flexibility) of nursing as vital to CT reminds nurses to remain aware of the art of practice as important to the total care of patients. Staib (2008) concluded that CT in nursing moves beyond the nursing process and identifies integration of affective dimensions as necessary for CT.

Common Themes from Student Reflections

Bransford and Schwartz (1999) discussed the importance of providing opportunities for students to use current learning to prepare for future learning. The theme Awareness of CT and its subthemes revealed how knowledge of the CT dimensions was important for application to problem solving in clinical practice. Also the emphasis on thinking about the process of thinking helped students remain alert to other situations in which their knowledge about CT could be applied. Learning the dimensions of CT in nursing provided more concrete concepts to recognize in their day-to-day practice as they planned care and solved problems. They were able to recognize and articulate the complexity of their practice through the language of the 17 dimensions of CT.

Delaney and Piscopo (2007) utilized interviews to describe the transition from RNs to BSNs with nurses at the completion of a RN-to-BSN program. Their theme of Recreating Everyday Practice (p. 172) described an ability to see the bigger picture that went beyond the patient and was described as the most powerful experience by the RN students. This theme is similar to one identified in the current study of Changes in Approach to Nursing, where the students were able to describe how use of the 17 dimensions improved their problem-solving skills. Delaney and Piscopo also identified a theme of Becoming Assertive Leaders and Advocates, which described interactions with physicians to impact patient care and outcomes. The themes identified in the current study of Better Patient Outcomes, Self-Image as a Professional Nurse, and Interactions with Peers similarly describe how the students applied dimensions of CT to positively impact care and advocate for patients.

The themes identified by this study demonstrate the goals of RN-to-BSN education as stated by the American Association of Colleges of Nursing:

> RN to BSN programs build on initial nursing preparation with course work to enhance professional development, prepare for a broader scope of practice, and provide a better understanding of the cultural, political, economic, and social issues that affect patients and influence care delivery. (2009, p. 2)

Exemplars written by the students suggest professional development by the students. They also describe how patient outcomes were positively impacted. These areas of growth were evident to the students by the end of the first semester in the nursing program.

Limitations of this study include the fact that it represents one nursing program in the time frame of a single semester. Future studies could evaluate student growth in CT and themes from reflection on responses to the CT Inventory using longitudinal and/or multiprogram data. A comparison of self-assessment with faculty evaluation would provide an additional perspective.

Conclusion

RN-to-BSN curricula must satisfy the interest and needs of students who may have worked as RNs for several years (Davidhizar & Vance, 1999). The results of this study support the value to the students of learning CT in the context of the 17 dimensions of CT in nursing and reflection on responses to the CT Inventory. The student descriptions of changes and growth in CT suggest this approach held meaning for the students. The themes identified in this study exemplify growth in the areas of Awareness of CT, Better Patient Outcomes, Changes in Approach to Nursing, Self-Image as a Professional Nurse, and Interactions with Peers resulting from an expanded understanding of CT. The dimensions help nurses understand and articulate the complexity of clinical reasoning required for professional nursing practice.

REFERENCES

American Association of Colleges of Nursing. (2009). Fact sheet: Degree completion programs for registered nurses: RN to master's degree and RN to baccalaureate programs. Retrieved from http://www.aacn.nche.edu/media-relations/fact-sheets/degree-completion-programs

American Nurses Association. (2010). *Scope and standards of practice: Nursing* (2nd ed.). Silver Spring, MD: Author.

Bransford, J. D., & Schwartz, D. L. (1999). Rethinking transfer: A simple proposal with multiple implications. *Review of Research in Education, 24,* 61–100. doi: 10.3102/0091732X024001061

Brunt, B. A. (2005). Critical thinking in nursing: An integrated review. *The Journal of Continuing Education in Nursing, 36*(2), 60–67.

Davidhizar, R., & Vance, A. (1999). Restructuring clinical time to professionalize the RN-BSN student. *The Health Care Supervisor, 17*(3), 26–32.

Delaney, C., & Piscopo, B. (2007). There really is a difference: Nurses' experiences with transitioning from RNs to BSNs. *Journal of Professional Nursing, 23*(3), 167–173. doi: 10.1016/j.profnurs.2007.01.011

Haffer, A. G., & Raingruber, B. J. (1998). Discovering confidence in clinical reasoning and critical thinking development in baccalaureate nursing students. *Journal of Nursing Education, 37*(2), 61–70.

Institute of Medicine. (2003). *Health professions education: A bridge to quality.* Washington, DC: National Academies Press.

Munhall, P. (1993). "Unknowing": Toward another pattern of knowing in nursing. *Nursing Outlook, 41*(3), 125–128.

Munhall, P. L. (2007). *Nursing research: A qualitative perspective* (4th ed.). Sudbury, MA: Jones and Bartlett.

Rubenfeld, M. G., & Scheffer, B. K. (2009). *Critical thinking TACTICS for nurses: Achieving the IOM competencies* (2nd ed.). Sudbury, MA: Jones and Bartlett.

Scheffer, B. K., & Rubenfeld, M. G. (2000). A consensus statement on critical thinking in nursing. *Journal of Nursing Education, 39*(8), 351–359.

Staib, S. (2003). Teaching and measuring critical thinking. *Journal of Nursing Education, 42*(11), 498–508.

Two Approaches to Assessing Critical Thinking: Vignette-Based and Free Responses

One way to assess critical thinking (CT) is the Assessing Critical Thinking (ACT) rubric-based method, the reliability of which was reported in the *Journal of Professional Nursing* (Allen, Rubenfeld, & Scheffer, 2004). We have used this method with its two approaches (vignette-based and free responses) to arrive at a numeric evaluation of nursing student thinking. For readers who may want to try one or both of these approaches in our method, we are providing the following:

- Student instructions for vignette responses
- Evaluator scoring instructions for vignette responses
- Sixteen vignettes for CT habits of the mind and skills
- Student instructions for free responses
- Evaluator scoring instructions for free responses
- Personal CT tracking form for free responses

The definitions of the habits of the mind and skills needed for these activities are available on your book tear-out card and in the reference citation, Scheffer and Rubenfeld (2000).

We have used these approaches primarily with baccalaureate students, and the instructions included in this appendix are specific to student situations. However, these two approaches for assessing CT could be adapted to specific patient situations so that nurses in practice or students in a specific course could be assessed with familiar patient situations. If you have multiple users, we recommend checking your interrater reliability as we did. To see our interrater reliability and examples of scoring for a vignette and a free response, see Allen, Rubenfeld, and Scheffer (2004). To see a second example of a free response, see Box 10-3 in Chapter 10.

Student Instructions for Vignette Responses

Please follow these instructions exactly:

1. Read the clinical vignette.
2. Read the definition of the CT skill or habit(s) that accompanies the vignette.

3. Describe how you would use the designated habit or skill to accomplish the proposed nursing intervention.
4. On a sheet of paper (or on a computer in about 200–300 words), describe the following:
   a. What you would do, including enough detail to show someone who was not there, to demonstrate the designated habit or skill.
   b. Why you believe your actions illustrate the designated habit or skill.
      You will be assessed for your ability to accurately represent the critical thinking skill or habit, your justification of how your actions demonstrate the skill or habit, and the specificity of the description.
5. You should do this assignment in 20–30 minutes.
6. Please be sure to write your name, the date, the title of vignette, and the habit or skill on your work.

Evaluator Scoring Instructions for Vignette Responses

Score each response for *identification*, *justification*, and *specification* as described in the following paragraphs. The three scores should be recorded at the top of the response sheet.

Identification

The purpose of *identification* is to assess students' ability to effectively match what they would do in the vignette situation with the definition of the designated skill or habit. Does the description of how they would use the skill or habit fit with the definition of that skill or habit, or does it represent some other habit or skill?

   2 = Clear representation of the identified skill or habit in the description of actions
   1 = Partial identification of the skill or habit
   0 = Misidentification of the skill or habit or no evidence of understanding the dimension they thought they were writing about

Justification

The purpose of *justification* is to assess students' ability to support their decision that their actions in this situation match this habit or skill. It is given fewer points because students typically devote less time to this part of the response.

   1 = Actions have been justified as representing the designated skill or habit
   0 = Actions have not been justified as representing the designated skill or habit

Specification

The purpose of *specification* is to assess students' ability to clearly explain what they would do to show the designated skill or habit in this situation. The teacher must judge the quality of the response relative to detail and level. *Detail* involves the ideas and facts the student brings together in the response; for example, does the student state that he or she will teach the patient, or does he or she describe how that teaching would be done? *Level* involves a judgment by the rater as to the ideas and facts that would be expected of students at that stage in their education or experience.

> 2 = Detailed, level-appropriate description of how the student would use the skill or habit in the situation
>
> 1 = Detailed description but inappropriate to level
>
> 0 = Unclear or inadequate description

Vignettes for Critical Thinking Habits of the Mind and Skills

Vignette 1: Charlotte and Mary's Adoption Plans

Critical Thinking Habit of the Mind: **Intellectual Integrity** (defined as: *seeking the truth through sincere, honest processes, even if the results are contrary to one's assumptions and beliefs*)

Charlotte Jones and Mary Kelly are partners who have lived together for 2 years. They are considering adopting a child. They are patients in the obstetrics/gynecology practice with another patient, Susan Simone, who is 11 weeks pregnant. Susan is unmarried and wishes to carry her child to term and consider adoption, even though her partner, Tom, would rather she had an abortion. Susan, a sophomore in college, is very close to her mother, who is supportive of the plan to offer the child for adoption. She has no health insurance and has income only from her part-time job as a waitress. When Susan was told that Charlotte and Mary were interested in adopting her baby, she immediately told the nurse that she wanted to go ahead with whatever was necessary to arrange the adoption.

Describe how you, as the nurse in this situation, would use the *Intellectual Integrity* habit of the mind to help Susan, Charlotte, and Mary prepare for and interact during their first meeting.

Vignette 2: Mr. Herman and His Diabetes Management

Critical Thinking Skill: **Predicting** (defined as: *envisioning a plan and its consequences*)

During a routine screening for diabetes at the automotive plant, Dan Herman was found to have a random blood glucose of 248. He was later diagnosed with Type 2 diabetes and was encouraged by his primary care physician to see the plant nurse every 2 weeks for assistance with his diet and activity plan. He is 5'9" and weighs 220 pounds, and he freely admits that his diet is made up primarily of meats and carbohydrates. He blames his weight on his love of sausage and beer. At the plant his job is to service the plumbing system, so he is fairly active each day. When asked about outside exercise, he laughed and asked, "Why would I do that when I'm active at work?"

Describe how you, as the plant nurse in this situation, would use the *Predicting* skill to help Mr. Herman with his diabetes management.

Vignette 3: Mrs. Bower's Thyroid Enlargement

Critical Thinking Habit of the Mind: **Confidence** (defined as: *assurance of one's reasoning abilities*)

Nancy Franklin is a nurse in a hemodialysis center to where she recently transferred after working her first year out of school on an inpatient medical unit. Working with Mrs. Bower, who started dialysis 4 weeks ago, Nancy has seen the patient get progressively sicker with each treatment. Last week Dr. Jones assessed Mrs. Bower and reported to Nancy that he thought the patient was having anxiety and would likely settle down once she adjusted to dialysis. This evening Mrs. Bower has been constantly nauseated and has vomited twice. Nancy decided to do a more thorough assessment to see if there were other issues besides anxiety. She started with questions about the patient's perception of the dialysis process, to which Mrs. Bower replied, "I really do hate it but if it means this is my only way to stay alive, I'll just have to adjust, won't I?" She continued with, "But I just feel so awful physically; I can't imagine why I'm so sick to my stomach each week. I'm losing weight and I feel really shaky." Nancy started collecting objective data and, when she palpated Mrs. Bower's neck, she thought she felt an enlarged thyroid gland. Because Dr. Jones was not due to come to the unit that afternoon, Nancy called him to report her findings. Dr. Jones was short in his response: "I assessed that patient last week and she's just anxious. It's so easy to palpate a thyroid wrongly. You'll get used to these patients after you've been here awhile. Just relax."

Put yourself in Nancy's place. Describe how you would use the *Confidence* habit of the mind to deal with Mrs. Bower's signs and symptoms and Dr. Jones.

Vignette 4: Mrs. Walters's Postpartum Stomachache

Critical Thinking Skill: **Information Seeking** (defined as: *searching for evidence, facts, or knowledge by identifying relevant sources and gathering objective, subjective, historical, and current data from those sources*)

The community health nurse is visiting the Walters family 4 days after the birth of their first child because Mrs. Walters asked for assistance with breastfeeding and bathing the baby. She reported feeling so nervous that she was afraid she might be doing things "all wrong." Upon arrival, the nurse asked Mrs. Walters how she was feeling physically, to which Mrs. Walters replied, "I feel pretty good except for a bad stomachache that I've had for the past 2 days." She pointed to her abdominal midsection.

Describe how you, as the community health nurse, would use the *Information Seeking* skill to deal with Mrs. Walters's stomachache.

Vignette 5: Mr. Franklin's Failure to Thrive

Critical Thinking Habit of the Mind: **Inquisitiveness** (defined as: *an eagerness to know by seeking knowledge and understanding through observation and thoughtful questioning to explore possibilities and alternatives*)

Mr. Franklin, an 82-year-old retired farmer, who was accompanied by his daughter, was admitted to the medical unit for failure to thrive. During the change of shift report, Jane Dore heard this: "Mr. Franklin is a new admit in 102. His daughter brought him in from his assisted living apartment. He hasn't said much; he's sitting up in bed and ate 25% of his lunch. He's incontinent of bladder and bowel and is unsteady on his feet. He needs contact guard for ambulation."

After the report, Jane reads the following medical admission note in the patient's chart: "82 yo male with evidence of anasarca admitted from assisted living apartment for failure to thrive. Per daughter, he has had vague complaints of being tired and appetite loss for the past month during which time he has lost 15 pounds. He has nonspecific stomach discomfort and difficulty attending to tasks but denies anhedonia. Mr. Franklin's wife was recently admitted to a nursing home for advanced dementia. ROS: Neuro: neg; CV: no chest pains, palpitations; GI: poss. obstipation, neg melena; GU: some urinary hesitation."

Describe how you, as nurse Jane Dore, would use the *Inquisitiveness* habit of the mind to plan your first encounter with Mr. Franklin.

Vignette 6: Mrs. O'Connor's Catheterization

Critical Thinking Habit of the Mind: **Contextual Perspective** (defined as: *consideration of the whole situation, including relationships, background, and environment relevant to some happening*)

Mrs. O'Connor is a 64-year-old woman with multiple sclerosis who recently was hospitalized for sepsis. It was determined that the source of infection was urinary retention secondary to a neurogenic bladder. Her postvoiding residuals consistently ranged from 200 to 250 ml. After the infection was under control and discharge was being planned, the nursing staff started to teach Mrs. O'Connor to perform self-intermittent catheterizations. The first attempts were unsuccessful. Mrs. O'Connor's response was, "I'd rather just live with the infections than do *that* to myself." On assessment, the nurse found that Mrs. O'Connor, a former corporate secretary, had been a widow for 17 years and lived alone. She had weak hand grasps, with the left being weaker than the right. She needed assistance to get up from a chair but could independently walk with a walker. She was 5'6" tall and weighed 126 pounds. Her eyesight was adequate for reading small print.

Describe how you would use the *Contextual Perspective* habit of the mind to help Mrs. O'Connor learn the catheterization procedure.

Vignette 7: Dolly and Monty's Ulcer Care

Critical Thinking Habit of the Mind: *Open-Mindedness* (defined as: *a viewpoint characterized by being receptive to divergent views and sensitive to one's biases*)

Dolly, a 63-year-old bartender, is a diabetic with peripheral vascular disease. She had an ulcer on her right ankle that would not heal. The area became gangrenous and she needed a below-the-knee amputation. She has been very quiet and refuses to wear her prosthetic leg to practice walking. The skin on her back is severely broken down. She has a nursing diagnosis of impaired skin integrity related to immobility.

Monty, a 26-year-old nurse, was in an automobile accident while he was stopped on the side of the road to fix a flat tire. A truck swerved as it came around a corner and hit him and his car. His 3-month-old baby, who was in a car seat, was also injured during the accident and is currently in the hospital. Monty has an amputated leg because his leg was pinned under the car during the accident. He has tried to use his prosthetic leg, but it has been rubbing on his stump. He has refused to get out of bed for the past 2 days and has two areas of skin breakdown on his back. He has a nursing diagnosis of impaired skin integrity related to immobility.

Describe how you would use the *Open-Mindedness* habit of the mind to provide care for the nursing diagnoses for these two patients.

Vignette 8: Mrs. Jones's Confusion

Critical Thinking Habit of the Mind: **Intuition** (defined as: *insightful sense of knowing without conscious use of reason*)

Mrs. Jones, who is 82 years old, has been a patient on the skilled unit of the nursing home for 3 days while recovering from a fractured hip. A Type 2 diabetic, she has been doing very well in therapies and has always been oriented x3. On Saturday morning at 6 a.m., you find her sitting in her chair mumbling. When you call her name, she looks up and asks, "Where am I?"

Describe how you would use the *Intuition* habit of the mind during this first encounter with Mrs. Jones.

Vignette 9: Ms. Chee's Home Care

Critical Thinking Habit of the Mind: **Creativity** (defined as: *intellectual inventiveness used to generate, discover, or restructure ideas; imagining alternatives*)

Bernie Chee is a 76-year-old Native American woman recently hospitalized for pneumonia. Her hospital stay progressed well, but she has lost about 10 pounds over the past 2 weeks. Although she has been participating in physical therapy, her strength and stamina are not back to her prehospitalization level. During her hospitalization she was diagnosed with osteoporosis and mild hypertension. She also has beginning cataracts in both eyes. Ms. Chee has convinced her doctor that she will progress better at home and has been discharged on the condition that a community health nursing referral be made to assess and plan care for her recovery at home. Ms. Chee's son lives close by and wants to be included in the plan of care for his mother.

Ms. Chee lives alone in a small two-story home with her bedroom and bathroom on the second floor. The downstairs includes a living room, dining room, kitchen, and small family room. There are five steps coming into the house at the front and the back entrances. Ms. Chee is an avid reader of magazines and newspapers and doesn't like to throw things out. The downstairs is filled with piles of reading materials stacked in numerous places on the floor. Ms. Chee stays busy during the day with her hobby of hooking small throw rugs. Because she has hardwood floors, many of her rugs are placed throughout the house. Her five cats have favorite rugs for sleeping.

Describe how you, as the community health nurse, would use the *Creativity* habit of the mind to develop a realistic plan of care for Ms. Chee's mobility and safety needs.

Vignette 10: Miss Bandy's Lasix Order

Critical Thinking Habit of the Mind: **Flexibility** (defined as: *capacity to adapt, accommodate, modify, or change thoughts, ideas, and behaviors*)

Miss Viola Bandy, age 93, has been a resident of the rural Hilltop Nursing Home for 3 years. The evening shift nurse receives the following report from the day shift: "Miss Bandy seems to be confused today and has been using her call light more frequently. She has gained 2.5 pounds since yesterday." While doing his rounds at 3:30 p.m., the nurse finds Miss Bandy to have an apical heart rate of 112. He calls the physician, who orders Lasix 80 mg for this evident episode of heart failure. The nurse calls the pharmacy and is told that the drug cannot be delivered until 9 or 10 p.m.

Describe how you, as the evening nurse, would use the *Flexibility* habit of the mind to care for Miss Bandy's episode of heart failure.

Vignette 11: Help for Hannah

Critical Thinking Habit of the Mind: *Perseverance* (defined as: *pursuit of a course with determination to overcome obstacles*)

Hannah is an 18-year-old single mom with newborn twins. She lives in an apartment that is neat and clean but sparsely furnished with attic and basement hand-me-downs from friends. Her older sister cares for the twins while she works afternoons and takes classes to become a dental hygienist. Her waitress income would have been adequate for herself and one child, but the extra food, clothing, diapers, and supplies for the twins are taxing her resources; also, her car just quit working and she now has no transportation. As her community health nurse, you have assessed that she has several needs:

■ Well-baby care and immunizations for the newborns
■ Financial assistance with her schooling, food, clothing, and formula
■ Transportation
■ Support group for mothers with twins

The babies are 3 months overdue for their immunizations. You have arranged several appointments at the Well-Baby Clinic, but Hannah has not been able to keep them for a variety of reasons.

Describe how you would use the *Perseverance* habit of the mind to help Hannah's twins get their immunizations.

Vignette 12: Steve's Decompensating Behavior

Critical Thinking Skill: *Applying Standards* (defined as: *judging according to established personal, professional, or social rules or criteria*)

Steve is a 24-year-old male on an inpatient psychiatric unit. His admission was involuntary, and his DSM-IV Axis I diagnosis is paranoid schizophrenia. You have been working with Steve for the past two evenings. Tonight after dinner he starts shouting at other patients, throws a chair at the window, threatens to kill his room-mate, and cannot be verbally redirected. Based on your assessment of the situation that Steve's behavior is placing himself, other patients, and the staff in danger, you quickly obtain an order from the doctor to place Steve in seclusion, including the use of four-point restraints. With the help of the other staff, the order is implemented and, because he is screaming, the door is closed. When it is time for you to attend a mandatory CPR in-service, Steve is temporarily assigned to Fran, another RN, until you return. When you return 45 minutes later, you find Steve still in the seclusion room with four-point restraints and the door closed. You ask Fran for a report on Steve's condition and are told, "I really have been pretty busy and since he couldn't get into any trouble in seclusion I haven't bothered to check on him. Once he quit screaming it was quiet and other patients kept asking me for things so I had to deal with their needs."

Describe how you would use the *Applying Standards* skill to deal with this situation.

Vignette 13: Jack's Delegation Dilemma

Critical Thinking Skill: *Analyzing* (defined as: *separating or breaking a whole into parts to discover their nature, function, and relationships*)

Jack is an RN working evenings on a step-down unit. He has one nurse aide working with him. He has not worked with this aide before. He delegates several tasks to the aide, including 4 p.m. blood pressures for five patients. At 6 p.m., after the aide has left for dinner break, he checks the flow sheet to assess the blood pressures on the five patients before passing meds. He discovers that none of the blood pressures have been recorded.

Describe how you, in Jack's position, could use the *Analyzing* skill to deal with this situation.

Vignette 14: Determining the Best Nursing Diagnosis

Critical Thinking Skill: *Discriminating* (defined as: *recognizing differences and simi-larities among things or situations and distinguishing carefully as to category or rank*)

David and Mack, university sophomores, visit the recreation center on campus daily to lift weights for an hour. On Monday afternoon, both students are on your schedule at the clinic because they need tetanus immunizations and physical exams before joining the wrestling team. While talking to David, who has Type 2 diabetes, you discover he has been trying to lose weight by eating a diet of eggs and bananas exclu-sively. He got on the scales and was quite happy to discover he had lost 4 pounds in 2 days. While talking to Mack, you discover he has been eating his usual diet, which, by his report, sounds balanced. When their lab tests are completed, Mack's serum albumin was 2.8 and David's was 4.8 (normal range 3.5–5.0 g/dL); Mack's fasting glucose was 178 and David's was 98 (normal range 70–105). You determine two nursing diagnoses: risk for imbalanced nutrition and imbalanced nutrition.

Describe how you would use the *Discriminating* skill to decide which of these diagnoses best matched with David and which with Mack.

Vignette 15: Validating a Nursing Diagnosis

Critical Thinking Skill: *Logical Reasoning* (defined as: *drawing inferences or conclusions that are supported in or justified by evidence*)

Trudy is a 15-year-old high school student. She has come to talk to you, the school nurse, about a stomachache. During your assessment you discover that she has been taking birth control pills with her parents' permission to deal with her very painful menses. She has also been sexually active for the past year and admits to not using condoms. Over the past year she has had three boyfriends, all of them seniors. You have a hunch that the following nursing diagnosis needs to be considered: deficient knowledge regarding safe sexual behavior.

Describe how you would you use the *Logical Reasoning* skill to validate your hunch.

Vignette 16: Tuberculosis Prevention Campaign

Critical Thinking Skill: *Transforming Knowledge* (defined as: *changing or converting the condition, nature, form, or function of concepts among contexts*)

Smallville has had an increased incidence of tuberculosis (TB) at its three homeless shelters over the past year. As a community health nurse responsible for working with the homeless population, you want to address this issue. You want to focus on preventing the development of new cases (primary prevention) and provide people who have the disease with effective ways to take care of themselves (secondary prevention). You know it is essential for individuals diagnosed with TB to have consistent follow-up care, take their medications regularly, avoid alcohol and other drugs while taking TB medication to prevent liver damage, and maintain good nutrition. You also know that important prevention strategies include avoiding close contact, not coughing on others, disposing of tissues properly, hand washing and general cleanliness, adequate ventilation in sleeping quarters, and so forth.

Describe how you would use the *Transforming Knowledge* skill to develop a campaign to share the basic principles of primary and secondary TB prevention with the homeless population and staff in the shelters.

Student Instructions for Free Responses

Nursing care is a combination of thinking, doing, and feeling. CT has both cognitive and affective dimensions, all of which are vital to quality nursing care. To become a great nurse, it is important to improve not only one's actions, but also one's thinking.

Thinking in nursing situations can be improved only when one reflects on one's thinking and considers how that thinking can be strengthened. These assignments will help you focus your thinking about your thinking.

Instructions:

1. Review the definitions of CT skills and habits of the mind. These 17 dimensions have been identified through research as collectively representing CT in nursing. Your Personal Tracking Form lists 16 of the 17 skills and habits. *Reflection* is not included in this assignment because the whole assignment is a lesson in reflection.

2. Reflect on your nursing situation for the day, focusing on your *thinking* rather than your *actions*.

3. Select one of the habits or skills from your Personal Tracking Form *that you have not previously written about*, and choose a situation that you believe best illustrates this component. Describe the following:

   a. That situation, including enough detail to show someone who was not there how you demonstrated that habit or skill. Do not include patient information (at the most, use initials). This will be scored from 0–2 for *identification*.

   b. Why you believe this situation illustrates the habit or skill you have chosen. This will be scored from 0–1 for *justification*.

   c. What you think you could have done better to use the habit or skill in this situation. This will be scored according to your experience level as *expansion* with the following scores: 5 = outstanding, comparable to a postbaccalaureate nurse; 4 = appropriate to a second-semester senior nursing student; 3 = appropriate to a first-semester senior nursing student; 2 = appropriate to a second-semester junior nursing student; 1 = appropriate to a first-semester junior nursing student; and 0 = insufficient for a junior-level nursing student.

4. Write approximately one page. If you work on a computer, aim for about 200–300 words.

5. You should do this assignment in 20–30 minutes.

6. Please be sure to include your name, the date, and the CT habit or skill you have chosen to describe.

7. On your Personal Tracking Form, mark the date you completed this task.

8. By the end of the semester, you should have written about each skill and habit of the mind at least once. Because there are 16 in total, some weeks you will describe two or more situations, each with a skill or habit. Four dimensions have been grouped into pairs because they are closely related. On the week you describe *Inquisitiveness*, you should also describe *Information Seeking*. On the

week you describe *Analyzing*, you should also describe *Discriminating*. Other combinations are at your discretion.

Evaluator Scoring Instructions for Free Responses

Score each response for *identification, justification,* and *expansion* as described in the following paragraphs. The three scores should be recorded at the top of the response sheet.

Identification

The purpose of *identification* is to assess students' ability to effectively demonstrate that their response represents the identified CT dimension.

> 2 = The description is a good representation of the dimension(s).
>
> 1 = The description was partially representative of the dimension(s).
>
> 0 = The description does not represent the dimension(s). (For example, the description seemed more like logical reasoning than creativity.)

Justification

The purpose of *justification* is to assess students' ability to support their decision that their response in this situation matches the CT dimension identified.

> 1 = Yes, there is support.
>
> 0 = No, there is insufficient support.

Expansion

The purpose of *expansion* is to assess students' ability to explain clearly what they would have done differently to improve the use of the designated dimension in the situation. The rater must judge the quality of the response relative to a normative level of performance. (What you would expect from senior students is different from what you would expect from first-semester junior students, for example.)

> 5 = Postbaccalaureate nurse
>
> 4 = Senior, second-semester nursing student
>
> 3 = Senior, first-semester nursing student
>
> 2 = Junior, second-semester nursing student
>
> 1 = Junior, first-semester nursing student
>
> 0 = Insufficient for junior-level nursing student

Personal CT Tracking Form for Free Responses

Name _____

These 16 alphabetically arranged dimensions include 9 habits of the mind and 7 skills of CT in nursing as defined by Scheffer & Rubenfeld (2000). One additional habit of the mind is *reflection*, defined as "contemplation upon a subject, especially one's assumptions and thinking or the purposes of deeper understanding and self-evaluation." This tracking form is to be used for weekly free response reflection assignments. See "Student Instructions for Free Responses" for details about how to proceed.

Date Submitted	*Dimension of Critical Thinking*
_____	*Analyzing*
	Separating or breaking a whole Into parts to discover their nature, function, and relationships
	and
	Discriminating
	Recognizing differences and similarities among things or situations and distinguishing carefully as to category or rank
_____	*Applying Standards*
	Judging according to established personal, professional, or social rules or criteria
_____	*Confidence*
	Assurance of one's reasoning abilities
_____	*Contextual Perspective*
	Consideration of the whole situation, including relationships, background, and environment, relevant to some happening
_____	*Creativity*
	Intellectual inventiveness used to generate, discover, or restructure ideas; imagining alternatives
_____	*Flexibility*
	Capacity to adapt, accommodate, modify, or change thoughts, ideas, and behaviors
_____	*Intellectual Integrity*
	Seeking the truth through sincere, honest processes, even if the results are contrary to one's assumptions and beliefs
_____	*Intuition*
	Insightful sense of knowing without conscious use of reason

Inquisitiveness

An eagerness to know by seeking knowledge and understanding through observation and thoughtful questioning to explore possibilities and alternatives

and

Information Seeking

Searching for evidence, facts, or knowledge by identifying relevant sources and gathering objective, subjective, historical, and current data from those sources

Logical Reasoning

Drawing inferences or conclusions that are supported in or justified by evidence

Open-Mindedness

A viewpoint characterized by being receptive to divergent views and sensitive to one's biases

Perseverance

Pursuit of a course with determination to overcome obstacles

Predicting

Envisioning a plan and its consequences

Transforming Knowledge

Changing or converting the condition, nature, form, or function of concepts among contexts

REFERENCES

Allen, G. D., Rubenfeld, M. G., & Scheffer, B. K. (2004). Reliability of assessment of critical thinking. *Journal of Professional Nursing, 20,* 15–22.

Scheffer, B. K., & Rubenfeld, M. G. (2000). A consensus statement on critical thinking in nursing. *Journal of Nursing Education, 39,* 352–359.

Note: Page numbers followed by *b*, *f*, or *t* indicate material in boxes, figures, or tables, respectively.